Dana
Carpender's
CARB GRAM
COUNTER

Dana Carpender's
CARB GRAM COUNTER

USABLE CARBS, PROTEIN, AND CALORIES—
PLUS TIPS ON EATING LOW-CARB!

DANA CARPENDER

FAIR WINDS
PRESS
GLOUCESTER, MASSACHUSETTS

Text © 2004 by Dana Carpender

First published in the USA in 2004 by
Fair Winds Press
33 Commercial Street
Gloucester, MA 01930

Library of Congress Cataloging-in-Publication Data available

ISBN 1-59233-077-0

10 9 8 7 6 5 4 3 2 1

Book design by Leslie Haimes and Tabula Rasa
Book production by Tabula Rasa

Printed and bound in Canada

*Although we have made every effort to publish a most comprehensive
and accurate directory, please be aware that these figures are frequently
updated.*

CONTENTS

CONTENTS (continued)

INTRODUCTION

Hello, low-carb dieter! Whether you're new to the low carb lifestyle, or have been doing this for a while, I hope you'll find this book a useful tool to achieving weight loss, abundant energy, and robust good health.

I've written a lot of words about the low-carbohydrate lifestyle in the past few years, and I won't try to repeat them all here. But I would like to offer the condensed version, as it were—what I feel are the most vital tips for low-carb success.

BASIC STUFF
- First, and perhaps most important, be clear on this: Whatever you do to lose weight is what you must do for the rest of your life to keep it off. And if carbs are a health problem for you now, they will continue to be a health problem for you until the day you die. Get it through your head that there is no finish line.
- Because you're in this for life, don't focus on losing your weight as quickly as possible. Instead, work on making low-carbing the enjoyable lifestyle it can be, while still achieving your goals. In particular, do not decide that if low carb is good, no carb is better, and cut out everything but eggs, meat, and cheese. You can't eat that way forever, and you know it. You need to incorporate the widest variety of low-carb foods you can, to add flavor and interest, not to mention vitamins, minerals, and fiber.

- It's important to know about "impact carbs," "usable carbs," "net carbs," or "effective carbs." These terms all refer to the grams of carbohydrate that you can actually digest and absorb. What carbohydrates can't you digest or absorb? Fiber! The carbohydrate chains that make up dietary fibers are just too big for the human gut to digest and absorb, which is why we can't live on grass like cows do. Accordingly, you can subtract the grams of fiber from the total grams of carbohydrate to get the number of grams of carbohydrate you actually need to worry about. In this book, we call this number "usable carbs." This approach dramatically increases the amount of vegetables, fruits, nuts, seeds, and other plant foods you can eat.

- It is my experience that a low-carbohydrate diet is a superb way to overcome genuine obesity and the health problems that come with it—but that it's not particularly useful for achieving that fashionably anorexic look. If you're a size 4 trying to become a size 0, I probably can't help you, and furthermore, I don't want to! It's about health, not about making yourself vanish!

- If you're new to low-carbing, be aware that the first week can be rough. If, like most people, you've been giving your body a little carbohydrate every few hours, your body is used to running on sugar, and probably hasn't been making much of the enzymes you need to burn fat for fuel. If you burn through your body's stores of sugar before your fat-burning enzyme levels increase, you may "bonk"—feel terribly tired and wrung-out for a day or two. Not everyone goes through this—I didn't—but if it happens to you, know that for most people it lasts no more than a few days. When it's over, you'll be burning fat for fuel, and have more energy than you ever imagined, because you're carrying your supply with you.

- If, along with feeling tired, you feel kind of achy, weak, or crampy, potassium loss—called "hypokalemia"—is likely to be your problem. And if this happens to you, get more potassium right away. Your heart needs potassium to run properly! Don't mess around. The best low-carb source of potassium is avocados; little black ones have 8 grams of usable carb apiece, and 1200 mg of potassium. Green leafy vegetables are also a good low-carb source of potassium, as are fresh pork, fresh fish, cantaloupe, and almonds. Indeed, it's best to include these things in your diet from Day One.

- You can also take potassium tablets, if you like, but be aware that the doses tend to be low—just 99 mg per tablet, when you need 2000–3000 mg of potassium per day. Another way to supplement is to use Morton's Lite Salt, which combines the usual sodium-based salt with potassium-based salt.

  CAUTION: If you are on blood pressure medication of any kind, check with your pharmacist or doctor before taking potassium supplements. Some blood pressure medications work by making your body hang on to potassium, and that makes it possible to get too much, which is as dangerous as too little.

- Potassium imbalance is a temporary problem, caused by your body's shifting over from a high-carb diet, which makes you throw off potassium and retain water, to a low-carb diet—which makes you dump all that excess water before your body stops throwing off the potassium. Just eat your good potassium sources, and your body will sort it all out in a week or two.

FINDING YOUR LOW-CARB LIFESTYLE

• There are many approaches to controlling carbohydrates in your diet. If all you've heard about is Atkins and/or *The South Beach Diet*, and you've been unhappy or uncomfortable on these diets, don't give up—do some research, and find the approach that works for your body and your life. To shamelessly plug my own book, in *How I Gave Up My Low Fat Diet and Lost 40 Pounds*, I outline more than a half a dozen different approaches to controlling your carbohydrate intake, and therefore your insulin levels. No need for a one-size-fits-all diet.

• Pay attention to your body to learn your "critical carbohydrate level"—the number of grams per day of carbohydrate you must stay below in order to lose weight. For most people this will be between 15 and 60 grams per day. Only time and attention will tell you your critical carbohydrate level.

• You can get an idea of where your critical carbohydrate level is likely to be by finding out how many of the signs of carbohydrate intolerance you have. Here's a list of indicators. How many of them apply to you?

☐ I have had a weight problem since I was quite young.
☐ I have bad energy slumps, especially in the late afternoon.
☐ I get tired and/or shaky when I get hungry.
☐ I'm depressed and irritable for no reason.
☐ I binge badly or frequently on carbohydrate foods.
☐ I carry most of my weight on my abdomen.
☐ I have high blood pressure.
☐ I have high triglycerides.
☐ I have high cholesterol.
☐ I have adult onset diabetes.
☐ I have heart disease.

☐ I have had a female cancer (breast, cervical, ovarian, uterine).
☐ I have had a stroke.
☐ I am an alcoholic.
☐ I have polycystic ovarian syndrome, or the symptoms of it.
☐ Obesity runs in my family.
☐ High blood pressure runs in my family.
☐ High triglycerides run in my family.
☐ High cholesterol runs in my family.
☐ Adult onset diabetes runs in my family.
☐ Heart disease runs in my family.
☐ Female cancers run in my family (breast, cervical, ovarian, uterine).
☐ Stroke runs in my family.
☐ Alcoholism runs in my family.
☐ Polycystic ovarian syndrome runs in my family.

- If your answer is "yes" to more than three of these, you're likely to be pretty carb-intolerant. The more yes answers, and the more people in your family have these problems, the more intolerant you're likely to be. Keep this in mind when choosing an approach.
- If you have any of the health problems listed above, it is imperative that you be under a doctor's supervision during at least the first few months of going low carb. Blood pressure can come down so quickly that if your medication isn't adjusted you'll get dizzy. Your customary dosage of diabetes medication may suddenly be enough to drop your blood sugar uncomfortably low. If you have trouble with high cholesterol and triglycerides you need a baseline to work from, or you won't know if you've gotten better or worse. Don't be stupid. If your doctor won't cooperate, find one that will, but don't fly blind.

- Most people see an across-the-board improvement in their coronary risk factors—cholesterol, triglycerides, and HDL/LDL ratio—on a low-carb diet, even when eating red meat and high fat dairy foods. However, a minority will see a decrease in triglycerides and an increase in HDL, which is good, but also see a jump in their LDL, which is not so good. If this happens to you, weigh your low-carb diet in favor of fish, poultry, and pork (which is now very lean), use lean cuts when eating beef or lamb, and choose olive oil, nuts, and avocados—sources of monounsaturated fats—over butter, sour cream, and cheese.

STAYING HAPPY

- In the pursuit of low-carb happiness, especially in the early stages, sit down and brainstorm a list of all of your favorite low-carb foods. What foods do you really love that you've been denying yourself because they were high fat and high calorie? Lobster with butter? Macadamia nuts? Deviled eggs? Brie? Really give this list some thought. Then buy or cook this stuff, and eat it! A great way to stave off feelings of deprivation.

- Buy at least one low-carb cookbook. Shamelessly plugging my own work again, *500 Low-Carb Recipes* is the most popular low-carb cookbook in the US. People tell me they like it because it doesn't call for a lot of weird ingredients, and has a lot of simple recipes that their families like. But there are plenty of other low-carb cookbooks on the market, many of them quite good. The point is, start exploring your kitchen options, instead of letting yourself get locked into fried eggs for breakfast, a bunless burger for lunch, and a plain steak for dinner.

- Make a list of ways to reward yourself that don't involve food. A massage, an hour in a hot bath with a good book, a manicure and pedicure, a phone call to an old friend you haven't talked to in forever—whatever you can think of that will make you feel rewarded, but won't make you fat, sick, and tired. When you've had a hard week, or reached a personal goal, give yourself one of these rewards, instead of carb-y garbage that will only hurt you in the long run.

- When you've lost your first ten or fifteen pounds, buy yourself something wonderful and new to wear—it's a terrific incentive. It's not a bad idea to do this every time you drop another size, if you can afford it, rather than waiting until you've reached your goal weight to buy new clothes. New clothes celebrate and show off your success, and keep you on track.

ABOUT LABELS

- Read the labels on everything you put in your mouth. Most people do far more research before buying a car or a DVD player than they do on what they put into their own bodies. "You are what you eat" is literally true. All your body has to make itself from is what you put in your mouth. If you give your body junk, you'll be made out of junk, and you'll feel and look like it. Read the labels even on things you've looked up in this book, or have purchased before—formulas change.
- Having read the labels, choose the products with the lowest carb counts. You can shave untold thousands of grams off of your yearly intake this way. For example, I have seen ham with 1 gram of carbohydrate per serving, and I have seen ham with 6 grams of carbohydrate per serving. That's a 600% difference!
- There is no such thing as good sugar! Obviously, sugar, brown sugar, and corn syrup are all bad for you. However, so are the "natural" and "healthy" alternatives like honey, concentrated fruit juice, Sucanat, dried sugar cane juice, malt syrup, rice syrup, turbinado, fructose, dextrose,

maltose, or anything else ending in "ose." All of it is sugar, and all of it will cause an insulin release.

- Many alcoholic beverages quote low-carb counts on the labels, and hard liquor, technically speaking, has none. However, alcohol, no matter how low carb, will slow your metabolism dramatically—you'll stop burning fat until your body has metabolized all of the alcohol. This doesn't mean that you can never have a light beer or a glass of dry wine, but it does mean that alcohol is always a major luxury on any kind of weight-loss diet.

- Keep a close eye on the portion sizes listed on labels. Often what you assume is one serving is really two or three—which means you'll get two or three times as much carbohydrate as you bargained for.

- It's important to know that just because a food says it has "0 grams of carbohydrate" per serving, doesn't mean that it's carbohydrate free. How can this be? Again, it has to do with portion size. The US federal government standards allow labels to say "0 grams" if the food contains 0.4 grams or less per serving, and "<1 gram" if the food contains 0.9 grams or less per serving. Yet we often use these foods in larger quantities, and the grams add up. A perfect example: A reader of mine wanted to know where the carbs in my Margarita Mix (*500 Low-Carb Recipes*) came from—after all, lime juice, lemon juice, and Splenda all had zero grams of carbohydrate. Only they don't, they all have carbs! They only look like they're carb-free because the serving sizes used on the labels are so small. When in doubt count 0.5 grams per serving for foods that say 0 grams on the label, and 1 gram for foods that say <1 gram.

- Be aware that there have been more than a few cases of mislabeled "low carb" products that turned out to be a lot higher in carbohydrate than the labels let on. If you add a new product to your diet and you bump up a pound or two, or find yourself hungry and craving, take a closer look—and remember that if it seems too good to be true, it just might be.

- This warning also applies to imported food products. Labeling laws vary from country to country, and much of the world does not include fiber counts in the total carb count on nutrition labels—so if you subtract the fiber count from the total carb count, you'll get an inaccurately low total, and eat more carbohydrate than you meant to.

COMMON SENSE

- The notion that you can eat unlimited quantities of food so long as you keep the carb count very low has been oversold. It does appear to be true that you can eat more calories on a low carb diet than you could on a carb-containing diet, and still lose weight, and you certainly never have to go hungry, but that doesn't mean you can eat 10,000 calories a day and still lose weight. Eat when you're hungry, eat enough to feel satisfied, then quit till you're physically hungry again. It's a shame that we even need to be told this, it's so basic, but our society has developed a bad habit of eating for the fun of it, regardless of hunger. Cut it out!

- Americans have been programmed to eat for entertainment—snacking for long periods of time on nutritionally empty junk food, whether they're hungry or not. Low carb foods are filling, and tend to be calorie-dense, and as a result, there are few low-carb foods that you can nosh on for hours without making yourself ill. If you really must have something to nibble on for hours and hours, your best bet is very low-carb vegetables, like celery and cucumber sticks. Pumpkin and sunflower seeds in the shell are another good choice, because having to open each individual shell slows down your consumption dramatically, and keeps your hands busy, to boot. Better yet, find something else to do for entertainment!

- The heart and soul of your nutritional program, for the rest of your life, should be meat, fish, poultry, eggs and cheese, healthy fats, low carbohydrate vegetables, low sugar fruits, and nuts and seeds. You know—food. A sugar-free candy bar or brownie or a bag of low-carb chips is never a substitute for a chicken Caesar salad for lunch. Got it?

LOW-CARBOHYDRATE/ SUGAR-FREE SPECIALTY PRODUCTS

- Roughly half of low-carbohydrate dieters find that diet soda and diet fruit flavored beverages like Crystal Light will slow or stop their weight loss. Many also find that these beverages act as a "trigger"—something that sets off their carb cravings. Why this should be so is controversial; some theorize that the aspartame is to blame, while others feel that citric acid, widely used as a flavoring in these products, interferes with ketosis. Still others claim that just the taste of sweetness can cause an insulin release, whether there's any sugar involved or not. The actual reason is unimportant—just know that if you're struggling, one of the first places to look is your diet soda consumption.

- Do not make low-carb specialty products a major part of your diet. Low-carb breads, pastas, candy, cookies, protein bars, etc. are flooding onto the market, and they do provide a nice variety. However, most of these products are not as nutritious, healthful, or filling as real food. Furthermore, they're all extremely expensive! And almost all of them have more carbohydrates than a hard-boiled egg or a chicken wing. So stop trying to make your low-carb diet look like your old high-carb diet—that's the diet that got you in trouble in the first place, remember?

- When you hit a plateau, lose the treats. The sugar-free chocolate bars, the low-carb baked goods, etc. are the first things to axe if you're not losing weight.

- Regarding those sugar-free chocolate bars, not to mention protein bars, jelly beans, brownies, etc: Just about all of them are sweetened with polyols, sometimes called sugar alcohols. These are carbohydrates, but they're carbohydrates that are slowly and incompletely absorbed, at most. Because of this, most low-carbers and all low-carb specialty food labels subtract out polyols from the total carb count, just like fiber. Polyol sweetened treats are easier on your body than the sugar sweetened kind, but it's optimistic to assume that none of that carbohydrate is absorbed. When low-carb sweets say you can subtract out all of the sugar alcohols from the carb count, take that with a grain of salt.

- Also be aware that polyols/sugar alcohols will cause gas and/or diarrhea if you eat them in any quantity. Be very careful with your portions—I rarely eat more than a half of a 1.5 ounce chocolate bar in a day. Don't eat sugar-free sweets at all before a big job interview, an important presentation, a hot date, or getting on a plane, or you may well be sorry.

- Don't be fooled by the fact that many alcoholic drinks have a low-carb count. Alcohol in any form will slow fat-burning dramatically. Doesn't mean you can't drink at all, just realize that alcohol is always a major luxury on a weight loss diet, and gauge your intake accordingly.

WHEN YOU'RE AWAY FROM HOME

• Make the best choice possible given any particular circumstance. What do I mean? If you're at work, and the vending machine has cookies, crackers, chips, candy, and peanuts, the peanuts are the best choice, even though they're relatively high carb for a nut (because, of course, they're really a legume!). When you're genuinely hungry, and faced with foods which are not ideal for the diet, choose the food that will screw you up the least. Don't be afraid to pick off breading, eat only the cheese and toppings off the pizza, ask for an extra salad in place of the potato, etc.

• Always remember that restaurants are in a service industry. Ask questions about ingredients, if you're not certain what's in a dish. Do not hesitate to ask for low-carb substitutions, within reason—steamed vegetables in place of the potato, a bed of lettuce instead of rice, whatever will make your meal low-carb, delicious, and satisfying. If the waiter or the kitchen gives you grief, go spend your money elsewhere. And if they're nice about it—as most restaurants are—be effusive with your praise, and tip well!

• Be polite but firm with people who want you to cheat on your diet. If you're embarrassed about asking for food exactly the way you want it at a restaurant, or about letting your friends know about your food restrictions before a dinner party, let me ask you this: If you had a deadly allergy, one that would cause you to go into anaphylactic shock and die at the mere taste of the wrong food, would you hesitate to bring it up to a waiter or a friend? Of course not, and no one would expect you to. Take care of yourself. [More people die of the effects of carbohydrate intolerance—heart disease, stroke, diabetes, cancer—than die of anything else! Your carbohydrate intolerance is just as deadly as the severest allergy.] It just takes longer, that's all. I find that it's often easier to say, "I'm afraid I can't have that" than to say, "Oh, no thanks, I'm on a diet." People are far less likely to argue if you make it sound medical—which it is!

- When you're traveling, carry some "friendly" food in your purse or carry-on bag. With transportation being as flukey as it is, and airlines rarely handing out anything more than pretzels, who knows how hungry you could get. Carry individually wrapped string cheese, a protein bar or two, some Just-The-Cheese Chips, a packet or two of nuts or seeds—anything that will get you through if the interval between meals gets stretched out unbearably.

10 GREAT SNACKS FOR 5 GRAMS OF USABLE CARB—OR LESS!

- **Cinnamon and Splenda flavored pork rinds,* 0.5 ounces:** 2 grams carb, 0 grams fiber, 2 grams usable carb, 6 grams protein, 80 calories.
* Gram's Gourmet and Katiedid's Pork Rinds make these.

- **Cheddar pork rinds,* 0.5 ounces:** 2 grams carb, 0 grams fiber, 2 grams usable carb, 6 grams protein, 80 calories.
* Gram's Gourmet calls them Cheddar Cheese Crunchies.

- **Hard-boiled egg:*** 0.5 grams carb, 0 grams fiber, 0.5 grams usable carb, 6 grams protein, 77 calories.
* Turning that egg into a deviled egg with a little mayo and mustard will add less than 1 gram of carbohydrate!

- **Frozen hot wings,* 4 pieces:** 1 gram carb, 0 grams fiber, 1 gram usable carb, 20 grams protein, 220 calories.
* Not barbecue wings—barbecue sauce is sugary.

- **⅓ cup smoke-flavored roasted almonds:** 8 grams carb, 4 grams fiber, 4 grams usable carb, 12 grams protein, 360 calories.

- **1 ounce blue cheese and 1 ounce cream cheese, mashed together and stuffed into 1 large celery rib:** 3 grams carb, 1 gram fiber, 2 grams usable carb, 9 grams protein, 205 calories.

- **1 ounce pumpkin seeds:*** 4 grams carb, 2 grams fiber, 2 grams usable carb, 9 grams protein, 150 calories.
* Pumpkorn brand comes in great flavors!

- **1 ounce deluxe mixed nuts (w/o peanuts):** 6 grams carb, 1 gram fiber, 5 grams usable carb, 4 grams protein, 174 calories.

- **String cheese, 2 snack-sized sticks:** 0 grams carb, 0 grams fiber, 0 grams usable carb, 14 grams protein, 160 calories.

- **Hot dogs (No bun of course!) The most common brand (Oscar Meyer):** 1 gram carb, 0 grams fiber, 1 gram usable carb, 5.1 grams protein, 147 calories.

10 TREATS FOR 10 GRAMS OR LESS

- *Sugar free ice pop, 1 stick:* 3.5 grams carb, 0 grams fiber, 3.5 grams usable carb, 0.4 grams protein, 17 calories.

- *6 large strawberries with ½ cup whipped cream (no sugar):* 7 grams carb, 2 grams fiber, 5 grams usable carb, 2 grams protein, 228 calories.

- *1 serving sugar free instant pudding made with half heavy cream, half water:* 2 grams carb, 0 grams fiber, 2 grams usable carb, 1 gram protein, 205 calories.

- *⅛ medium cantaloupe, sprinkled with 1 tablespoon lime juice and ½ tablespoon Splenda:* 8 grams carb, 1 gram fiber, 7 grams usable carb, 1 gram protein, 31 calories.

- *Sugar free fudge pop, 1 stick:* 9 grams carb, 0 grams fiber, 9 grams usable carb, 2 grams protein, 45 calories.

- *Popcorn, 2 cups:* 12 grams carb, 2 grams fiber, 10 grams usable carb, <1 gram protein, 55 calories (assuming oil popped).

- *½ bag Keto brand low carb Nacho Cheese Tortilla Chips:* 16 grams carb, 8 grams fiber, 24 grams protein, 300 calories.

- *¾ cup plain yogurt with ½ teaspoon vanilla extract, 1 tablespoon Splenda, and ¼ cup Gram's Flax 'n Nut Crunchies* stirred in:* 8 grams carb, 3 grams fiber, 5 grams usable carb, 12 grams protein, 301 calories.
* This is a low carb granola-like product made of nuts and seeds.

- *5 Reese's miniature sugar-free peanut butter cups:* 23 grams carb, 1 gram fiber, 19 grams polyols, 3 grams usable carb, 2 grams protein, 170 calories.

- *17 Jelly Belly sugar free jelly beans:** 18 grams carb, 0 grams fiber, 16 grams polyols, 2 grams usable carb, 0 grams protein, 60 calories.
*This is half of what the Jelly Belly company lists as a serving size, but since these are so polyol-rich, I fear that eating 35 jelly beans would cause gastric upset in many people. Be warned!

LOWEST-CARB FAST FOOD MEALS

For a more complete list of fast food that will work for a low carb diet, see page 206—these are just the very lowest-carb choices at each of the biggest chains. At all of these chains, your beverage choices will be coffee, tea, iced tea, diet soda, or water.

McDonalds:
- Side Salad with Low-Fat Balsamic Vinaigrette dressing, plus a Quarter Pounder, no bun, no toppings: 7 grams carb, 1 gram fiber, 6 grams usable carb, 24 grams protein, 285 calories.

- Side Salad with Caesar dressing, plus a Quarter Pounder, no bun, no toppings: 7 grams carb, 1 gram fiber, 6 grams usable carb, 26 grams protein, 435 calories.

- Side Salad with Ranch dressing, plus a Quarter Pounder, no bun, no toppings: 7 grams carb, 1 gram fiber, 6 grams usable carb, 25 grams protein, 535 calories.

Burger King:
- Side Garden Salad with Ranch Dressing, plus a Chicken Whopper Filet, no bun, no toppings: 8 grams carb, 3 grams fiber, 5 grams usable carb, 30 grams protein, 395 calories.

- Side Garden Salad with Ranch Dressing, plus a Whopper, no bun, no toppings: 7 grams carb, 2 grams fiber, 5 grams usable carb, 22 grams protein, 510 calories.

Wendy's:
- BLT Salad, no croutons, Caesar dressing: 11 grams carb, 4 grams fiber, 7 grams usable carb, 34 grams protein, 510 calories.

Subway:
- Roast Beef Salad, no dressing: 10 grams carb, 3 grams fiber, 7 grams usable carb, 12 grams protein, 120 calories.

Pizza Hut:
- Hot Wings, 4 pieces: 2 grams carb, 0 grams fiber, 2 grams usable carb, 22 grams protein, 220 calories.
- Mild Wings, 4 pieces: <2 grams carb, 0 grams fiber, <2 grams usable carb, 2 grams protein, 220 calories.

Arby's:
- Chicken Caesar Salad with Caesar dressing: 9 grams carb, 3 grams fiber, 6 grams usable carb, 34 grams protein, 540 calories.

Taco Bell:
- Taco Salad, no beans, no shell, double chicken: 15 grams carbs, 4 grams fiber, 11 grams usable carb, 43 grams protein, 350 calories.
- Taco Salad, no beans, no shell, double taco meat: 21 grams carb, 10 grams fiber, 11 grams usable carb, 30 grams protein, 452 calories.

KFC:
I'm sorry to say that since KFC discontinued their Tender Roast rotisseried chicken there is simply nothing for us on their menu, with the possible exception of a side of green beans, at 5 grams of carb per serving. All of KFC's chicken is breaded, and simply will not do. If you're stuck at a highway exit that has no other option, pick all the breading off the chicken, and eat some green beans, and you should be okay—but if you have any other option, take it.

Boston Market:
- Marinated Grilled Chicken: 1 gram carb, 0 grams fiber, 1 gram usable carb, 33 grams protein, 230 calories,

OR,

- ¼ Chicken, dark meat, no skin: 1 gram carb, 0 grams fiber, 1 gram usable carb, 22 grams protein, 190 calories.

For some reason I don't pretend to understand, the dark meat without the skin is listed in the Boston Market nutrition tables as having one gram of carb less than the dark meat with the skin. I have no idea why, since the same does not hold true for the white meat, and you'd figure that whatever they sprinkle on the skin (which undoubtedly is the source of any carbs) would be on the breast as well as the leg and thigh. However, since I was going for the "very lowest" carb count for a meal at each place, I took the tables at their word.

Me, I'd have the skin, and the 1 gram of carb be damned.

WITH

- Steamed Vegetable Medley: 6 grams carb, 2 grams fiber, 4 grams usable carb, 2 grams protein, 30 calories,

OR,

- Caesar Side Salad, no croutons: 4 grams carb, <1 gram fiber, >3 grams usable carb, 5 grams protein, 240 calories.*

* The nutritional figures for these items are approximate, working from figures available from Boston Market for the values of these items, and the calorie and fat contents of a portion of croutons.

A DOZEN LOW-CARB THINGS
YOU CAN BUY AT MINI-MARTS

After years of buying low-carb snacks at mini-marts in many regions, I can state with confidence that anyone who says that they have to eat high-carb junk food because they're on the road a lot, and that's all that is available, is making excuses, plain and simple.

Of course, different mini-marts carry different stock, so you can't count on a particular item, or a particular brand of something, being available. Still, in every store I have found a reasonable selection of low-carb items amidst the piles of candy and chips. The chances are nearly 100% that you'll be able to find at least one or two of these items.

Remember to look not only with the chips and other snacks, but in the refrigerator case—many convenience stores have sliced deli meats and cheese snacks, which are pretty ideal low-carb food—and you can usually find mustard and mayo to go with them. Look in the grocery section, as well; frequently you'll find canned tuna, Vienna sausage, and/or canned sardines, as well.

With all of the foods listed, but especially nuts, seeds, and jerky, pay attention to the suggested serving size. Often a small bag of peanuts or jerky looks like one serving to you—but the manufacturer's carb count assumes that the package contains 3, 4, or even 5 servings.

- **Sunflower seeds* (roasted, salted, no shells), 1 ounce bag:** 4.2 grams carb, 1.9 grams fiber, 2.3 grams usable carb, 6 grams protein, 174 calories.

- **Sunflower seeds* (roasted and salted in the shell), 1.75 ounce bag:** 4 gram carb, 2 grams fiber, 2 grams usable carb, 6 grams protein, 160 calories.

* Sunflower seeds even come in nifty flavors, like Ranch, Barbecue, and Nacho Cheese.

- **Peanuts, 1 ounce:** 5.6 grams carb, 2.5 grams fiber, 3.1 grams usable carb, 7.3 grams protein, 164 calories.

- **Almonds, 1 ounce:** 5 grams carb, 2.9 grams fiber, 2.1 grams usable carb, 6 grams protein, 172 calories.

- **Smoke flavored almonds, 30 grams (just over an ounce):** 4 grams carb, 2 grams fiber, 2 grams usable carb, 6 grams protein, 180 calories.

- **Pistachios, 1 ounce:** 7 grams carb, 3.1 grams fiber, 3.9 grams usable carb, 6 grams protein, 164 calories.

- **Pumpkin seeds:*** 0.75 ounce bag: 2 grams carb, 1 gram fiber, 1 gram usable carb, 5 grams protein, 90 calories
* *These figures assume you shell the pumpkin seeds before eating them. If you, like me, like to chew up the shells, look for David brand pumpkin seeds. If only Planter's brand pumpkin seeds are available, shell them and discard the shells—Planter's puts flour on them! If you can find David brand, the shells will be virtually all fiber and salt.*

- **Slim Jim Original beef jerky,* 1 stick:** 2 grams carb, 1 gram fiber, 1 gram usable carb, 9 grams protein, 210 calories.
* *Read the labels on different brands of beef jerky—the carb counts vary radically, from just 1 gram per serving to 8 grams or more!*

- **Plain pork rinds, 1 ounce:** 0 grams carb, 0 grams fiber, 0 grams usable carb, 17.4 grams protein, 154.5 calories.

- **Barbecue flavor pork rinds, most brands,* 1 ounce:** 0.5 grams carb, 0 g. fiber, 0.5 grams usable carb, 16.4 grams protein, 152.5 calories.
**There are a few brands of barbecue flavored pork rinds that have a lot more carb added—read the labels!*

- **Sliced deli meats—ham, turkey, chicken, roast beef, and the like:** These vary, but most have between 1 and 2 grams of carbohydrate per serving, with 3 or 4 grams of protein, and 70 to 90 calories.

■ *Cheese snacks—mostly sticks of cheddar and/or string cheese.* 1 ounce will have between 0.5 and 1 gram of carbohydrate, no fiber, 7 grams of protein, and 80 to 120 calories.

13 LOW-CARB CONVENIENCE FOODS

I would have said a baker's dozen, but none of them are baked goods! Carb counts may vary some from brand to brand, so read the labels.

■ *Rotisseried chicken 3 ounces:* 0 grams carb, 0 grams fiber, 0 grams usable carb, 19 grams protein, 160 calories.

■ *Frozen cooked shrimp (not breaded!), 3 ounces:* 0 grams carb, 0 grams fiber, 0 grams usable carb, 18 grams protein, 84 calories.

■ *Frozen grilled fish fillets, most flavors, 1 fillet:* 1 gram carb, 0 grams fiber, 1 gram usable carb, 17 grams protein, 100 calories.

■ *Pre-cooked chicken strips, 3 ounces:* 0 grams carb, 0 grams fiber, 0 grams usable carb, 20 grams protein, 90 calories.

■ *Frozen pre-formed hamburgers (make sure they're 100% beef), 3 ounces:* 0 grams carb, 0 grams fiber, 0 grams usable carb, 21 grams protein, 240 calories.

■ *Pre-cooked ham:* these vary a great deal, so read the label!

■ *Canned tuna in water, 3 ounces:* 0 grams carb, 0 grams fiber, 0 grams usable carb, 22 grams protein, 98 calories.

■ *Canned tuna in oil, 3 ounces:* 0 grams carb, 0 grams fiber, 0 grams usable carb, 25 grams protein, 168 calories.

■ *Canned crab meat, 3 ounces:* 0 grams carb, 0 grams fiber, 0 grams usable carb, 17 grams protein, 84 calories.

■ *Canned salmon, 3 ounces:* 0 grams carb, 0 grams fiber, 0 grams usable carb, 17 grams protein, 130 calories.

- **Canned shrimp, 3 ounces:** <1 gram carb, 0 grams fiber, < 1 gram usable carb, 20 grams protein, 102 calories.

- **Bagged salad:** depends on type, read the label!

- **Pre-cut broccoli and cauliflower florets, 2 cups mixed florets:** 8.5 grams carb, 5 grams fiber, 3.4 grams usable carb, 4 grams protein, 40 calories.

EXTRANEOUS FAST FOOD DATA

Here is a bunch of data regarding fast food that I dug up while figuring out the lowest-carb choices at each chain. You'll find things like the stats for burgers without buns, and salads without high-carb toppings like croutons.

McDonald's:

- Side Salad, no dressing, plus a Quarter Pounder with Cheese, no bun, no toppings: 4 grams of carb, 1 gram fiber, 3 grams usable carb, 29 grams of protein, 365 calories.

- California Cobb Salad with Grilled Chicken, no dressing: 11 grams carb, 3 grams fiber, 8 grams usable carb, 30 grams protein, 280 calories.

- Bacon Ranch Salad with Grilled Chicken, no dressing: 11 grams carb, 3 grams fiber, 8 grams usable carb, 28 grams protein, 270 calories.

- Chicken Caesar Salad with Grilled Chicken, no dressing: 11 grams carb, 3 grams fiber, 8 grams usable carb, 26 grams protein, 210 calories.

- Paul Newman's Caesar Dressing: 4 grams carb, 0 grams fiber, 4 grams usable carb, 2 grams protein, 190 calories.

- Paul Newman's Cobb Dressing: 9 grams carb, 0 grams fiber, 9 grams usable carb, 1 gram protein, 120 calories.

- Paul Newman's Low-Fat Balsamic Vinaigrette: 4 grams carb, 0 grams fiber, 4 grams usable carb, 0 grams protein, 40 calories.

- Paul Newman's Ranch Dressing: 4 grams carb, 0 grams fiber, 4 grams usable carb, 1 gram protein, 290 calories.

- 2 scrambled eggs: 1 gram carb, no fiber, 1 gram usable carb, 13 grams protein, 160 calories.

- Sausage: 0 grams carb, 0 grams fiber, 0 grams usable carb, 6 grams protein, 170 calories.

- Quarter Pounder, no bun, with toppings:, 5 grams carb, 0 grams fiber, 5 grams usable carb, 24 grams protein, 260 calories.

- Quarter Pounder, no bun, no toppings: 0 grams carb, 0 grams fiber, 0 grams usable carb, 18 grams protein, 230 calories.

- Quarter Pounder with Cheese, no bun, with toppings: 6 grams carb, 0 grams fiber, 6 grams usable carb, 24 grams protein, 360 calories.

- Quarter Pounder with Cheese, no bun, no toppings: 1 gram carb, 0 grams fiber, 1 gram usable carb, 23 grams protein, 340 calories.

Burger King:
- Chicken Caesar Salad, no croutons, Caesar dressing: 9 grams carbs, 3 grams fiber, 6 grams usable carbs, 37 grams protein, 360 calories.

- KRAFT® Light Italian Salad Dressing: 4 grams carb, 0 grams fiber, 4 grams usable carb, 0 grams protein, 40 calories.

- KRAFT® Ranch Salad Dressing: 2 grams carb, 0 grams fiber, 2 grams usable carb, 0 grams protein, 220 calories.

- KRAFT® Creamy Caesar Salad Dressing: 4 grams carb, 0 grams fiber, 4 grams usable carb, 1 gram protein, 135 calories.

- Whopper with cheese, patty and cheese only: 1 gram carb, 0 grams fiber, 1 gram usable carb, 26 grams protein, 355 calories.

- Chicken Whopper, filet only: 1 gram carb, 1 gram fiber, 0 grams usable carb, 29 grams protein, 150 calories.

Wendy's:
- Spring Mix Salad, no honey roasted pecans, Caesar dressing: 13 grams carb, 5 grams fiber, 8 grams usable carb, 11 grams protein, 330 calories.

- Classic Single, no bun (but with pickle, ketchup, lettuce, tomato, mustard, mayo, onion): 6 grams carb, 1 gram fiber, 5 grams usable carb, 19 grams protein, 250 calories.

- Classic Single with Cheese, no bun (but with everything else): 6 grams carb, 1 gram fiber, 5 grams usable carb, 23 grams protein, 320 calories. (Omit the ketchup and the onion on either of these, and you'll drop your total to 3 grams carb, <1 gram fiber.)

- Caesar Side Salad, no croutons, no dressing: 2 grams carb, 1 gram fiber, 1 gram usable carb, 6 grams protein, 70 calories.

- Side Salad, no dressing: 7 grams carb, 3 grams fiber, 4 grams usable carb, 2 grams protein, 35 calories.

- Caesar Dressing: <1 gram carb, 0 grams fiber, <1 gram usable carb, <1 gram protein, 150 calories.

- Blue Cheese Dressing: 3 grams carb, 0 grams fiber, 3 grams usable carb, 2 grams protein, 260 calories.

- Caesar Dressing: <1 grams carb, 0 grams fiber, <1 gram usable carb, <1 gram protein, 150 calories.

- Creamy Ranch Dressing: 5 grams carb, 0 grams fiber, 5 grams usable carb, 1 gram protein, 230 calories.

Subway:
- Tuna Salad, no dressing: 11 grams carb, 3 grams fiber, 8 grams usable carb, 13 grams protein, 240 calories.

- Roasted Chicken Breast Salad, no dressing: 12 grams carb, 3 grams fiber, 9 grams usable carb, 16 grams protein, 140 calories.

- Subway Club Salad, no dressing: 12 grams carb, 3 grams fiber, 9 grams usable carb, 17 grams protein, 150 calories.

- BMT Salad, no dressing: 12 grams carb, 3 grams fiber, 9 grams usable carb, 16 grams protein, 280 calories.

- Subway Melt Salad, no dressing: 12 grams carb, 3 grams fiber, 9 grams usable carb, 18 grams protein, 200 calories.

Arby's:

- Turkey Club Salad with Caesar dressing: 10 grams carb, 3 grams fiber, 7 grams usable carb, 34 grams protein, 660 calories.

- Caesar Dressing: 1 gram carb, 0 grams fiber, 1 gram usable carb, 1 gram protein, 310 calories.

- Buttermilk Ranch Dressing: 3 grams carb, 0 grams fiber, 3 grams usable carb, 1 gram protein, 290 calories.

Boston Market:

- ¼ Chicken, white meat, with skin and wing: 2 grams carb, 0 grams fiber, 2 grams usable carb, 40 grams protein, 280 calories.

- ¼ Chicken, white meat, no skin or wing: 2 grams carb, 0 grams fiber, 2 grams usable carb, 33 grams protein, 170 calories.

- ¼ Chicken, dark meat, with skin: 2 grams carb, 0 grams fiber, 2 grams usable carb, 30 grams protein, 320 calories.

- Skinless Rotisserie Turkey Breast: 3 grams carb, 0 grams fiber, 3 grams usable carb, 36 grams protein, 170 calories.

- Chunky Chicken Salad: 4 grams carb, 0 grams fiber, 4 grams usable carb, 25 grams protein, 480 calories.

- Green Beans: 6 grams carb, 2 grams fiber, 4 grams usable carb, 1 gram protein, 70 calories.

- Grilled Chicken Caesar Salad, no croutons: 9 grams carb, 3 grams fiber, 6 grams usable carb, 47 grams protein, 650 calories. (The nutritional figures for these items is approximate, working from figures available from Boston Market for the values of these items, and the calorie and fat contents of a portion of croutons.)

- California Cobb Salad with Grilled Chicken: 11 grams carb, 3 grams fiber, 8 grams usable carb, 30 grams protein, 280 calories.

- Bacon Ranch Salad with Grilled Chicken: 11 grams carb, 3 grams fiber, 8 grams usable carb, 28 grams protein, 270 calories.

- Chicken Caesar Salad with Grilled Chicken: 11 grams carb, 3 grams fiber, 8 grams usable carb, 26 grams protein, 210 calories.

NOTE ON USING THIS BOOK:

We've put items with less than 5 grams of usable carbohydrate per serving in **bold italics** so that they are easy to spot.

	Calories	Total Carb	Fiber	Usable Carb	Protein
MILK					
COW MILK					
Average All Brands					
Whole (3.5% fat):					
2 Tbsp, 1 fl. oz.	*20*	*1.5*	*0*	*1.5*	*1.1*
1 Glass, 6 fl. oz.	110	8.5	0	8.5	6.3
1 Cup, 8 fl. oz.	150	12	0	12	8.4
1 Pint, 16 fl. oz.	300	23	0	23	16.8
1 Quart, 946 ml	600	46	0	46	33.1
Reduced-fat (2% fat):					
2 Tbsp, 1 fl. oz..	*15*	*1.5*	*0*	*1.5*	*1.2*
1 Glass, 6 fl. oz.	90	8.5	0	8.5	7.2
1 Cup, 8 fl. oz.	130	13	0	13	9.6
1 Pint, 16 fl. oz.	260	26	0	26	19.2
1 Quart, 946 ml	520	52	0	52	37.8
Light/Lowfat (1% fat):					
2 Tbsp, 1 fl. oz.	*12*	*1.5*	*0*	*1.5*	*1.3*
1 Glass, 6 fl. oz.	75	8.5	0	8.5	8.1
1 Cup, 8 fl. oz.	120	14	0	14	10.8
1 Pint, 16 fl. oz.	240	28	0	28	21.6
1 Quart, 946 ml	480	56	0	56	42.6
Fat-free/Skim:					
2 Tbsp, 1 fl. oz.	*10*	*1.5*	*0*	*1.5*	*1.1*
1 Cup, 8 fl. oz.	90	13	0	13	8.4
1 Pint, 16 fl. oz.	180	26	0	26	16.8
Protein-Fortified:					
2% fat, 1 cup	140	14	0	14	9.6
1% fat, 1 cup	120	14	0	14	9.6
Skim, 1 cup	100	14	0	14	9.6
Acidophilus: Average All Brands					
Reduced Fat (2%), 1 cup	130	13	0	13	8
Lowfat (1%), 1 cup	100	13	0	13	7.2
Buttermilk: Average All Brands					
Reduced Fat (2%), 1 cup	120	10	0	10	9.6
Low Fat (1%), 1 cup	100	12	0	12	8.4
Lactose-Reduced:					
Reduced Fat:					
Lactaid, 1 cup	130	12	0	12	7.9
Lowfat, Lactaid, 1 cup	110	13	0	13	7.9
Fat Free:					
Lactaid/Lucerne, 1 cup	80	13	0	13	7.9

	Calories	Total Carb	Fiber	Usable Carb	Protein
CANNED & DRIED MILK					
Condensed:					
Reg. 2 Tbsp, 1fl. oz.	130	22	0	22	3
Lowfat (Eagle), 2 Tbsp.	120	23	0	23	3
Fat Free (Eagle), 2 Tbsp.	110	24	0	24	3
Dried: Whole, ¼ cup, 1 oz.	150	11	0	11	7.5
Skim/Nonfat,					
Made-up, 1 cup, 8 fl. oz.	80	12	0	12	43.2
WHEY DRINK					
Nutri Mil:					
Orig./Low Fat 8 fl. oz.	80	11	0	11	2
Chocolate, 8 fl. oz.	110	19	0	19	2
Fat Free	60	11	0	11	2

FLAVORED MILK DRINKS

	Calories	Total Carb	Fiber	Usable Carb	Protein
CHOCOLATE MILK					
Average All Brands:					
Per Cup, 8 fl. oz.					
Whole Milk (3.3%): 1 cup	225	26	0	26	9.6
1 Pint	450	52	0	52	19.2
Reduced Fat (2%), 1 cup	190	26	0	26	9.6
Lowfat (1%), 1 cup	160	26	0	26	9.6
BRANDS-CHOCOLATE MILK					
Ready-To-Drink:					
Per 8 fl. oz. cup					
Meadow Gold (3.5%)	210	25	0	25	8
Nesquik Chocolate:					
Regular, 1 cup, 8 fl. oz.	230	31	0.5	30.5	8
16 fl. oz. bottle	460	62	1	61	16
Fat Free, 1 cup, 8 fl. oz.	160	31	0.5	30.5	8
16 fl. oz. bottle	320	62	1	61	16
Double Chocolate,					
1 cup, 8 fl. oz.	230	30	0.5	29.5	8
16 fl. oz. bottle	460	60	1	59	16
Quik: (Nestle)					
Chocolate Milk	230	30	0.5	29.5	8
Strawberry Milk	220	31	0	31	7
SHAKES & SMOOTHIES					
McDonald's Thick Creamy Shakes:					
16 fl. oz., avg. all flavors	570	92	1.3	90.7	14.7

	Calories	Total Carb	Fiber	Usable Carb	Protein
Burger King:					
Vanilla, medium	720	73	1	72	15
Chocolate w/ Syrup,					
Medium	790	89	2	87	15

COCOA-CHOCOLATE MIXES

	Calories	Total Carb	Fiber	Usable Carb	Protein
Carnation Cocoa Mixes:					
Chocolate Rich,					
3 Tbsp/1 pkt	110	24	0.7	23.3	1.3
Milk Chocolate, 3 Tbsp.	110	24	0.7	23.3	1.3
w/ Mini Marshmallows	110	24	0.5	23.5	1.3
No Sugar, 1 pkt	50	8	0.8	7.2	4.3
Swiss Miss Cocoa Mixes:					
Milk Chocolate, 1 oz. pkt	110	22	0	22	2
w/ Marshmallows,					
1.2 oz. pkt	140	22	0	22	6.5
Choc. Sensation,					
1.25 oz. pkt	150	27	0	27	1.5
Lite, 1 pkt	70	18	0	18	0
Diet Cocoa Mix, 1 pkt	*20*	*4*	*0*	*4*	*1*
Hot Cocoa Mix, 1 pkt					
no added sugar	60	10	1	9	2
Sugar Free	60	10	0	10	5
Fat Free, 0.53 oz.	50	9	0	9	3.5
Vending Machine,					
1.34 oz. pkt	145	24	0	24	8

SOY & NON-DAIRY DRINKS
(PER 1 CUP SERVING, 8 FL. OZ)

EDEN BLEND

	Calories	Total Carb	Fiber	Usable Carb	Protein
1 cup	120	18	0	18	6.7

EDENSOY

	Calories	Total Carb	Fiber	Usable Carb	Protein
Original, 1 cup	130	13	1.9	11.1	10.6
Extra, Vanilla	150	23	1	22	7
Carob	170	27	0	27	6.7
Light: Original, 1 cup	95	14	0	14	4.8
Vanilla	120	21	0	21	3.8

8TH CONTINENT

	Calories	Total Carb	Fiber	Usable Carb	Protein
Chocolate, Lowfat	140	23	1	22	5.5
Original, Lowfat	80	8	0	8	5.5
Vanilla, Lowfat	90	11	0.5	10.5	7

	Calories	Total Carb	Fiber	Usable Carb	Protein
HARMONY FARMS					
Regular, 1 cup	80	10	0	10	3.2
Enriched; Vanilla, 1 cup	100	14	0	14	4.2
HEALTH SOURCE					
Soy Protein Shake					
All Flavors	*100*	*4*	*0*	*4*	*20*
IT'S SOY DELICIOUS					
Vanilla	110	22	0	22	3.5
Awesome; Chocolate	120	22	0	22	3.5
LIFEWAY					
Soy Treat, Apple, Caramel	160	23	0	23	7
NAKED JUICE					
Chocolate Soy Shake	210	38	0	38	9
Vanilla Soy Shake	170	33	0	33	8
ODWALLA FUTURE SHAKE					
Chocolate	160	27	0	27	6.5
Vanilla al'Monde	190	24	0	24	10
SILK (WHITE WAVE)					
Plain, regular	100	8	0	8	7
Plain, unsweetened	90	5	0	5	8.5
Chai, Mocha	140	20	0	20	8.5
Chocolate	140	23	0	23	4
Coffee Soylatte, 1 cup	170	29	0	29	5.5
11 oz bottle	220	38	0	38	7.6
Spice Soylatte, 11 oz bottle	200	27	0	27	9.5
Vanilla	100	10	0	10	6
Silk Creamer, 1 Tbsp	*15*	*1*	*0*	*1*	*0.5*
SOYDREAM					
Orig./Enriched 8 fl. oz	130	17	0	17	7
Carob/Chocolate Enriched	210	37	0	37	7
Vanilla; Vanilla Enriched	150	22	0	22	7
SOY NICE					
Natural, 8 fl. oz	*70*	*2*	*0*	*2*	*7*
Original	80	6	0	6	6
Chocolate, 1 cup	110	17	0	17	6
Vanilla	100	11	0	11	6
SUNSOY					
Chocolate, 1 cup	140	23	0	23	5

	Calories	Total Carb	Fiber	Usable Carb	Protein
Creamy Original	80	7	0	7	7
Vanilla	110	15	0	15	6
VITASOY					
Refrigerated, Creamy Orig.	110	12	0	12	7
Rich Chocolate	160	24	0	24	7
Low Fat Vanilla Delite	90	13	0	13	4
Long Life: Creamy Original	110	9	0	9	9
Creamy Unsweetened	80	5	0	5	6
Carob Supreme; Rich Cocoa	150	20	0	20	8
Vanilla Delite	120	14	0	14	7
Light: Original	60	7	0	7	4
Cocoa	110	18	0	18	5
Vanilla	90	14	0	14	4
Enriched: Original	90	9	0	9	4
Light Original	60	7	0	7	4
Vanilla	110	14	0	14	4
Light Vanilla	90	13	0	13	4
WESTSOY					
Plus, Plain	130	18	3	15	6
Plus, Vanilla	140	19	3	16	7
100% Organic:					
Original (2% fat)	140	18	3	15	7
Unsweetened, Plain	***90***	***4***	***4***	***0***	***9***
Unsweetened, Vanilla	***100***	***5***	***4***	***1***	***9***
Nonfat: Plain	80	16	1	15	3
Vanilla	90	17	1	16	3
Lite: Plain, 1 cup	100	15	2	13	2
Cocoa	120	28	2	26	2
Vanilla	120	21	0	21	3
Lowfat: Plain	90	14	2	12	4
Chocolate	180	32	3	29	6
Vanilla	110	20	2	18	4
Smart Lite: Plain	120	19	1	18	7
Vanilla	150	25	1	24	7
Café: Coffee; Mocha; Fr. Van	130	24	0.5	23.5	2
Chai: Orig./Green Tea, avg	140	26	0.5	25.5	1
Smoothies, all flavors	140	28	2	26	3
Soy Shakes: Choc; Vanilla	170	30	4	26	7
Vigor Aid: French Vanilla	260	44	7	37	10
Choc Mocha, Creamy Choc.	240	38	7	31	10
Juice Bar, Average all flavors	120	24	2	22	3

	Calories	Total Carb	Fiber	Usable Carb	Protein
WILD OATS					
Original, 1 cup, 8 fl. Oz	100	12	3	9	7

YOGURT & YOGURT DRINKS

AVERAGE ALL BRANDS: PER 8 OZ. CUP					
Plain Yogurt:					
Whole, 8 oz.	180	11	0	11	18.6
Lowfat	140	16	0	16	19.9
Nonfat	110	18	0	18	14.6
Fruit Flavored:					
Whole, 8 oz.	250	38	0	38	11
Lowfat	230	32	0	32	31.2
Nonfat, regular	150	32	0	32	16.8
Nonfat, No sugar added	120	32	0	32	13.2
ALTA DENA					
Fruit on the bottom:					
Cherry Vanilla	270	55	0	55	7
BREYERS					
Light n' Lively, 4.4 oz.	135	27	0.2	26.8	4
Lowfat: 1% fat,					
All flavors, 8 oz.	220	41	0.5	40.5	8.4
1.5% fat, plain, 8 oz.	125	22	0	22	7.7
Smooth & Creamy, 8 oz.	230	45	0.7	44.3	8.6
BROWN COW: PER 8 OZ.					
Cream Top: Chocolate	250	39	0	39	7
Creamy Coffee, Vanilla	210	25	0	25	7
Fruit Flavors, Average	230	35	0	35	7
Lowfat Flavors, average	220	41	0	41	9
Non Fat Fruit Flavors, Average	190	39	0	39	9
CASCADE FRESH					
Lowfat, 6 oz.	140	23	0	23	8
Fat Free, all flavors,					
6 oz. carton	110	20	0	20	7
Whole Milk, 8 oz.	170	12	0	12	13
COLUMBO					
Light, all flavors, 8 oz.	110	20	0	20	7
Classic, avg. all types, 8 oz.	220	41	0	41	7
Fat Free, Plain, 8 oz.	110	16	0	16	10

	Calories	Total Carb	Fiber	Usable Carb	Protein
CONTINENTAL NONFAT, 8 OZ. CTN					
Fruit on the bottom	190	38	0	38	11
Plain	200	38	0	38	12
CROWLEY					
Lowfat Blueberry, 8 oz.	240	48	0	48	7
DANNON					
Plain					
Natural, 8 oz.	170	14	0	14	9
Danimals:					
Super Creamy, 4 oz.	120	18	0	18	5
Squeezable, 2 oz.	140	20	0.5	19.5	2
Drinkable, 3.3 fl. oz.	120	22	0	22	4
Fruit Blends:					
Blueberry, 6 oz.	170	33	0	33	6
Strawberry, Blueberry, 4 oz.	110	21	0	21	4
Fruit on the Bottom:					
Avg. all flavors, 6 oz. ctn	160	29	0	29	6
Frusion Smoothie:					
10 fl. oz. bottle	280	53	0	53	8
la Crème:					
Avg. all flavors, 4 oz.	150	21	0	21	5
Mousse, all flavors, 2.6 oz.	120	15	0	15	3
Light 'n Fit (0% Fat):					
Average, all flavors, 6 oz.	90	17	0	17	6
Creamy, avg.					
all flavors, 6 oz.	120	16	0	16	8
Smoothie, 7 fl. oz. bottle	80	15	0	15	5
Natural:					
Avg. all flavors, 6 oz.	160	22	0	22	7
Sprinkl'ins:					
All flavors, 4.1 oz. ctn	120	22	0	22	4
Whipped:					
Avg. all flavors, 4.6 oz.	160	28	0	28	6
GROCER'S PRIDE					
Lowfat, 4.4 oz.	140	28	0	28	5
IMPERIAL SUPREME					
Lowfat, 6 oz.	140	26	0	26	6
JELL-O:					
Kid Pack, All flavors, 125g	130	25	0	25	4.4

	Calories	Total Carb	Fiber	Usable Carb	Protein
MOUNTAIN HIGH					
Original: Plain, 8 oz.	190	18	0	18	11
Fat Free, Plain, 8 oz.	120	20	0	20	11
Fat Free: Plain, 8 oz.	110	19	0	19	10
Flavors, average, 6 oz. ctn	110	29	0	29	7.5
SILK (SOY)					
Vanilla, 6 oz. ctn	120	23	1	22	2.5
Other flavors, average, 6 oz.	170	31	1	30	4
SNACKWELL'S					
Nonfat, 6 oz.	160	36	0	36	5
STONYFIELD FARM, ORGANIC					
Whole Milk:					
Plain, 1 cup, 8 oz.	180	16	3	13	9
French Vanilla, 8 oz.	250	36	4	32	8
6 oz. cups:					
Vanilla, Mocha	190	27	3	24	7
Other flavors, avg	170	24	2	22	5
Lowfat:					
Plain, 6 oz.	90	13	1.5	11.5	5.2
Flavors, average, 6 oz.	140	25	3	22	6
4 oz. cup pkg	100	19	2	17	4
Nonfat: Plain, 8 oz. cup	100	15	0	15	9
Other flavors, avg. 8 oz.	160	32	0.5	31.5	8
YoBaby, 4 oz. ctn	120	17	0	17	4
YoSqueeze, 2 oz. tube	60	11	1	10	2
TRADER JOE'S					
Nonfat: Regular, 8 oz.	190	40	0	40	9
French Village, Vanilla, 8 oz.	170	32	0	32	10
Organic Vanilla, 8 oz.	160	27	0	27	11
Lowfat, average, 8 oz.	230	44	0	44	8
Organic Low Fat, Average, 6 oz.	*150*	*24*	*21*	*3*	*7*
Cultured Soy, all varieties, 6 oz.	140	28	0.5	27.5	5
YOCRUNCH					
Lowfat w/ Toppings, 6.5 oz. cup					
Oreo Cookies	190	35	1	34	5
Peach/Strawb./Rasp. w/ granola	220	46	1	45	6

	Calories	Total Carb	Fiber	Usable Carb	Protein
Strawberry					
w/ Nestlé Crunch	240	41	1	40	6
Vanilla					
w/ Choc Crunch/Reese's	240	39	1	38	5
YOPLAIT					
Fat Free: Plain, 3.5 oz.	45	7.5	0	7.5	4
Vanilla, 3.5 oz.	70	14	0	14	3.5
Original 99%: 6 oz.	180	34	0	34	7.5
Multi Pack, container, 4 oz.	120	22	0	22	6
Go-Gurt, 2.25 oz. tube	80	13	0	13	2
Lowfat,					
Crmy Strawberry, 3.5 oz.	110	21	0	21	4
Original, Plain, 8 oz.	80	5.3	0	5.3	14.7
Cherry; Peach, 8 oz.	151	29	0	29	5.3
Avg. other flavors, 8 oz.	220	44	0	44	6.7
Trix, Avg., all flavors, 4 oz.	120	23	0	23	4
Custard Style, 6 oz.	190	32	0	32	7
Light, avg., all flavors, 6 oz.	100	19	0	19	6
Yumsters, 4 oz.	120	21	0	21	5
YOGURT DRINKS & PROBIOTICS					
Actimel (Dannon)					
Probiotic, 3.3 fl. oz.	90	16	0	16	3
Alta Dena, Drinkables, 1 cup	220	46	0	46	9
Carbolite, 8 fl. oz.	85	8	0	8	6
Dannon, Danimals,					
3.4 fl. oz. bottle	90	16	0	16	4
Glen Oaks,					
all flavors, avg, 1 cup	250	46	0	46	7.5
Nouriche, all flavors, 11 fl. oz.	290	60	0	60	12.5
Stonyfield Farm, 10 fl. oz.	240	44	0	44	9
Wow Cow, 8 fl. oz.	80	16	0	16	2
Yonique, 6 fl. oz.:					
Pina Colada	190	30	0	30	8.5
Peach; Banana; Guava	170	30	0	30	8

ICE CREAM & FROZEN YOGURT

ICE CREAM					
Vanilla: Average All Brands					
Regular Ice cream (10% fat):					
3 fl. oz. scoop	100	12	0	12	0.8

	Calories	Total Carb	Fiber	Usable Carb	Protein
½ cup, 4 fl. oz.	130	16	0	16	1
1 Pint, 16 fl. oz.	520	62	0	62	4
½ Gallon (4 Pints)	2100	248	0	248	16
Rich (16% fat):					
3 fl. oz. scoop	130	12	0	12	2.2
½ cup, 4 fl. oz.	170	17	0	17	3
1 Pint	690	68	0	68	12
Super-Rich (20% fat):					
3 fl. oz.	200	16	0	16	4.5
½ cup, 4 fl. oz.	270	21	0	21	6
1 Pint	1100	84	0	84	24
Reduced Fat/Light (6% fat):					
3 fl. oz. scoop	100	14	0	14	6
½ cup, 4 fl. oz.	140	18	0	18	8
1 Pint	560	72	0	72	32
Low Fat (less than 4% fat):					
3 fl. oz. scoop	90	17	0	17	1.9
½ cup, 4 fl. oz.	120	22	0	22	2.5
1 Pint	480	88	0	88	10
Fat Free:					
3 fl. oz. scoop	75	17	0	17	2.2
½ cup, 4 fl. oz.	100	22	0	22	3
1 Pint	400	88	0	88	12
Soft Serve:					
Regular, ½ cup	140	20	0	20	4
Regular, 1 cup	280	40	0	40	8
Nonfat, ½ cup	90	23	0	23	0.5
Nonfat, 1 cup	180	46	0	46	1

FROZEN YOGURT

	Calories	Total Carb	Fiber	Usable Carb	Protein
Average All Brands:					
Hard:					
Lowfat, ½ cup	140	26	0	26	2.5
Nonfat, ½ cup	110	29	0	29	2.5
Soft:					
Lowfat, ½ cup	120	28	0	28	0.5
Nonfat, ½ cup	100	30	0	30	1
Ben & Jerry's					
Frozen Yogurt: Per ½ cup					
Cherry Garcia Yogurt	170	32	0	32	4
Choc. Fudge Brownie Yogurt	190	36	1	35	6
Half Baked Yogurt	210	39	0.5	38.5	5

	Calories	Total Carb	Fiber	Usable Carb	Protein
Phish Food Yogurt	230	42	1	41	4
Sorbet:					
Average, All flavors	120	30	0	30	0
Scoop Shop: Per ½ cup					
Coconut Almond Fudge	260	20	1	19	5
Coffee Buzz;					
Marble Mint Chip	240	22	0.5	21.5	3
Mint Chocolate Chunk	240	23	0	23	3
S'Mores	180	34	1	33	4
Southern Peach;					
Strawberry	180	20	0	20	3
Sweet Cream & Cookie	230	23	0.5	22.5	4
White Russian	200	18	0	18	3

GELATO/ICES

	Calories	Total Carb	Fiber	Usable Carb	Protein
Gelato: Per ½ cup					
Milk base:					
Vanilla	200	18	0	18	0.5
Choc. Hazelnut	370	26	0	26	1.5
Water base: ½ cup	100	25	0	25	0

SUNDAES

	Calories	Total Carb	Fiber	Usable Carb	Protein
Denny's Sundaes:					
Single scoop, No topping	190	14	0	14	3
Double scoop, No topping	375	29	0	29	6
Banana Split	895	112	6	106	15
Butterfinger, Hot Fudge	780	106	1	105	9
Toppings:					
Blueberry, 2 oz.	70	17	7.4	9.6	0
Chocolate, 2 oz.	320	27	0	27	2
Fudge, 2 oz.	200	30	1	29	1
Strawberry, 2 oz.	*80*	*17*	*12.7*	*4.3*	*0.7*
McDonald's Sundaes:					
Hot Fudge Sundae, 6.3 oz.	340	52	1	51	8
Oreo Cookie, McFlurry	570	82	0	82	15
Toppings:					
Nut/Sundae, ¼ oz.	*40*	*2*	*0*	*2*	*2*

ICE CREAM CONES & CUPS

	Calories	Total Carb	Fiber	Usable Carb	Protein
Wafer Cone/Cup, Average	*20*	*4*	*0*	*4*	*1*
Sugar Cone, Average	40	9	0	9	1
Waffle Cone: Small	60	11	0	11	0.5
Large	100	22	0	22	2

	Calories	Total Carb	Fiber	Usable Carb	Protein
Brands:					
Oreo, Chocolate Cone	50	10	0.5	9.5	0
Comet, Sugar Cone	50	11	0	11	3
Keebler, Sugar Cone	45	11	0	11	1
ALTA DENA: PER ½ CUP					
Golden Honey, Vanilla	160	17	0	17	2
Honey Chocolate	160	19	0	19	2
BEN & JERRY'S: PER ½ CUP					
Apple Crumble	280	33	0	33	3
Butter Pecan	290	20	1	19	4
Cherry Garcia; Vanilla	260	26	0	26	5
Choc. Chip Cookie Dough	270	31	0	31	4
Choc. Fudge Brownie	280	33	2	31	5
Chubby Hubby	330	32	1	31	7
Chunky Monkey;					
Coffee Heath Bar	310	32	1	31	4
Concession Obsession	310	32	1	31	4
Fudge Central	300	31	0.5	30.5	4
Honey, I'm Home!	260	29	0	29	4
Karamel Sutra	280	32	1	31	4
Makin' Whoopie Pie	270	33	2	31	4
Mint Chocolate Cookie	270	28	0.5	27.5	4
New York Super					
Fudge Chunk	310	30	2	28	5
Nutty Waffle Cone	310	31	0	31	5
Peanut Butter Cup	310	32	2	30	6
Peanut Butter Me Up	330	25	2	23	6
Peanut Butter Truffle	300	30	2	28	6
Phish Food	280	38	2	36	4
Pistachio Pistachio	280	21	0	21	6
S'mores	260	34	1	33	3
The Full Vermonty	260	27	0	27	4
Triple Caramel Chunk	290	32	0	32	4
World's Best Chocolate	280	27	0	25	5
World's Best Vanilla	250	21	0	21	4
2-Twisted: Half Baked	280	33	1	32	4
Everything But The...	320	30	1	29	5
From Russia With Buzz	270	26	0.5	25.5	4
Jerry's Jubilee	260	29	0.5	28.5	4
S.N.A.F.U.	250	28	0.5	27.5	4
Vanilla Caramel Fudge	280	32	0	32	4

	Calories	Total Carb	Fiber	Usable Carb	Protein
Vanilla Heath Bar Crunch	300	29	0	29	4
BLUE BUNNY:					
Health Smart	80	18	0	18	2
Sweet Freedom: Sugar Free	*15*	*4*	*0*	*4*	*0*
Icecream Lites; Krunch Lites	105	11	0	11	2
Vanilla Icecream Sandwich	155	25	0.5	24.5	4
Vanilla Sundae Cone	255	30	0.5	29.5	5
Ice Cream Fat Free,					
No Added Sugar: Chocolate;					
Mint Fudge Swirl; Vanilla	95	20	0	20	4
Average Other flavors	105	23	0	23	3
Icecream Reduced Fat,					
No Added Sugar:					
Banana Split	135	20	0	20	3
Butter Pecan	135	16	0	16	4
Cherry Vanilla	125	18	0	18	3
Neopolitan	115	16	0	16	3
Rocky Road	155	21	0	21	4
Tin Roof Sundae	145	19	0	19	4
Vanilla	120	16	0	16	3
BREYERS: PER ½ CUP					
Fat Free: Average	*90*	*2*	*0*	*2*	*20.5*
Lactose-Free: Vanilla	130	14	0	14	2
Light: Average	*130*	*0*	*0*	*0*	*4.5*
All Natural: Butter Pecan	165	14	0	14	3
Cherry Vanilla; Coffee	150	16	0	16	2
Chocolate; French Vanilla	160	15	0.5	14.5	2
Choc. Chip;					
Mint Choc. Chip;	165	17	0	17	2
Cookies 'n Cream	165	18	0	18	3
Dulche de Leche	155	21	0	21	2
Extra Creamy					
Chocolate/Vanilla	160	19	0.5	18.5	2
Peach; Strawberry	130	18	0	18	2
Peanut Butter & Fudge	175	17	0.5	16.5	4
Vanilla & Chocolate;					
Vanilla Fudge Twirl	160	18	0	18	2
Vanilla & Chocolate					
Fudge Checks	160	17	0	17	3
Vanilla; Vanilla/Choc./Strwb.	150	16	0	16	2
Wild Berry Swirl	145	16	0	16	2

	Calories	Total Carb	Fiber	Usable Carb	Protein
Light: Average all flavors,					
½ cup	120	18	0	18	3
Icecream Parlor:					
Chips Ahoy	160	18	0	18	3
Heath English Toffee; Reese's	180	22	0	22	2
Hershey's; Almond Joy	170	21	0.5	20.5	3
Klondike Icecream Sandwich	160	21	0	21	3
Mint w/ Oreo	165	20	0	20	2
Homemade:					
Double Choc Fudge	180	23	0.5	22.5	2
Neopolitan	150	17	0	17	3
Viennetta: All flavors, avg.,					
1 Slice	180	20	0	20	3
Frozen Yogurt:					
Average, ½ cup	140	22	0.5	21.5	3
No Sugar Added	105	13	0	13	3
DOLEWHIP (SOFT SERVE):					
Per 4 fl. oz., ½ cup					
Chocolate; Vanilla	100	18	1	17	0.5
Fruit flavors, Average	80	16	0	16	0
DREYERS: PER ½ CUP					
No Sugar Added:					
Average All flavors	90	12	0	12	3
Fat Free:					
Average All flavors	110	25	0	25	3
No Sugar Added	95	20	0	20	4
Grand:					
Cracker Jack	170	20	0	20	3
Scooby Doo!	160	16	0	16	3
Dexter's Lab.,					
Amazing Creation	160	21	0	21	2
Grand Light:					
Vanilla	100	15	0	15	3
Cookie Dough;					
P'nut Butter Cup	130	17	0	17	3
Other varieties, Average	120	18	0	18	3
DREAMERY					
Black Raspberry Avalanche	270	27	0	27	4
Caramel Toffee Bar;					
Heaven Vanilla	290	32	0	32	4

	Calories	Total Carb	Fiber	Usable Carb	Protein
Cherry Chip ba da Bing	280	33	0	33	3
Chocolate Almond Bar	300	32	0	32	5
Choc P'nut Butter Chunk	310	29	0	29	7
Cool Mint	300	32	0	32	4
Dulce de Leche, Caramel	270	32	0	32	4
Grandma's Cookie Dough	300	32	0	32	4
Strawberry Fields	220	26	0	26	3
New York Strawberry					
Cheesecake	260	27	0	27	4
Nothing But Chocolate	280	34	0	34	5
Tiramisu	270	33	0	33	4
Homemade:					
Butter Pecan, 71g	160	16	0	16	3
Cracker Jack; Scooby Snack	170	20	0	20	3
Vanilla, ½ cup, 71g	140	16	0	16	2
frozen Yogurt:					
Vanilla	90	19	0	19	2
Chips Supreme, ½ cup	120	19	0	19	2
Fat Free, average All flavors	90	20	0	20	0
Starburst Sherbet:					
Avg. All flavors	150	30	0	30	1
Whole Fruit Sorbet:					
Boysenberry	150	37	1	36	0
Strawberry, Peach;					
Raspberry	130	33	0	33	0
EDY'S: PER ½ CUP					
Banana Split;					
Choc Fudge Mousse	160	19	0	19	3
Cherry Choc; Van/Choc;					
Espresso	150	17	0	17	2
Choc Fudge Sundae/					
Dble Fudge	170	19	0	19	2
Ice Cream Sandwich	140	14	0	14	3
Grand Light:					
Vanilla	100	15	0	15	3
Butter Pecan; Choc Almond	120	16	0	16	3
Chiquita 'N Chocolate	110	13	0	13	3
Choc Fudge Mousse	110	17	0	17	3
Cookie Dough;					
P'nut Butter Cups	130	18	0	18	3

	Calories	Total Carb	Fiber	Usable Carb	Protein
Cookies 'n Cream;					
Rocky Road	110	16	0	16	3
French Silk	120	18	0	18	3
Fat Free:					
Average All Flavors	115	25	0	25	3
Reduced Fat: Butter Pecan	140	16	1	15	4
Choc Marshmallow	130	23	1	22	4
Neopolitan; Vanilla	110	18	0	18	4
Fudge Ripple	120	19	0	19	4
FROSTLINE (SOFT SERVE):					
Chocolate	90	20	0	20	1
Vanilla, ½ cup	90	18	0	18	1
GODIVA: PER ½ CUP					
Belgian Dark Chocolate	280	26	2	24	5
Choc Hazelnut Truffle	350	31	3	28	5
Choc Raspberry Truffle	290	32	2	30	4
Chocolate Cheesecake	310	36	0	36	4
Chocolate					
w/ Chocolate Hearts	330	32	0	32	5
Classic Milk Chocolate	290	28	1	27	5
Pecan Caramel Truffle	320	32	2	30	5
Vanilla Caramel Pecan	290	33	0	33	5
Vanilla w/ Chocolate					
Caramel Hearts	310	32	0	32	5
White Choc Raspberry	260	32	0	32	5
HEALTHY CHOICE: PER ½ CUP					
Brownie Bliss	130	25	1	24	2
Cookies 'N Cream	130	24	1	23	3
Double Karma	140	28	0.5	27.5	2
Happy Together	150	29	0.5	28.5	2
Jumpin' Java	140	25	0.5	24.5	3
Peanut Butter	110	19	0.5	18.5	3
Praline & Caramel	130	25	1	24	3
Rocky Road	130	25	2	23	3
Vanilla; Mint Choc Chip	100	18	0	18	4
Other flavors, average	120	22	0.5	21.5	3
Lowfat, No Sugar Added:					
Vanilla	90	16	0	16	3
No Sugar Added:					
Coffee Almond Fudge	110	20	0	20	3

	Calories	Total Carb	Fiber	Usable Carb	Protein
Chocolate Fudge Brownie	110	20	0	20	4
Mint Chocolate Chip	100	28	0	28	3

HOOD: PER ½ CUP SERVING

	Calories	Total Carb	Fiber	Usable Carb	Protein
Regular Ice cream:					
Average all flavors	150	17	0	17	4
No Sugar Added,					
Lowfat Ice cream:					
Vanilla Dream; Classic Trio	100	14	0	14	3
Chocolate Frenzy;					
Mocha Madness, avg	120	19	0	19	3
Chocolate Chip	120	16	0	16	3
frozen Yogurt:					
Nonfat: Strawberry,					
Old Fashioned Vanilla	110	24	0	24	1.9
Other flavors, average	120	27	0	27	2.9
Regular: Avg All flavors	150	17	0	17	1.9

SOY DREAM (NON-DAIRY)

	Calories	Total Carb	Fiber	Usable Carb	Protein
Per ½ Cup					
Butter Pecan	160	17	2	15	1
Chocolate Fudge Brownie	150	20	2	18	1
Mint Chocolate Chip	150	19	1	18	1
Average other flavors	140	20	2	18	1
Rocket Bars: Choc/Vanilla	220	29	2	27	1
Heavenly Pies: Mocha/Vanilla	290	40	2	38	3

STONYFIELD FARM (ORGANIC): PER ½ CUP SERVING

	Calories	Total Carb	Fiber	Usable Carb	Protein
Ice cream: Chocolate	265	22	1	21	3
Decaf Coffee; Vanilla, avg	260	21	0	21	3
Other flavors, average	260	26	0	26	2
frozen Yogurt:					
Nonfat Choc; Raspberry	100	21	0	21	3
Nonfat Vanilla; Decaf Coffee	90	19	0	19	4
Nonfat Vanilla Fudge Swirl	110	23	0	23	4
Lowfat: Crème Caramel	120	23	0	23	4
Choc Mint; Mocha Almond	130	22	1	21	5

TOFUTTI NON-DAIRY DESSERT:

	Calories	Total Carb	Fiber	Usable Carb	Protein
Per ½ Cup					
Premium: Vanilla	190	20	0	20	2
Better Pecan; Alm Bark	220	22	0	22	1
Choc Cookie Crunch	210	26	1	25	3
Chocolate Supreme	180	18	0	18	3

	Calories	Total Carb	Fiber	Usable Carb	Protein
Van Fudge; Wildberry	190	24	0	24	2
Low Fat Supreme: Average	110	25	0	25	2
Cutie Pies: Average, 67g bar	250	18	0	18	2
Too Toos: Vanilla S'wich	215	28	0.	28	3
Van Choc Swirl/Chip S'wich	230	30	0	30	3
Teddy Fudge: 52g bar	70	19	0	19	1

ICE CREAM BARS & POPS
(PER BAR/SERVING)

BEN & JERRY'S

	Calories	Total Carb	Fiber	Usable Carb	Protein
Cherry Garcia: Ice Cream Bar	240	23	1	22	3
Yogurt Bar	250	35	2	33	6
Cookie Dough: 89ml Bar	330	36	0.5	35.5	4
110ml Bar	410	45	0.6	44.4	4.9
Cookie Dough Pop	410	45	0	45	5
One Sweet Whirled	260	27	0.5	26.5	4
Phish Stick: 89ml Bar	260	29	2	27	3
Vanilla Heath Crunch	320	32	0	32	4

BREYERS

	Calories	Total Carb	Fiber	Usable Carb	Protein
Fruit Bars:					
All Natural, 1.75 fl. oz.	45	11	0	11	0
No Sugar Added, 1.75 fl. oz.	20	5	0	5	0
Natural Strawberry					
Fruit Juice	120	30	0.5	29.5	0
Soft Caramel Magnum Bar	375	38	0.5	37.5	4
Soft frozen Lemonade Cup	295	74	0	74	0
Soft frozen Strawberry Cup	265	66	0	66	0

CREAMSICLE

	Calories	Total Carb	Fiber	Usable Carb	Protein
Sugar-free pops	25	15	0	15	0
Orange, 2.8 fl. oz.	110	20	0	20	1

DOVE BAR

	Calories	Total Carb	Fiber	Usable Carb	Protein
Almond	340	30	1	29	6
Bite Size, 5 pcs, avg	350	36	1	35	4
Vanilla Dark Choc; Cookie	340	35	2	33	4
Vanilla Milk Choc	350	29	1	28	4

ESKIMO PIE

	Calories	Total Carb	Fiber	Usable Carb	Protein
Arctic Madness, 2.5 oz.	230	23	0	23	1
Bars:					
Milk/Dark Chocolate, 50g	160	15	0	15	2

	Calories	Total Carb	Fiber	Usable Carb	Protein
Fudge Bar, 55g	60	11	0	11	2
Reduced Fat varieties	120	13	0	13	3
Crispy Bar, 47g	130	13	0	13	3
Big Bar, 99g	300	26	0	26	4
Ice Cream Sandwich, 65g	160	27	1	26	4
Cones, 74g	210	24	0	24	3
No Sugar Added: Bar, 49g	120	13	0	13	0
Pudding Bar, 59g	90	16	0	16	3
FUDGESICLE					
Fudge Bar (1)	45	9	0	9	1
Fat Free (1)	60	13	0.5	12.5	2
GOOD HUMOR					
Bubble Play	105	26	0	26	0
Candy Center Crunch	315	24	0.5	23.5	3
Chocolate Éclair	225	30	0.5	29.5	2
Great White	70	18	0	18	0
Hyper Stripe	85	21	0	21	0
Number 1	190	21	0.5	20.5	2
Premium Vanilla	255	23	0.5	22.5	3
Reese's P'nut Butter Cup	335	33	1	32	4
Strawberry Shortcake;					
Toasted Almond	235	30	0.5	29.5	2
Cones: Giant King	395	44	0.5	43.5	7
King	275	33	1	32	4
Premium Sundae	265	29	0.5	28.5	4
Strawberry Shortcake	235	34	0.5	33.5	2
Sundae Twist	165	33	0	33	2
Sandwiches: Giant Vanilla	250	36	0	36	4
Giant Mississippi Mud	300	37	1	36	6
Giant Neapolitan	260	37	0.5	36.5	5
Premium Cookie	295	41	1	40	3
Premium Vanilla	190	29	0.5	28.5	3
KLONDIKE					
Choco Taco, 4 fl. oz.	300	35	1	34	4
Dark Choc. Crunch, 2.5 fl. oz.	140	15	0.5	14.5	2
Heath, 5 fl. oz.	295	26	0	26	3
Krunch, 4 fl. oz.	275	26	0.5	25.5	4
Movie Bites, 4.5 fl. oz.	320	26	0	26	4
Original, 5 fl. oz.	285	25	0	25	4
Planters Caramel & Peanut	310	28	0.5	27.5	4

	Calories	Total Carb	Fiber	Usable Carb	Protein
Cones:					
Big Bear Sundae Kone	315	36	0.5	35.5	5
Big Bear Vanilla					
Sundae Kone	300	31	0.5	30.5	5
Cup, Sundae, 6 fl. oz.	280	26	0.5	25.5	6
Sandwich: Big Bear, 7 fl. oz.	295	42	1	41	5
Giant Cookie w/					
Hershey's Chips	470	66	2	64	7
Oreo, 4.2 fl. oz.	230	34	2	32	3
M&M'S: COOKIE					
Ice Cream Sandwich	240	32	1	31	3
MILKY WAY					
Caramel Swirl, 1 bar	180	21	0	21	2
NESTLÉ CRUNCH					
Reduced Fat, 2.5 oz.	130	14	0	14	2
OREO					
Big Stuf, 1 sandwich	240	33	0	33	4
Cookies n' Cream, 1 bar, 59g	180	18	0	18	2
POPS					
(water/juice), Average	60	14	0	14	0
POPSICLES					
Fudgesicle Fudge Pop	90	16	0.5	15.5	3
Juice Pops, 2 pieces	60	16	0	16	0
Sprinklers Ice Cream, 1 bar	130	18	0	18	1
Pokémon Ice w/ Candy, 1 pc	80	19	0	19	0
Sugar-Free, 1 piece	*15*	*3*	*0*	*3*	*0*
SILHOUETTE (SKINNY COW)					
Lowfat Ice Cream Sandwich:					
Vanilla/Chocolate	130	23	2	21	3
SLIM-FAST					
Fudge Bar	110	22	0.5	21.5	3
Ice Cream Sandwich,					
Vanilla	130	27	0.5	26.5	3
Chocolate	130	27	0.5	26.5	3
SMART ONES (WEIGHT WATCHERS)					
Chocolate Mousse	40	9	1	8	2
Chocolate Treat	100	20	1	19	3
English Toffee Crunch	110	12	1	11	2

	Calories	Total Carb	Fiber	Usable Carb	Protein
Mocha Java	80	15	1	14	3
Orange Vanilla Treat	40	10	0	10	2
Vanilla Lowfat Sandwich	150	28	1	27	3
SNACKWELL					
Ice Cream Sandwich	90	18	1	17	2
Yogurt Bars, 1 bar, 80g	120	22	0	22	3.5
SNICKERS: ICE CREAM BAR					
The Big One	251	25	1	24	4
SOY DREAM (NON-DAIRY)					
Dreamwich Vanilla	130	15	1	14	1
Heavenly Pies: Mocha; Vanilla	290	40	2	38	3
Lil' Dreamers: Choc; Vanilla	60	7	0.5	6.5	0
Rocket Bars: Choc; Vanilla	220	29	2	27	1

CREAM & CREAMERS

CREAM

	Calories	Total Carb	Fiber	Usable Carb	Protein
Average All Brands					
Half & Half Cream:					
1 Tbsp, 0.5 oz.	*20*	*0.5*	*0*	*0.5*	*0.5*
Light, coffee/table					
(20% fat): 1 Tbsp	*30*	*0.5*	*0*	*0.5*	*0.4*
Medium (25% fat), 1 Tbsp	*40*	*0.5*	*0*	*0.5*	*0.5*
SOUR CREAM					
Regular, 1 Tbsp, 0.5 oz.	*30*	*0.5*	*0*	*0.5*	*0.4*
1 cup, 8 oz.	490	8	0	8	6.9
Lowfat/Light,					
1 Tbsp 0.5 oz.	*20*	*1.5*	*0*	*1.5*	*0.5*
Half & Half, Fat Free,					
2 Tbsp, 1 oz.	*20*	*3*	*0*	*3*	*0.5*
Fat Free:					
Heluva Good, 2 Tbsp	20	6	0	6	0
Knudsen, 2 Tbsp, 1 oz.	35	6	0	6	2
Sour Cream Substitute:					
Albertson's/IMO,					
2 Tbsp, 1 oz.	*60*	*2*	*0*	*2*	*0*
Tofutti Sour					
Supreme, 1 oz.	*50*	*1*	*0*	*1*	*0.3*

	Calories	Total Carb	Fiber	Usable Carb	Protein
WHIPPING CREAM					
Heavy (37% fat):					
1 Tbsp fluid/2 Tbsp					
Whipped	50	1	0	1	0.5
¼ cup whipped	100	2	0	2	1.1
½ cup fluid/1 cup whipped	400	8	0	8	4.2
Light (30% fat):					
1 Tbsp fluid/2 Tbsp					
whipped	45	0.5	0	0.5	0.5
½ cup fluid/1 cup					
whipped	350	4	0	4	4.4
COCONUT CREAM/MILK					
Coconut Cream (Canned),					
Plain/unsweetened,					
2 Tbsp, 1 oz.	70	4	0.8	3.2	1.0
½ cup, 4 oz.	280	16	3.3	12.7	4.0
Coconut Milk (Canned),					
Natural Value: Reg,					
¼ cup, 2 fl. oz.	90	1	0	1	1.5
Lite, ¼ cup, 2 fl. oz.	55	1	0	1	1
Thai Kitchen:					
Reg, ¼ cup, 2 fl. oz.	125	3	0	3	12.5
Lite, ¼ cup, 2 fl. oz.	50	2	0	2	3.5
Coconut Water (center),					
1 cup	45	9	2.6	6.4	1.7
WHIPPED TOPPINGS					
Average All Brands					
Cream (Pressurized):					
2 Tbsp	20	1	0	1	0.2
¼ cup	45	2	0	2	0.5
CREAM TOPPINGS					
Cool Whip:					
Extra Creamy, 1 Tbsp	25	2	0	2	1
Lite, 2 Tbsp, 9g	20	2	0	2	1
Free, 2 Tbsp, 9g	15	3	0	3	0
Non Dairy, 2 Tbsp	22	2	0	2	0
Kraft:					
Whipped, 2 Tbsp	20	1	0	1	0.5
Real Cream, 2 Tbsp	20	1	0	1	0.5

	Calories	Total Carb	Fiber	Usable Carb	Protein
Reddi-Wip:					
Original, 2 Tbsp, 8g	*20*	*0*	*0*	*0*	*0*
Original Light, 2 Tbsp	*15*	*2*	*0*	*2*	*0*
Non-Dairy, 2 Tbsp, 8g	*20*	*2*	*0*	*2*	*0*
Extra Creamy, 2 Tbsp	*30*	*0.5*	*0*	*0.5*	*0*
Fat Free, 2 Tbsp, 8g	*10*	*2*	*0*	*2*	*0*
NON-DAIRY COFFEE CREAMERS					
Powder Coffee-Mate/					
Cremora/N-Rich:					
Regular, 2 tsp	*20*	*1*	*0*	*1*	*0*
Fat Free, 1 tsp	*10*	*2*	*0*	*2*	*0*
Lite, 1 tsp	*10*	*2*	*0*	*2*	*0*
Liquid/Refrigerated: Per Tbsp					
Coffee-Mate Non-Dairy					
Creamer: Plain:					
Regular, 1 Tbsp	*20*	*2*	*0*	*2*	*0*
Fat Free, 1 Tbsp	*10*	*2*	*0*	*2*	*0*
Lite, 1 Tbsp	*10*	*1*	*0*	*1*	*0*
all flavors, 1 Tbsp	40	5	0	5	0
Fat Free, all flavors, 1 Tbsp	25	5	0	5	0

FATS, SPREADS & OILS

BUTTER & MARGARINE					
Average All Brands					
Regular: 1 tsp (5g)	*35*	*0*	*0*	*0*	*0*
1 Pat (5g)	*35*	*0*	*0*	*0*	*0*
1 Tbsp, approx ½ oz.	*100*	*0*	*0*	*0*	*0*
1 Stick, ½ cup, 4 oz.	*810*	*0*	*0*	*0*	*0*
Light (Regular) 40 % Fat:					
1 tsp, 5g	*17*	*0*	*0*	*0*	*0*
1 Tbsp, ½ oz.	*50*	*0*	*0*	*0*	*0*
Whipped Butter (Regular):					
1 tsp (4g)	*27*	*0*	*0*	*0*	*0*
1 Tbsp (10g)	*70*	*0*	*0*	*0*	*0*
1 Stick, ½ cup	*570*	*0*	*0*	*0*	*0*
Whipped Light Butter 40% Fat:					
1 tsp, 5g	*10*	*0*	*0*	*0*	*0*
1 Tbsp, 9g	*35*	*0*	*0*	*0*	*0*
Unsalted: Same as Regular					

	Calories	Total Carb	Fiber	Usable Carb	Protein
CLARIFIED BUTTER					
100% Fat: 1 Tbsp, ½ oz.	130	0	0	0	0
FLAVORED BUTTER/SPREAD					
Average All Brands:					
Honey Butter (60% Fat):					
1 Tbsp, ½ oz.	90	4	0	4	3
Garlic Butter (80% Fat):					
1 Tbsp, ½ oz.	100	0	0	0	0
Sweet Cream Butter:					
Regular, 1 Tbsp	100	0	0	0	0
Stick (70% Fat), 1 Tbsp	90	0	0	0	0
Tub (60% Fat), 1 Tbsp	80	0	0	0	0
OTHER SPREADS & FATS					
Copha, Dripping, Lard,					
Suet, Shortening:					
1 Tbsp, ½ oz.	120	0	0	0	0.7
Chicken, Duck, Goose Fat:					
1 Tbsp, ½ oz.	115	0	0	0	0
LIGHT & REDUCED FAT SPREADS					
Per 1 Tbsp, ½ oz. (Unless Stated)					
Benecol:					
Spread, 1 Tbsp	80	0	0	0	0
Light, Spread, 1 Tbsp	45	0	0	0	0
Brummel & Brown: Spread	45	0	0	0	0
Country Crock (Shedd's):					
Regular	60	0	0	0	0
Light; Calcium & Vitamins	50	0	0	0	0
I Can't Believe It's Not Butter!:					
Regular	90	0	0	0	0
Light; Sweet Cream	50	0	0	0	0
Kraft: 'Touch of Butter'					
(bowl)	50	0	0	0	0
Land O' Lakes:					
Fresh Buttery Taste	80	0	0	0	0
Honey Butter	90	4	0	4	3
Light Butter Whipped	35	0	0	0	0
Light Butter	50	0	0	0	0
Nucoa: Heartbeat					
Margarine	25	0	0	0	0

	Calories	Total Carb	Fiber	Usable Carb	Protein
Parkay:					
Squeeze, 1 Tbsp	80	0	0	0	0
Stick, ⅓ Less Fat	70	0	0	0	0
Tub, 1 Tbsp	60	0	0	0	0
Tub, Light/Soft Diet	50	0	0	0	0
Whipped	70	0	0	0	0
Smart Balance:					
Regular, 1 Tbsp	80	0	0	0	0
Light, 1 Tbsp	45	0	0	0	0
Smart Beat: Fat Free	10	3	0	3	0
Take Control:					
Regular Spread	80	0	0	0	0
Light Spread	45	0	0	0	0
Weight Watcher's:					
Light, all types	45	2	0	2	0.5
BUTTER SUBSTITUTES					
Butter Buds: 1 serving, ½ tsp	4	0	0	0	0
Earth Balance,					
Non GMO, 1 tsp	35	0	0	0	0
Molly McButter: ½ tsp	5	0	0	0	0
SPREADS COMPARISON					
Mayonnaise:					
Regular, 1 Tbsp	100	0.5	0	0.5	0
Light, average, 1 Tbsp	50	1	0	1	0
Fat Free, 1 Tbsp	12	3	0	3	0
Miracle Whip (Kraft):					
Light, 1 Tbsp	40	3	0	3	0
Free, 1 Tbsp	15	3	0.3	2.7	0
SmartBeat Dressing:					
1 Tbsp	12	2	0	2	0
Peanut Butter, 1 Tbsp	100	3.5	1	2.5	3.5
Avocado, mashed, 1 Tbsp	25	2	0.7	1.3	0.3
Birdseye:					
No Fat Veggie Dip, 2 Tbsp	25	5	0	5	1.5
ANIMAL FATS/LARDS					
Average All Types:					
Beef Tallow/Drippings,					
Lard (Pork), Chicken, Duck,					
Goose, Turkey					
1 Tbsp, 13g	115	0	0	0	0.7

	Calories	Total Carb	Fiber	Usable Carb	Protein
Ghee/Butter Oil					
1 Tbsp 13g	110	0	0	0	0

VEGETABLE SHORTENING

Average All Types:					
1 Tbsp	113	0	0	0	0
2¼ Tbsp, 1 oz.	250	0	0	0	0
1 cup, 7¼ oz.	1810	0	0	0	0

VEGETABLE OILS

Includes almond, avocado, canola, corn, coconut, flaxseed, grapeseed, linseed, mustard, olive, palm, peanut, rice-bran, safflower, sesame, sunflower, soybean, wheatgerm: Note: Oil is 100% fat.					
1 tsp, 5g	45	0	0	0	0
1 Tbsp, ½ oz.	120	0	0	0	0
1 cup, 7¾ oz.	1930	0	0	0	0

FISH OILS

Average All Types (Includes cod liver, herring, salmon, sardine):					
1 Tbsp, ½ oz.	125	0	0	0	0

COOKING SPRAYS/SQUEEZES

Cooking Sprays (Pam, Mazola, Weight Watchers, Wesson):					
Per serving	2	0	0	0	0
I Can't Believe It's Not Butter!	0	0	0	0	0
Parkay Buttery Spray	0	0	0	0	0

OLESTRA (OLEAN)

Olestra (Olean)	0	0	0	0	0

CHEESES

FIRM/HARD CHEESES

(American, Cheddar, Colby, Coon, Swiss) Regular Cheese:					
1 oz. slice/piece	110	0.5	0	0.5	6.5
8 oz. package	880	4	0	4	52

	Calories	Total Carb	Fiber	Usable Carb	Protein
Cubes: 1" cube, ¾ oz.	55	0.5	0	0.5	4.8
Diced: 1 cup, 4½ oz.	500	2	0	2	28.8
Grated: 1 Tbsp, ¼ oz.	27	0	0	0	1.8
Shredded: ¼ cup, 1 oz.	110	0.5	0	0.5	7
Sliced: 1 thin (3½ sq), ¾ oz.	85	0.5	0	0.5	5.3
Light:					
Average All Brands	80	0.5	0	0.5	8
Fat Free:					
Average All Brands, 1 oz.	50	2	0	2	10.5
Lowfat:					
Average All Brands, 1 oz.	50	1	0	1	8

CHEESE

	Calories	Total Carb	Fiber	Usable Carb	Protein
Per 1 oz. (Unless Stated)					
American:					
Regular, 1 slice, 1 oz.	110	1	0	1	6.5
Kraft Deluxe, 0.7 oz. slice	70	0.5	0	0.5	3
Grated, 1 Tbsp, ¼ oz.	23	0	0	0	1
Light (Borden), 1 oz.	70	0.5	0	0.5	8
Fat Free:					
Single, 0.75 oz.	30	3	0	3	4.5
Weight Watchers,					
All types, ¾ oz.	30	3	0	3	4.5
Brie, 1 oz.	95	1	0	1	5.9
Camembert, 1 oz.	90	1	0	1	6
Cheddar:					
Regular, 1 oz.	110	0.5	0	0.5	7.1
Weight Watchers, 1 oz.	80	1	0	1	8
Fat Free:					
Alpine Lace, 1 oz.	45	2	0	2	9.5
Weight Watchers,					
1 slice, ¾ oz.	30	3	0	3	4.5
Cheese Balls, 1 oz.	100	0.5	0	0.5	4.5
Colby, Regular, 1 oz.	110	0.5	0	0.5	6.7
Cottage Cheese:					
Average All Brands					
Creamed (4% milk fat):					
2 Tbsp, 1 oz.	30	1	0	1	4.2
½ cup, 4 oz.	120	4	0	4	17
w/ fruit, ½ cup, 4 oz.	130	15	0	15	9
Reduced Fat (2%),					
2 Tbsp, 1 oz.	25	1	0	1	3.9

	Calories	Total Carb	Fiber	Usable Carb	Protein
½ cup, 4 oz.	100	4	0	4	16
Low Fat (1%),					
2 Tbsp, 1 oz.	20	1	0	1	3
½ cup, 4 oz.	80	3	0	3	12
Fat Free/Non Fat,					
2 Tbsp, 1 oz.	20	1	0	1	3.9
½ cup, 4 oz.	80	3	0	3	16
Cottage Doubles,					
Average, 5.5 oz. ctn	150	18	0	18	14
Knudsen:					
Free, Non Fat, ½ cup,					
4.3 oz.	80	7	0	7	13
Low Fat, 2% Milk Fat,					
½ cup, 4.3 oz.	100	5	0	5	14
4% Milk Fat, ½ cup, 4.3 oz.	120	5	0	5	13
Edam: Regular, 1 oz.	100	0	0	0	7
Feta: Regular,					
Frigo, 1 oz.	100	1	0	1	6
Crumbled, ½ cup, 2½ oz.	190	2.5	0	2.5	11.3
Reduced Fat, (Alpine Lace)	60	1	0	1	5
Goat's Milk Cheese:					
Semi-Soft: 1 oz.	100	1	0	1	5
Hard: Sargento, 1 oz.	130	0.5	0	0.5	9.5
Monterey, 1 oz.	105	0	0	0	7.1
Monterey Jack:					
Regular, 1 oz.	110	0	0	0	7.3
Light Naturals (Kraft), 1 oz.	80	0	0	0	7.8
Weight Watchers, 1 oz.	90	1	0	1	8
Mozzarella:					
Regular: Kraft/					
Dorman's, 1 oz.	90	0.5	0	0.5	5.5
Shredded, ¼ cup, 1 oz.	80	0.5	0	0.5	5.4
Part Skim					
(Alpine Lace), 1 oz.	70	0.5	0	0.5	6.9
Neufchatel:					
Philadelphia, 1 oz.	70	0.5	0	0.5	3
Parmesan:					
Fresh/Block, 1 oz.	110	1	0	1	12
Shredded/Grated, 1 Tbsp	22	0	0	0	2.3
Grated (Packaged): 1 Tbsp	26	0	0	0	2.2
1 oz. quantity	130	1	0	1	11.5

	Calories	Total Carb	Fiber	Usable Carb	Protein
½ cup, 1¾ oz.	230	2	0	2	20.2
w/ Romano (Frigo), grated, 1 oz.	130	1	0	1	11.5
Pizza, shredded:					
Frigo, ¼ cup, 1 oz.	90	1	0	1	6
Lowfat (Frigo), 1 oz.	65	1	0	1	8.5
Provolone:					
Regular, 1 oz.	100	1	0	1	6
Reduced Fat, Alpine Lace, 1 oz.	70	1	0	1	5.5
Quark: 40% fat, 1 oz.	47	1	0	1	4
20% fat, 1 oz.	32	1	0	1	3.5
Skim, 1 oz.	22	1.5	0	1.5	4
Ricotta Cheese:					
Whole Milk,					
2 Tbsp, 1 oz.	50	1	0	1	3.3
½ cup, 4½ oz.	225	4.5	0	4.5	14.9
Part Skim,					
2 Tbsp, 1 oz.	40	1	0	1	3.2
½ cup, 4½ oz.	180	4.5	0	4.5	14.5
Light/Low Fat,					
2 Tbsp, 1 oz.	30	1.5	0	1.5	2
½ cup, 4½ oz.	140	6	0	6	9
Fat Free (Polly-O),					
½ cup, 4½ oz.	100	4	0	4	20.2
Baked Ricotta,					
1 oz. portion	130	3	0	3	5.5
Romano:					
Block/Loaf, 1 oz.	110	1	0	1	8.5
Grated (Pkg), 1 oz.	120	1	0	1	9
String (Frigo/Kraft/ Sargento), 1 oz.	80	1	0	1	8
String Lite (Frigo), 1 oz.	60	1	0	1	9.5
Swiss:					
Regular, 1 oz.	110	1	0	1	6.5
Reduced Fat:					
Alpine Lace, 1 oz.	90	1	0	1	8
Weight Watchers,					
¾ oz. slice	30	2	0	2	5.5
Taco, shredded, ¼ cup (Frigo/Kraft/Sargento)	110	1	0	1	6.5

	Calories	Total Carb	Fiber	Usable Carb	Protein
CHEESE PRODUCTS					
Cheese Food:					
Average all flavors,					
¾ oz. slice	70	1.5	0	1.5	4.8
1 oz. slice	90	2	0	2	6.5
Jalapeno:					
Average all brands, 1 oz.	90	2	0	2	1.9
Kraft:					
American grated,					
1 Tbsp, 0.2 oz.	25	1	0	1	1.1
Singles, 1 slice, ¾ oz.	70	1	0	1	3
Free Singles, 1 slice, 0.7 oz.	40	3	0	3	4.8
Pimento Spread,					
2 Tbsp, 1.1 oz.	80	3	0	3	3.5
Velveeta (Process					
Cheese Spread):					
Regular, ⅜" slice, 1 oz.	100	3	0	3	4.6
Light, ⅜" slice, 1 oz.	60	3	0	3	5.6
Precious: String					
Cheese Stuffsters, 1 oz.	70	1	0	1	7
SmartBalance:					
Crmy Cheddar, 1 slice	40	2	0	2	4
SmartBeat: All flavors,					
1 slice, 0.6 oz.	35	2	0	2	4
Velveeta: Cheese,					
1 slice, 1 oz.	100	3	0	3	8.5
Light, 1 oz.	60	3	0	3	5.5
Shredded, ¼ cup, 1.3 oz.	130	3	0	3	11
CHEESE WHIZ (SAUCE)					
Regular, 2 Tbsp, 33g	90	2	0	2	5.8
Light, 2 Tbsp, 33g	80	6	0	6	7.5
Squeezable, 2 Tbsp, 33g	100	4	0	4	4
CHEESE SUBSTITUTES					
Per 1 oz. (Unless Stated)					
Formagg:					
American Wh/Yellow,					
1 slice, 0.7 oz.	60	0.5	0	0.5	5.5
Cheddar, 1 slice, 0.7 oz.	60	0.5	0	0.5	5.5
Mozzarella (Old World),					
1 oz.	60	1	0	1	7.5

	Calories	Total Carb	Fiber	Usable Carb	Protein
Parmesan Grated,					
1 Tbsp, ¼ oz.	22	1.5	0	1.5	0.5
Provolone (Vintage), 1 oz.	60	1	0	1	7.5
Swiss White, 1 slice, 0.7 oz.	60	0.5	0	0.5	5.5
Frigo: Cheddar;					
Mozzarella, 1 oz.	90	1	0	1	6
Harvest Moon:					
Per ¼ cup, 1.3 oz.					
Shredded: American;					
Cheddar	120	3	0	3	7
Mozzarella	110	3	0	3	4.5
Smart Beat, all varieties,					
0.6 oz. slice	35	2	0	2	4
Tofu Rella: Per 1 oz.					
Tofu Rella,					
Average all varieties	180	39	0	39	6
Zero-Fat Rella, All varieties	45	3	0	3	8.5
Almond/Hemp/Rice Rella,					
Average all varieties	70	3	0	3	6
Tofutti Better Than					
Cream Cheese	80	1	0	1	1
Weight Watchers:					
Fat Free Slices,					
All varieties, ¾ oz. slice	30	3	0	3	4.5
Grated Italian Topping,					
1 Tbsp	20	2	0	2	3
Yves Good Slice,					
¾ oz. slice, average	35	1	0	1	4
CREAM CHEESE					
Regular/Soft:					
2 Tbsp, 1 oz.	100	1	0	1	1.5
3 oz. package	300	2	0	2	4.5
w/ Chives/Herbs/					
Pimento, 1 oz.	90	0.5	0	0.5	1.8
w/ Fruit/Strawberry/					
Pineapple, 1 oz.	90	5	0	5	0
Lox, 1 oz.	90	0.5	0	0.5	1.8
Philadelphia Brand:					
Plain/Soft, 2 Tbsp, 1 oz.	100	1	0	1	2
⅓ Less Fat, 1 oz.	70	1	0	1	3
Light, 1 oz.	70	2	0	2	2.7

64

	Calories	Total Carb	Fiber	Usable Carb	Protein
Fat Free, 2 T, 1 oz.	*30*	*3*	*0*	*3*	*4*
Flavored/Herbs/Fruit/					
Salmon, 1 oz.	*100*	*2*	*0*	*2*	*1*
Light Blueberry, 2 Tbsp	70	5	0	5	1
Snack Bars: Average,					
All types	190	20	1	19	3
Whipped, 3 Tbsp, 1 oz.	*110*	*1*	*0*	*1*	*1.4*
Weight Watchers,					
2 Tbsp, 1 oz.	*40*	*1*	*0*	*1*	*3.5*

SNACK & CHEESE DIPS, SPREADS
AVOCADO/GUACOMOLE
Per 2 Tbsp (1 oz.)	*50*	*4*	*0*	*4*	*0*

BIRDSEYE
No Fat Veggie Dip, 1.1 oz.	25	5	0	5	1.5

FRENCH ONION DIP
Average all brands	*60*	*3*	*0*	*3*	*0*
Frito Lay: French Onion	*60*	*4*	*0.9*	*3.1*	*0.9*
Heluva Good Cheese:					
Clam/French Onion	*50*	*2*	*0*	*2*	*0*

HUMMUS
2 Tbsp, 1 oz.	*50*	*5*	*1.7*	*3.3*	*1.5*
½ cup, 4.5 oz.	*220*	*23*	*7.7*	*15.3*	*7*
Kraft:					
Average all flavors, 2 Tbsp	*60*	*4*	*0*	*4*	*1*
Premium: Bacon & Onion/					
Nacho Cheese	*60*	*2*	*0*	*2*	*1*
Other flavors	*50*	*2*	*0*	*2*	*1*

OLD EL PASO
Black Bean	*25*	*5*	*1*	*4*	*1*
Cheese 'n Salsa: Mild;					
Medium	*40*	*3*	*0*	*3*	*0*
Lowfat, medium	*30*	*3*	*0*	*3*	*0*
Chunky Salsa varieties	*15*	*3*	*0*	*3*	*1*
Jalapeno Dip	*30*	*4*	*2*	*2*	*1*

OLYS BAGEL SPREAD:
Berry	*100*	*3*	*0*	*3*	*4*
Honey Cinnamon; Raisin	100	6	0	6	1

	Calories	Total Carb	Fiber	Usable Carb	Protein
Garden Veg; Garlic & Herb	90	1	0	1	1.5
RUFFLES					
French Onion; Ranch	70	4	0.5	3.5	1
TGI FRIDAY'S					
Spinach, Cheese, Artichoke	45	2	2	0	2
TOSTITOS DIP					
Con Queso	40	5	0.1	4.9	0.5
Medium/Mild/Hot	15	3	1	2	0.5

EGG & EGG DISHES

CHICKEN EGGS

	Calories	Total Carb	Fiber	Usable Carb	Protein
Fresh Eggs:					
Raw (weight with shell):					
Small, 40g	65	0	0	0	5
Medium, 44g	70	0	0	0	5.5
Large, 50g	75	0	0	0	6.3
Extra Large, 56g	80	0	0	0	7
Jumbo, 63g	90	0	0	0	7.9
Egg Yolk, 1 extra large	63	0	0	0	2.7
Egg White, 1 extra large	16	0	0	0	3.5
Dried Egg Powder:					
Whole Egg: ¼ cup, 1 oz.	170	0	0	0	13.6
1 Tbsp	30	0	0	0	2.4
Egg White, ¼ cup, 1 oz.	105	0	0	0	23.3
Egg Yolk, ¼ cup, 1 oz.	195	0	0	0	9.7

EGG SUBSTITUTES

	Calories	Total Carb	Fiber	Usable Carb	Protein
¼ cup (Equivalent to 1 Egg) — Zero Cholesterol.					
Better 'n Eggs (Papetti),					
¼ cup, 2 oz.	30	0	0	0	6.2
Egg Beaters (Fleischmann's):					
Regular, ¼ cup	30	1	0	1	6
Cheese Omelete, ½ cup	110	2	0	2	14.5
Vegetable Omelete, ½ cup	50	5	0	5	7.5
Egg Watchers (Tofutti), 2 oz.	30	1	0	1	6.5
Scramblers (Morn Star),					
¼ cup	35	0	0	0	0

OTHER EGGS

	Calories	Total Carb	Fiber	Usable Carb	Protein
Duck, 1 large, 2½ oz.	130	0	0	0	11

	Calories	Total Carb	Fiber	Usable Carb	Protein
Goose, 1 large, 5 oz.	**280**	**0**	**0**	**0**	**27**
Quail, 3 eggs, 1 oz.	**42**	**0**	**0**	**0**	**3.8**
Turkey, 1 large, 3 oz.	**135**	**0**	**0**	**0**	**12**
Turtle, 1 egg, 1¾ oz.	**75**	**0**	**0**	**0**	**7.5**
OMEGA-3 FAT ENRICHED					
Eggs Land's Best, 1 large	**70**	**0**	**0**	**0**	**6**
Eggs Plus (Pilgrim's Pride), 1 large	**70**	**0**	**0**	**0**	**6**
COOKED EGGS					
Boiled Egg: Same as raw egg					
Fried Egg:					
With fat: 1 large egg	**100**	**0.5**	**0**	**0.5**	**6.5**
2 small eggs	**175**	**1**	**0**	**1**	**13.5**
No fat/nonstick pan, 1 large	**80**	**0**	**0**	**0**	**7.5**
Deviled Egg, 2 halves	**145**	**0.5**	**0**	**0.5**	**6.5**
Eggs Benedict (2) on toast Or English muffin	860	25	0	25	64
Eggs Florentine (2) on toast Or English muffin	890	25	0	25	65
Pickled Egg, 1 large	**80**	**0**	**0**	**0**	**7.5**
Poached Egg: 1 large	**80**	**0**	**0**	**0**	**7.5**
Scotch Egg, 1 egg	300	16	0	16	12
Scrambled Eggs:					
1 large egg:					
w/ 1 Tbsp milk + 1 Tsp fat	**120**	**1**	**0**	**1**	**9**
w/ 1 Tbsp skim milk/ no fat	**85**	**1**	**0**	**1**	**8**
2 large eggs:					
w/ 2 Tbsp milk + 2 Tsp fat	**260**	**2**	**0**	**2**	**18**
w/ 2 Tbsp skim milk/ no fat	**180**	**2**	**0**	**2**	**19**
OMELETS					
1 Egg:					
Plain (w/ 1 Tsp fat)	**125**	**0.5**	**0**	**0.5**	**8.5**
With ½ oz. cheese	**175**	**0.5**	**0**	**0.5**	**9.5**
W/ ½ oz. cheese + ½ oz. ham	**200**	**0.5**	**0**	**0.5**	**13.5**

	Calories	Total Carb	Fiber	Usable Carb	Protein
Extras:					
Tomato/Onion/Veges	**20**	**4.5**	**0**	**4.5**	**0.9**
Egg Substitute (Egg Beaters):					
2 eggs (2 cup) + 1 Tsp fat	**100**	**2**	**0**	**2**	**14**
3 eggs (¾ cup) + 2 Tsp fat	**160**	**3**	**0**	**3**	**21**
Extras: 1 oz. cheese	**110**	**1**	**0**	**1**	**6.5**
1 oz. ham	**50**	**1**	**0**	**1**	**6.4**
Tom/Onion/Veges	**20**	**4.5**	**0**	**4.5**	**0.9**

EGG NOG

	Calories	Total Carb	Fiber	Usable Carb	Protein
Per ½ Cup (4 Fl oz.):					
Regular: Borden	160	16	0	16	4
Hood (Golden)	180	22	0	22	5
Light/Lowfat: Borden	120	23	0	23	2.5
Horizon; Hood	140	23	0	23	2.5
Fat Free: Hood	100	21	0	21	4

BREAKFAST SIDES

	Calories	Total Carb	Fiber	Usable Carb	Protein
Toast: Plain, 1 thick slice	85	13	1	12	3.4
English Muffin: Plain, 2 oz.	130	26	1.5	24.5	4.4
Bacon, 2 strips	**70**	**0**	**0**	**0**	**3.8**
Ham: Lean, 2 oz.	100	0	0	0	12.5
Hash Browns: ½ cup	125	14	0	14	2.3
Sausages, 2 links (1 oz. each)	**180**	**1.5**	**0**	**1.5**	**11.4**

FROZEN EGG DISHES

	Calories	Total Carb	Fiber	Usable Carb	Protein
Pillsbury Toaster Scrambles:					
Cheese, Egg & Bacon/Ham	180	14	0	14	4
Cheese, Egg & Sausage	180	14	0	14	4
Swanson Great Starts:					
Per Package:					
Egg, Sausage & Cheese	510	35	3	32	15
Muffin Sandwich	290	26	2	24	14
Pancakes w/ Sausage	490	52	3	49	14
Scrambled Eggs:					
w/Burrito	200	25	0	25	7
w/ Bacon & Home Fries	290	17	1	16	11
w/ Sausage & Hash Browns	360	21	3	18	12

FROZEN EGG ROLLS

	Calories	Total Carb	Fiber	Usable Carb	Protein
Chun King/La Choy:					
Average All Brands:					
Chicken Egg Rolls:					
Mini, 6 rolls	210	25	2	23	6

	Calories	Total Carb	Fiber	Usable Carb	Protein
Restaurant Style, 1 roll, 3 oz.	210	25	2	23	6
Pork & Shrimp Egg Rolls:					
Mini, 6 rolls, 3 oz.	210	27	2	25	6
Shrimp Egg Rolls:					
Mini, 6 rolls	190	28	2	26	5
Restaurant Style, 1 roll, 3 oz.	180	25	2	23	5

FAST FOOD/RESTAURANTS

	Calories	Total Carb	Fiber	Usable Carb	Protein
Bojangles:					
Bacon/Egg/Cheese S'wich	550	27	1	26	17
Burger King:					
Croissan'wich Sausage/					
Egg/Cheese	520	24	1	23	19
Carl's Jr: Scrambled Eggs	*180*	*1*	*0*	*1*	*13*
Denny's:					
Two Egg Breakfast	825	24	2	22	31
Omelette:					
Ham 'n Cheddar	*580*	*4*	*0*	*4*	*37*
Veggie-Cheese	480	9	2	7	26
Sirloin Steak & Eggs	*620*	*1*	*1*	*0*	*43*
Hardee's:					
Bacon, Egg, Cheese Bisc	520	45	0	45	17
Sausage & Egg Bisc	620	45	0	45	19
McDonald's:					
Egg McMuffin	300	29	2	27	18
Bacon, Egg & Cheese Biscuit	480	31	1	30	20
Scrambled Eggs (2)	*160*	*1*	*0*	*1*	*13*
Perkins: Country Club Omelet	930	6	0	6	47
Roy Rogers:					
Ham & Egg Biscuit	470	44	0	44	14
Sausage & Egg Biscuit	560	44	0	44	18

BEEF

STEAK

	Calories	Total Carb	Fiber	Usable Carb	Protein
Sirloin (Choice Grade):					
External fat trimmed to ¼"					
Broiled, Edible Portion					
(no bone), Small Serving					
(3 oz. cooked, from					
4–4½ oz. raw)					
Lean + fat (¼"), 3 oz.	*230*	*0*	*0*	*0*	*26*
Lean + marbling, 3 oz.	*195*	*0*	*0*	*0*	*26.3*

	Calories	Total Carb	Fiber	Usable Carb	Protein
External fat trimmed before cooking,					
Lean only, 3 oz.	170	0	0	0	26.8
No external fat or marbling, Medium/Regular Serving, 5 oz. (from approx. 7 oz. raw)					
Lean + fat (¼"), 5 oz.	470	0	0	0	52.5
Lean + marbling, 5 oz.	400	0	0	0	80
Lean only, 5 oz.	350	0	0	0	56
Large Serving, 8 oz. (from 11–12 oz. raw)					
Lean + fat, 8 oz.	610	0	0	0	67
Lean + marbling, 8 oz.	520	0	0	0	71.5
Lean only, 8 oz.	454	0	0	0	73
Extra Large Serving, 12 oz. (from approx 16–17 oz. raw)					
Lean + fat (¼"), 12 oz.	915	0	0	0	100.5
Lean + marbling, 12 oz.	780	0	0	0	107
Lean only, 12 oz.	680	0	0	0	84.3
Pan Fried Sirloin (choice), medium serving:					
Lean + fat, 5 oz.	450	0	0	0	40.5
Lean only, 5 oz.	330	0	0	0	49

OTHER STEAKS

	Calories	Total Carb	Fiber	Usable Carb	Protein
Filet Mignon (Tenderloin): 1 medium steak, 6 oz. raw weight Broiled, with ¼" fat trim					
Lean + fat (¼"), 4 oz.	340	0	0	0	28.4
Lean only, 3½ oz.	210	0	0	0	27.8
Broiled, (¼" fat removed before cooking)					
Lean + marbling, 3¼ oz.	220	0	0	0	24.9
Lean only, 3 oz.	180	0	0	0	23.9
New York/Club Steak: Top Loin/Short Loin, 1 steak, regular (9¼ oz. raw, ¼" fat) Broiled:					
Lean + fat (¼"), 6¼ oz.	510	0	0	0	45.3
Lean + marbling, 5½ oz.	330	0	0	0	44.7

	Calories	Total Carb	Fiber	Usable Carb	Protein
Lean only, 5¼ oz.	310	0	0	0	42.6
Porterhouse Steak:					
1 medium, 6 oz. raw weight					
(no bone), Broiled:					
Lean + fat (¼"), 4¼ oz.	370	0	0	0	27.4
Lean only, 3½ oz.	220	0	0	0	25.8
T-Bone Steak:					
1 medium, 8 oz. raw weight					
Broiled:					
Lean + fat	380	0	0	0	35.8
Lean only	220	0	0	0	29.5
BEEF-AVERAGE ALL CUTS					
Average All Retail Cuts					
Edible weight (no bone) Raw:					
(1 lb raw yields approx					
11–12 oz. cooked)					
Lean + fat (¼" trim), 1 oz.	70	0	0	0	5
½ pound, 8 oz.	560	0	0	0	40
Lean only, 1 oz.	40	0	0	0	8
½ pound, 8 oz.	320	0	0	0	64
Fat only, 1 oz.	190	0	0	0	0
Cooked (No Added Fat)					
Lean + fat (¼"), 1 oz.	86	0	0	0	8
Small serving, 3 oz.	260	0	0	0	24.2
Lean + marbling,					
(no ext fat), 1 oz.	78	0	0	0	9.5
Small serving, 3 oz.	235	0	0	0	28.8
Lean only, 1 oz.	60	0	0	0	8.3
Small serving, 3 oz.	180	0	0	0	25
Fat only, 1 oz.	193	0	0	0	3
BEEF-INDIVIDUAL CUTS					
Average All Grades					
Edible Weight (no bone)					
Brisket, whole, braised:					
Lean + fat (¼"), 3 oz.	330	0	0	0	20
Lean only, 3 oz.	205	0	0	0	25.3
Chuck, blade, braised:					
Lean + fat (¼"), 3 oz.	290	0	0	0	22.6
Lean only, 3 oz.	210	0	0	0	26.4
Flank: Raw, 4 oz.	200	0	0	0	22.4

	Calories	Total Carb	Fiber	Usable Carb	Protein
Ribs, whole (ribs 6–12):					
Average all grades, roasted					
(1 lb raw yields					
10 ¼ oz. roasted)					
Lean + fat (¼")					
(3.6 oz. w/ bone,					
3 oz. no bone)	300	0	0	0	18.7
Lean only, 3 oz.					
(no bone)	200	0	0	0	22.2
Round, bottom, braised:					
Lean + fat (¼"), 3 oz.	235	0	0	0	22.8
Lean only, 3 oz.	180	0	0	0	26.8
Round, eye/tip, roasted:					
Lean + fat (¼"), 3 oz.	200	0	0	0	22.8
Lean, 3 oz.	150	0	0	0	24.7
Round, top: Per 3 oz.					
Braised, Lean + fat	210	0	0	0	29
Lean only	175	0	0	0	30.7
GROUND BEEF					
Raw:					
Regular					
(73% fat free), 4 oz.	350	0	0	0	20
Lean					
(80% fat free), 4 oz.	300	0	0	0	22
Extra lean					
(85% fat free), 4 oz.	250	0	0	0	25
Healthy Choice					
(97% lean), 4 oz.	130	0	0	0	23.6
Baked/Broiled:					
Regular, 3 oz.	250	0	0	0	18.8
Lean, 3 oz.	230	0	0	0	20.4
Extra lean, 3 oz.	200	0	0	0	22.7
Pan-fried:					
Regular, 3 oz.	260	0	0	0	21.2
Lean, 3 oz.	230	0	0	0	20.4
Extra lean, 3 oz.	200	0	0	0	23
Ground Beef Patties:					
Average					
Frozen, raw, 4 oz.	320	0	0	0	21.9
Broiled, 3 oz.	240	0	0	0	22.7

	Calories	Total Carb	Fiber	Usable Carb	Protein
ROAST BEEF					
Round (Eye/Tip, average)					
Average All Cuts					
Small Serving, 3 oz.					
(2 thin slices/1 thick slice)					
Lean + fat (¼"), 3 oz.	200	0	0	0	26.5
Lean only, 3 oz.	150	0	0	0	27.3
Medium Serving, 5 oz.					
(3–4 thin slices)					
Lean + fat, 5 oz.	330	0	0	0	43.8
Lean only, 5 oz.	250	0	0	0	45
Large Serving, 8 oz.					
(3 thick slices)					
Lean + fat, 8 oz.	530	0	0	0	69.9
Lean only, 8 oz.	400	0	0	0	71.9
ROAST DINNER EXTRAS					
Gravy:					
Thin, 2 Tbsp	20	0.5	0	0.5	0
Thick, 2 Tbsp	50	0.5	0	0.5	0
1 Ladle/4 Tbsp	100	1	0	1	0
Vegtables:					
Beans, green, ½ cup	20	5	1.9	3.1	1.1
Corn, kernels, ¼ cup	35	9	1	8	1.2
Carrots, ¼ cup	20	3	1	2	0.3
Peas, ¼ cup	35	6	0	6	1.9
Pumpkin baked:					
w/ fat, 4 oz.	90	5	0	5	2
No added fat, 2 pces, 4 oz.	25	5	0	5	1.5
Potato: Baked in skin,					
1 large	220	50	0	50	5
Sweet Potato/Yam, 1 med.	80	20	3.4	16.6	1.9

LAMB, VEAL, PORK

LAMB

	Calories	Total Carb	Fiber	Usable Carb	Protein
Choice Grade					
Leg (Whole), roasted:					
Lean + fat, 3 oz.	220	0	0	0	21.7
Lean only, 3 oz.	160	0	0	0	24.2
Leg (Sirloin Half), roasted:					
Lean + fat, 3 oz.	250	0	0	0	20.8

	Calories	Total Carb	Fiber	Usable Carb	Protein
Lean only, 3 oz.	*175*	*0*	*0*	*0*	*24.2*
Leg (Shank Half), roasted:					
Lean + fat, 3 oz.	*190*	*0*	*0*	*0*	*22.5*
Lean only, 3 oz.	*155*	*0*	*0*	*0*	*23.8*
Loin Chop, broiled:					
1 chop (raw weight, 4¼ oz.):					
Lean + fat (2¼ oz. edible)	*200*	*0*	*0*	*0*	*16*
Lean only (1.6 oz. edible)	*100*	*0*	*0*	*0*	*13.6*
Rib Chop, broiled/roasted:					
1 chop (raw weight 3½ oz.)					
Lean + fat (2½ oz. edible)	*255*	*0*	*0*	*0*	*15.6*
Lean only (1¾ oz. edible)	*120*	*0*	*0*	*0*	*13.7*
Shoulder (Arm/Blade):					
Braised:					
Lean + fat, 3 oz.	*290*	*0*	*0*	*0*	*25.9*
Lean only, 3 oz.	*240*	*0*	*0*	*0*	*30.2*
Broiled:					
Lean + fat, 3 oz.	*240*	*0*	*0*	*0*	*20.8*
Lean only, 3 oz.	*180*	*0*	*0*	*0*	*23.4*
Roasted: Similar to Broiled					
Cubed Lamb (Leg/Shoulder):					
For stew or kabob					
Raw, lean only, 8 oz.	*310*	*0*	*0*	*0*	*45.4*
Braised, lean only, 3 oz.	*190*	*0*	*0*	*0*	*28.6*
Broiled, lean only, 3 oz.	*160*	*0*	*0*	*0*	*23.8*
New Zealand Lamb (Imported):					
Similar calories and fat to domestic.					
VEAL					
Edible Weights					
Leg (Top Round):					
Braised:					
Lean + fat, 3 oz.	*180*	*0*	*0*	*0*	*30.8*
Lean only, 3 oz.	*170*	*0*	*0*	*0*	*31.3*
Pan-fried, breaded:					
Lean + fat, 3 oz.	195	9	0.3	8.7	23.3
Lean only, 3 oz.	175	9	0.2	8.8	24.2
Pan-fried, not breaded:					
Lean + fat, 3 oz.	*180*	*0*	*0*	*0*	*27*
Lean only, 3 oz.	*155*	*0*	*0*	*0*	*28.2*
Roasted:					
Lean + fat, 3 oz.	*135*	*0*	*0*	*0*	*23.6*

	Calories	Total Carb	Fiber	Usable Carb	Protein
Lean only, 3 oz.	130	0	0	0	23.9
Loin Chop: 1 chop, 7 oz. raw weight					
Braised:					
Lean + fat	230	0	0	0	24.2
Lean only	155	0	0	0	23.1
Roasted:					
Lean + fat	175	0	0	0	20.4
Lean only	125	0	0	0	19.7
Rib, roasted:					
Lean + fat, 3 oz.	195	0	0	0	20.4
Lean only, 3 oz.	150	0	0	0	21.9
Shoulder, Arm/Blade, roasted:					
Lean + fat, 3 oz.	155	0	0	0	21.6
Lean only, 3 oz.	145	0	0	0	22.2
Sirloin, roasted:					
Lean + fat, 3 oz.	170	0	0	0	21.4
Lean only, 3 oz.	145	0	0	0	22.4
Cubed for Stew, braised:					
Leg/Shoulder,					
lean only, 3 oz.	160	0	0	0	29.7
(1 lb raw yields approximately 9¼ oz. cooked)					

PORK

	Calories	Total Carb	Fiber	Usable Carb	Protein
Fresh Pork:					
(Cooked Weight, no bone)					
(4 oz. raw weight = approximately 3 oz. cooked weight)					
Blade Steak, broiled:					
Lean + fat, 3 oz.	220	0	0	0	21.7
Lean only, 3 oz.	190	0	0	0	22.7
Country Style Ribs, broiled:					
Lean + fat, 3 oz.	270	0	0	0	19.9
Lean only, 3 oz.	205	0	0	0	22.7
Spareribs, braised:					
lean + fat, 6 oz.					
(from 1 lb raw weight)	700	0	0	0	51.3
Leg (Ham), roasted:					
Lean + fat, 3 oz.	250	0	0	0	22.8

	Calories	Total Carb	Fiber	Usable Carb	Protein
Lean only, 3 oz.	**180**	**0**	**0**	**0**	**25**
Loin Chops, broiled:					
Average (From 1 chop:					
5 oz. raw weight w/ bone					
or 4 oz. raw weight,					
no bone)					
Lean + fat, 3 oz.	**200**	**0**	**0**	**0**	**24.5**
Lean only, 3 oz.	**165**	**0**	**0**	**0**	**25.7**
Rib Chops, broiled:					
Lean + fat, 3 oz.	**215**	**0**	**0**	**0**	**24.5**
Lean only, 3 oz.	**180**	**0**	**0**	**0**	**26.2**
Rib Roast, roasted:					
Lean + fat, 3 oz.	**210**	**0**	**0**	**0**	**23.3**
Lean only, 3 oz.	**175**	**0**	**0**	**0**	**24.5**
Loin Roast, roasted:					
Lean + fat, 3 oz.	**190**	**0**	**0**	**0**	**24.5**
Lean only, 3 oz.	**160**	**0**	**0**	**0**	**25.7**
Sirloin Chop, broiled:					
Lean + fat, 3 oz.	**175**	**0**	**0**	**0**	**25.9**
Lean only, 3 oz.	**155**	**0**	**0**	**0**	**26.3**
Sirloin Roast, roasted:					
Lean + fat, 3 oz.	**215**	**0**	**0**	**0**	**22.9**
Lean only, 3 oz.	**180**	**0**	**0**	**0**	**24.6**
Tenderloin, roasted:					
Lean + fat, 3 oz.	**147**	**0**	**0**	**0**	**23.7**
Lean only, 3 oz.	**140**	**0**	**0**	**0**	**23.9**
Ground Pork					
Raw: Average,					
¼ lb, 4 oz.	**300**	**0**	**0**	**0**	**19.2**
Broiled, 3 oz.	**245**	**0**	**0**	**0**	**21.9**
Pan-fried, drained,					
3 oz.	**250**	**0**	**0**	**0**	**21.9**

BACON, HAM, GAME

BACON

	Calories	Total Carb	Fiber	Usable Carb	Protein
Raw: (1 lb raw yields					
approximately 5 oz. cooked)					
1 medium slice, ¾ oz.	**125**	**0**	**0**	**0**	**2**
1 thick slice, 1⅓ oz.	**210**	**0**	**0**	**0**	**3.3**
Broiled/Pan-Fried:					
1 medium slice, 6g	**36**	**0**	**0**	**0**	**1.9**

	Calories	Total Carb	Fiber	Usable Carb	Protein
3 medium slices, 18g	110	0	0	0	5.8
2 thin slices, ½ oz.	80	0	0	0	4.3
1 thick slice, 12g	70	0	0	0	3.7
Canadian-style:					
Cooked, 1 slice	43	0	0	0	5.6
As purchased, 1 slice, 1 oz.	45	1	0	1	5.9
Bacon Bits, 1 Tbsp, ¼ oz.	20	0	0	0	5.3
Breakfast Strips:					
Broiled, 1 slice, 12g	50	0	0	0	3.3

HAM

	Calories	Total Carb	Fiber	Usable Carb	Protein
Boneless Ham, cooked:					
Regular (approx 11% fat):					
Unheated					
(as purchased), 1 oz.	52	0	0	0	5.2
Roasted, 3 oz.	150	0	0	0	19.3
Extra Lean (5% fat):					
Unheated, 1 oz.	37	0	0	0	5.2
Roasted, 3 oz.	125	0	0	0	17.9
Whole Ham, cooked:					
Lean + fat (as purchased)					
Unheated, 1 oz.	70	0	0	0	5.3
Lean only, unheated, 1 oz.	40	0	0	0	6.3
Ham Patties, cooked,					
1 patty, 2¼ oz.	205	1	0	1	8.3
Ham Steak, extra lean, 2 oz.	70	0	0	0	11.1

GAME & OTHER MEATS

	Calories	Total Carb	Fiber	Usable Carb	Protein
Bison Steak,					
Lean, 6 oz. (raw)	210	0	0	0	36.8
Boar (wild), roasted, 3 oz.	140	0	0	0	24.1
Buffalo Steak					
(New West Foods), 4 oz.	70	0	0	0	11
Caribou, roasted, 3 oz.	140	0	0	0	25.3
Deer/Venison,					
roasted, 3 oz.	135	0	0	0	25.7
Goat (Capretto):					
Raw, 3 oz.	110	0	0	0	17.6
Roasted, 3 oz.	150	0	0	0	23.1
Ostrich:					
Blackwing Ostrich Meats,					
Sport Jerky, ½ oz. pce	25	0	0	0	5
Sausage Patties, (2), 2 oz.	60	0	0	0	12

	Calories	Total Carb	Fiber	Usable Carb	Protein
New West Foods:					
Ground Ostrich, 4 oz.	*110*	*0*	*0*	*0*	*24*
Ostrich Steak, 4 oz.	*130*	*0*	*0*	*0*	*28*
Rabbit:					
Roasted, 3 oz.	*130*	*0*	*0*	*0*	*24.8*
Stewed, 1 cup, diced, 5 oz.	*300*	*0*	*0*	*0*	*43*
VARIETY & ORGAN MEATS					
Brains:					
Braised, 3 oz.	*130*	*0*	*0*	*0*	*10.6*
Pan-fried, 3 oz.	*200*	*0*	*0*	*0*	*14.4*
Chitterlings, pork,					
simmered, 3 oz.	*260*	*0*	*0*	*0*	*8.7*
Ears, pork,					
simmered, 1 ear	*180*	*0*	*0*	*0*	*17.8*
Feet, pork:					
Simmered, 3 oz.	*165*	*0*	*0*	*0*	*16.4*
Cured, pickled, 3 oz.	*170*	*0*	*0*	*0*	*11.5*
Head Cheese (Pork Snouts/					
Ears/Vinegar/Spices):					
1 oz. slice	*50*	*0*	*0*	*0*	*4.5*
Jowl, pork, raw, 4 oz.	*750*	*0*	*0*	*0*	*7.2*
Kidneys, simmered, 3 oz.	*130*	*0*	*0*	*0*	*20*
Liver:					
Braised, 3 oz.	*140*	*3*	*0*	*3*	*25.9*
Pan-fried, 3 oz.	*200*	*3*	*0*	*3*	*21.7*
Pork Cracklins, 0.5 oz.	*80*	*0*	*0*	*0*	*7*
Scrapple, pork, 1 oz.	*60*	*4*	*0*	*4*	*2*
Tripe, beef, raw, 4 oz.	*110*	*0*	*0*	*0*	*17.9*

FRANKS, SAUSAGES

FRANKS & WEINERS

	Calories	Total Carb	Fiber	Usable Carb	Protein
Beef: Average All Brands					
Regular/Smoked: Per Frank					
4 oz. link	280	5	0	5	13.6
2.6 oz. link	*240*	*2*	*0*	*2*	*8.9*
2 oz. link					
(8/16 oz. pkg)	*180*	*2*	*0*	*2*	*5.8*
1.6 oz. link					
(10/16 oz. pkg)	*140*	*1*	*0*	*1*	*5.4*
1.5 oz. link					
(8/12 oz. pkg)	*135*	*1*	*0*	*1*	*5.2*

	Calories	Total Carb	Fiber	Usable Carb	Protein
1.2 oz. link					
(10/12 oz. pkg)	**110**	**1**	**0**	**1**	**4.1**
1 oz. link					
(16/16 oz. pkg)	**90**	**0.5**	**0**	**0.5**	**3.4**
Small/Cocktail, Each	**30**	**0.5**	**0**	**0.5**	**1.1**
Beef Light/Reduced Fat Franks:					
Oscar Mayer, 2 oz. link	**110**	**2**	**0**	**2**	**6.1**
Hebrew National:					
97% Fat Free	**50**	**2**	**0**	**2**	**6**
Reduced Fat	**120**	**0**	**0**	**0**	**6**
Healthy Choice,					
Lowfat, 1.75 oz.	70	6	0	6	6
Beef Fat-Free Franks:					
Ball Park (1), 1.76 oz.	50	5	0	5	6
Oscar Mayer (1)	**40**	**3**	**0**	**3**	**6.6**
Pork Franks:					
Oscar Mayer (2),					
1.7 oz. cooked	**170**	**1**	**0**	**1**	**5**
Light, 2 oz. link	**110**	**2**	**0**	**2**	**6.9**
Turkey Franks:					
Louis Rich: Original,					
Lower Fat (1)	**100**	**2**	**0**	**2**	**6**
FRESH SAUSAGES					
Pork/Beef:					
Average All Brands:					
Small: Raw, 4" link, 1 oz.	**120**	**1.5**	**0**	**1.5**	**1.5**
Broiled/Pan-Fried	**50**	**1.5**	**0**	**1.5**	**1.8**
Medium: Raw, 2 oz.	**235**	**2.5**	**0**	**2.5**	**4.5**
Broiled/Pan-Fried	**100**	**2.5**	**0**	**2.5**	**2**
Large: Raw, 3 oz.	**360**	**3.5**	**0**	**3.5**	**5.5**
Broiled/Pan-Fried	**150**	**3.5**	**0**	**3.5**	**7**
Italian: Raw, 3.2 oz.	**315**	**1.5**	**0**	**1.5**	**13.2**
Cooked, 2.4 oz.	**215**	**1.5**	**0**	**1.5**	**13.4**
SMOKED SAUSAGES					
Ball Park:					
Knockwurst (1), 4 oz.	**360**	**4**	**0**	**4**	**12**
Beef Corn Dog (1), 2.6 oz.	220	21	8	13	4
Healthy Choice, 2 oz.	80	6	0	6	7

	Calories	Total Carb	Fiber	Usable Carb	Protein
BREAKFAST SAUSAGES/BISCUITS					
Healthy Choice					
Breakfast Sausage,					
2 patties, 1.6 oz.	**50**	**3**	**0**	**3**	**5.3**
Breakfast Sausage					
3 Links, 1.6 oz.	**50**	**3**	**0**	**3**	**8**
Jimmy Dean Sausage Biscuit, 2	400	29	1.4	27.6	9.5
CHORIZO-REYNALDO'S					
Beef Chorizo, 2.5 oz. piece	**320**	**3**	**0**	**3**	**17**

HOT DOGS, DELI MEATS

CORN & HOT DOGS					
Hot Dogs, Ready-To-Go					
(Includes Ketchup/Relish;					
No Mayo):					
Small (1 oz. frank/1 oz. roll)	200	24	0	24	8
Regular (1½ oz. frank/					
2 oz. roll)	310	39	0	39	9.3
Large (2 oz. frank/2 oz. roll)	360	40	0	40	9.5
Super/Giant (3 oz. frank/					
3 oz. roll)	540	59	0	59	37.5
Corn Dogs					
Beef/Pork Frank:					
Average, 2.6 oz.	250	21	0	21	3.3
Mini, each	65	5	0	5	1
Mini Corn Dogs,					
(4) 2.68 oz.	210	18	1	17	7
State Fair w/Ball Park Franks,					
Corn Dogs, 1 dog,					
2.68 oz. (76g)	170	16	1	15	5
Beef, 1 dog, 2.68 oz. (76g)	180	15	8	7	4
Mini Corn Dogs,					
(4) 2.68 oz. (76g)	230	22	3	19	7
Toppings/Extras					
American Cheese, 1 slice	**110**	**1**	**0**	**1**	**6.5**
Catsup, 1 Tbsp	**16**	**4**	**0.2**	**3.8**	**0.2**
Chili (w/ beans), ¼ cup	70	9	2	7	5
Mustard, 1 Tbsp	**20**	**1**	**0.5**	**0.5**	**0.6**
Pickle Relish, 1 Tbsp	20	5	0	5	0
Sauerkraut, ½ cup	20	5	0	5	1

	Calories	Total Carb	Fiber	Usable Carb	Protein
DELI & LUNCHEON MEATS					
Beef Jerky:					
Beef Stick					
(5.5 oz. stick), 1 oz.	140	0	0	0	8.1
Pepperoni Sticks,					
(2), 1 oz.	140	0	0	0	6
Pepperoni					
(1" diameter), 1 oz.	130	0	0	0	6
Berliner (pork/beef),					
1 oz.	65	0.5	0	0.5	4.4
Beerwurst (Beef):					
Small (2.75" diameter),					
1⁄16" slice	20	0	0	0	0.8
Large (4" diameter),					
1⁄8" slice	75	0.5	0	0.5	3.2
Bologna, Beef & Pork:					
Regular: 1 thin slice, 1 oz.	90	1	0	1	3.3
1 thick slice, 1.6 oz.	145	1	0	1	5.2
Light (Oscar Mayer),					
1 slice, 1 oz.	60	2	0	2	3.3
Reduced Fat					
(Hebrew National), 1 oz.	65	0	0	0	4
Fat Free (Oscar Mayer),					
2 slices, 1.6 oz.	40	1	0	1	5.7
Healthy Choice, 1 oz.	35	3	0	3	3.5
Turkey, average, 1 oz.	60	0.5	0	0.5	3.8
Blood Sausage, 1 oz.	100	0.5	0	0.5	4.1
Bratwurst: Average, 1 oz.	90	0.5	0	0.5	4
Braunschweiger					
(Pork/Liver/Sausage),					
Oscar Mayer, 1 oz. slice	100	1	0	1	3.8
Chicken Roll, 1 slice, 1 oz.	90	1.5	0	1.5	11.1
Corned Beef:					
Average, full fat, 1 oz.	70	1.5	0	1.5	5
Healthy Choice,					
Hillshire Farm, 1 oz.	30	0.5	0	0.5	5.1
Loaf, jellied, 1 oz.	45	0	0	0	6.5
Hash, canned,					
average, 1 oz.	50	2	0.2	1.8	2.9
Dutch Brand Loaf,					
Average, 1 oz.	70	1.5	0	1.5	3.8

	Calories	Total Carb	Fiber	Usable Carb	Protein
Ham, Luncheon:					
Armour, canned, 1 oz.	35	0.5	0	0.5	5
97% Fat Free, 1 oz.	25	1.5	0	1.5	2.5
Healthy Choice					
Deli Traditions:					
Baked, 2 slices, 2 oz.	60	1	0	1	9.8
Larger Slice, 1 sl, 1 oz.	30	1	0	1	5
Oscar Mayer, 1 oz. slice	60	1	0	1	10.4
Honey/Brown Sugar,					
average, 1 oz.	30	0.5	0	0.5	4.7
Healthy Choice Deli					
Traditions: 2 slices, 2 oz.	60	2	0	2	9
Prosciutto, average, 1 oz.	70	1	0	1	5.5
Ham & Cheese Loaf,					
Average, 1 oz.	70	0.5	0	0.5	4.7
Head Cheese					
(Oscar Mayer), 1 oz. slice	50	0	0	0	4.5
Honey Loaf					
(Oscar Mayer), 1 oz. slice	35	2	0	2	5.2
Italian Sausage, 2.6 oz.	270	1	0	1	14.8
Kielbasa					
(Polish Sausage), 1 oz.	85	0.5	0	0.5	3.8
Knackwurst, 1 oz.	90	0.5	0	0.5	3.4
Liverwurst, 1 oz.	95	0.5	0	0.5	4
Liver Pate, fresh,					
Average, 1 oz.	110	3.5	0	3.5	1
Luncheon Loaf					
(Foods Co), 1 oz.	80	2	0	2	4.1
Mortadella, 1 oz.	90	0.5	0	0.5	4.7
Olive Loaf, average, 1 oz.	70	3	0	3	3.4
Oscar Mayer, 1 oz. slice	70	2	0	2	2.8
Pastrami (Beef),					
average, 1 oz.	99	0.9	0	0.9	4.8
Turkey Pastrami,					
1 slice, 1 oz.	30	1	0	1	5.2
Peppered Beef,					
1 oz. slice	40	1	0	1	5
Pepperoni:					
5 slices, 1 oz.	135	0	0	0	6
Pickle Loaf, average, 1 oz.	80	1	0	1	3.3

	Calories	Total Carb	Fiber	Usable Carb	Protein
Pickle & Pimento Loaf,					
(Oscar Mayer), 1 oz.	80	3	0	3	2.7
Roast Beef, lean, 1 oz.	40	0.5	0	0.5	8
Healthy Choice,					
all types, 2 oz.	60	1	0	1	10
Salami: Beef,					
Average, 1 oz.	80	1	0	1	4.3
Beer, average, 1 oz.	70	0.5	0	0.5	2.9
Cotto: Oscar Mayer,					
1 slice, 1 oz.	70	1	0	1	4
Dry: Hard, average,					
3 slices, 1 oz.	110	0.5	0	0.5	6.5
Oscar Mayer, 2 slices,					
1.6 oz.	120	1	0	1	7.4
Genoa: Average, 1 oz.	110	0	0	0	5.6
Stick (Best's Kosher),					
2, 1.75 oz.	180	2	0	2	9.5
Turkey, average, 1 oz.	55	1	0	1	4.7
Spam (Hormel):					
Regular, ¼" slice, 1 oz.	90	0	0	0	3.5
Lite: ¼" slice, 1 oz.	55	0	0	0	4.6
Turkey: ¼" slice, 1 oz.	40	0.5	0	0.5	5.1
Treet (Armour),					
canned, 1 oz.	100	1.5	0	1.5	3.5
Turkey: Average,					
1 oz. slice	30	0.5	0	0.5	6.4
¾ oz. slice	22	0.5	0	0.5	4.8
Turkey Breast:					
Butterball					
Fat Free, 4 slices, 2 oz.	50	2	0	2	10
Deli Thin Smoked,					
1 slice, 1 oz.	25	2	0	2	4
Louis Rich					
Carvery Board, 2 slices,					
1.8 oz. (52g)	50	2	0	2	10
Free, 2 slices, 2 oz.	50	2	0	2	8.5
Healthy Choice,					
2 slices, 2 oz.	60	2	0	2	9.8
Hearty Deli Roasted,					
2 slices, 2 oz.	50	1	0	1	10

	Calories	Total Carb	Fiber	Usable Carb	Protein
Honey Roasted,					
2 slices, 2 oz.	*70*	*2*	*0*	*2*	*9.8*
Oven Roasted,					
2 slices, 2 oz.	*45*	*1*	*0*	*1*	*9.8*
Honey Roasted &					
Smoked, 2 oz.	*60*	*2*	*0*	*2*	*9.8*
Turkey Ham, 1 slice, 1 oz.	*35*	*0.5*	*0*	*0.5*	*5.4*
Turkey Pastrami, 1 oz.	*35*	*0.5*	*0*	*0.5*	*5.2*
Turkey Roll, 1 oz.	*40*	*0.5*	*0*	*0.5*	*5.1*

MEAT SPREADS

Average All Brands:
Per ¼ Cup (2 oz.)

	Calories	Total Carb	Fiber	Usable Carb	Protein
Chicken	*120*	*2*	*0*	*2*	*10*
Ham, deviled	*160*	*0*	*0*	*0*	*7*
Liverwurst	*170*	*3*	*0*	*3*	*8*
Roast Beef	*140*	*0*	*0*	*0*	*10*
Sandwich Spread	140	8	0	8	4.5
Turkey	*110*	*2*	*0*	*2*	*10*

PÂTÉ

CANNED

Average All Brands

	Calories	Total Carb	Fiber	Usable Carb	Protein
Chicken Liver, 1 Tbsp, ½ oz.	*30*	*1*	*0*	*1*	*1.8*
Foie Gras, goose liver, 1 oz.	*130*	*2*	*0*	*2*	*3.3*

FRESH (REFRIGERATED)

	Calories	Total Carb	Fiber	Usable Carb	Protein
Average all types, 1 oz.	*110*	*4*	*0*	*4*	*1*
Marcel Henri, 2 oz. serving	*220*	*2*	*0*	*2*	*8*
Pate de Champagne, 1 oz.	*105*	*1*	*0*	*1*	*5*
Chicken Liver w/					
Port Wine, 1 oz.	*105*	*1*	*0*	*1*	*4*
Duck Truffle w/					
Port Wine, 1 oz.	*120*	*1*	*0*	*1*	*2*

LUNCH PACKS

FUNNY BAGELS (STONYFIELD FARM)

Per Package:

	Calories	Total Carb	Fiber	Usable Carb	Protein
Ham Sandwich,					
2 bagels & juice	350	66	3	63	13
Pizza Bagel,					
2 bagels & juice	420	71	3	68	15

	Calories	Total Carb	Fiber	Usable Carb	Protein
PB & J, 2 bagels & juice	490	79	4	75	14
Turkey Bologna, 2 bagels & juice	370	66	3	63	12
Turkey Breast, 2 bagels & juice	400	67	3	64	14
LUNCHABLES (OSCAR MAYER)					
Per Package:					
Ham & American Cheese	450	54	0.5	53.5	15
Ham & Cheddar	360	21	1	21	17
CRACKER STACKERS					
Per Package w/ Drink, Dessert:					
Bologna & American Cheese	520	64	0.5	63.5	12
Ham & American Cheese	420	60	0.5	59.5	15
Ham & Cheddar	390	56	1	55	17
Ham & Swiss	350	52	1	51	17
Turkey & American Cheese	420	60	1	59	15
Turkey & Cheddar	420	61	0	61	15
FUN FUEL					
Per Package:					
Chicken/Ham Wraps, 2 wraps	440	64	2	62	16
Ham/Turkey bagels, 2 bagels	420	64	2	62	16
MEGA LUNCHABLES					
Per Package:					
2 Pepp Pizza/ Reese's PB Cup/Cola	760	105	4	101	22
Soft Pizzastix + Twix	680	118	3	115	19
Ultimate Nachos	800	107	6	101	9
SMUCKERS					
Snackers, 3.96 oz. package	610	88	3	85	12

CHICKEN & TURKEY

CHICKEN

	Calories	Total Carb	Fiber	Usable Carb	Protein
From 3lb ready-to-cook chicken					
Breast/Wing Quarter					
Roasted:					
With skin	*300*	*0*	*0*	*0*	*60*
Without skin	*190*	*0*	*0*	*0*	*36*

	Calories	Total Carb	Fiber	Usable Carb	Protein
Fried, batter dipped	480	18	0	18	44
Leg Quarter:					
Thigh & Drumstick					
Roasted:					
With skin	**265**	**0**	**0**	**0**	**33**
Without skin	**180**	**0**	**0**	**0**	**27**
Fried, batter dipped	430	16	0	16	33

AVERAGE-ALL MEATS

	Calories	Total Carb	Fiber	Usable Carb	Protein
Average of Light & Dark Meats					
Per 4 oz. Serving (no bone)					
Roasted:					
With skin	**270**	**0**	**0**	**0**	**34**
Without skin	**215**	**0**	**0**	**0**	**36**
Stewed:					
With skin	**250**	**0**	**0**	**0**	**31**
Without skin	**200**	**0**	**0**	**0**	**32**
Fried: Batter dipped	330	11	0.3	10.7	28.4
Flour coated	**305**	**3.5**	**0.1**	**3.4**	**36.4**

CHICKEN PARTS

	Calories	Total Carb	Fiber	Usable Carb	Protein
Broilers or Fryers:					
Edible Weights (no bone)					
Breast: Per ½ Breast					
Raw:					
With skin, 5 oz.	**245**	**0**	**0**	**0**	**29.8**
Without skin, 4¼ oz.	**130**	**0**	**0**	**0**	**27.8**
Roasted:					
With skin, 3½ oz.	**195**	**0**	**0**	**0**	**29.8**
Without skin, 3 oz.	**140**	**0**	**0**	**0**	**26.7**
Stewed:					
With skin, 4 oz.	**210**	**0**	**0**	**0**	**30.7**
Without skin, 3¼ oz.	**140**	**0**	**0**	**0**	**27.7**
Fried: Batter-dipped, 5 oz.	370	12	0.4	11.6	35.5
Flour coated,					
w/ skin, 3½ oz.	**222**	**1.6**	**0.1**	**1.5**	**32**
Drumstick: Per Drumstick					
Roasted:					
With skin, 2 oz.	**125**	**0**	**0**	**0**	**17.1**
Without skin, 1½ oz.	**75**	**0**	**0**	**0**	**13.6**
Fried: Batter-dipped, 2½ oz.	195	7	0.2	6.8	17.8
Flour coated, 1¾ oz.	**120**	**1**	**0**	**1**	**15.9**

	Calories	Total Carb	Fiber	Usable Carb	Protein
Stewed:					
With skin, 2 oz.	115	0	0	0	15.3
Without skin, 1½ oz.	80	0	0	0	12.8
Thigh Portion:					
Edible Weight (no bone)					
Roasted:					
With skin, 2¼ oz.	155	0	0	0	19.2
Without skin, 2 oz.	110	0	0	0	18.1
Stewed:					
With skin, 2½ oz.	160	0	0	0	19.5
Without skin, 2 oz.	105	0	0	0	16.1
Fried: Batter-dipped, 3 oz.	240	8	0.3	7.7	21.3
Flour coated, 2¼ oz.	165	2	0.1	1.9	20.4
Roasters					
Average of Light & Dark Meat:					
Roasted:					
With skin, 4 oz.	250	0	0	0	34
Without skin, 4 oz.	190	0	0	0	36
Chicken Offal & Stuffing					
Liver:					
Raw, 4 oz.	140	3.5	0	3.5	20.4
Simmered, 1 cup	220	1	0	1	34.3
Liver Pate Fresh,					
1 Tbsp, ½ oz.	60	2	0	2	0.5
Stuffing: Average,					
½ cup	200	22	0	22	2.5

CHICKEN PRODUCTS

	Calories	Total Carb	Fiber	Usable Carb	Protein
Tyson					
Chicken Chunks:					
Regular, (6)	280	19	0	19	6
Breast, (6)	220	11	0	11	1.5
Southern Fried, (6)	260	11	0	11	11.5
Breast Patties:					
Regular, each	190	11	0	11	9.5
Chick 'n Quick/Chedd,					
74g each	220	12	0	12	11.5
Crispy Baked, each	80	9	0	9	11
Thick 'n Crispy, each	200	10	0	10	12.5
Southern Fried, each	180	8	0	8	10
Nuggets: Breaded					
White Meat, (6)	250	12	0	12	10

	Calories	Total Carb	Fiber	Usable Carb	Protein
Wings: Flavored,					
Average, (3)	**170**	**1**	**0**	**1**	**19**
BBQ Style, (3)	**200**	**2**	**0**	**2**	**19**
Stir Fry Kit:					
Chicken, 2¾ cup, frozen	430	73	0	73	24.5
Wraps:					
Southwest Black, 1½	560	82	0	82	31
Mandarin Sesame, 1½	560	82	0	82	31
Microwave Sandwiches:					
Breast, 119g	320	33	0	33	13.5
Stove Top: Per Serving					
Chicken Stuffing Mix: 1 oz.	110	20	0	20	5.5
½ cup prepared	170	20	0	20	2.5
DUCK, GOOSE, QUAIL					
Goose: Roast,					
With skin, 3 oz.	**260**	**0**	**0**	**0**	**22**
Without skin, 3 oz.	**200**	**0**	**0**	**0**	**25**
TURKEY					
Fryer-Roasters:					
Per 3 oz. Serving					
Roasted:					
Light Meat,					
With skin	**140**	**0**	**0**	**0**	**26**
Without skin	**120**	**0**	**0**	**0**	**28**
Dark Meat:					
with skin	**155**	**0**	**0**	**0**	**25**
Without skin	**140**	**0**	**0**	**0**	**26**
Ground Turkey,					
Raw: (4 oz. raw wt=3 oz. ckd wt)					
Regular (85% lean), 4 oz.	**180**	**0**	**0**	**0**	**10**
Lean (90% lean), 4 oz.	**160**	**0**	**0**	**0**	**22**
Breast, no skin, 4 oz.	**115**	**0**	**0**	**0**	**26.5**
TURKEY PARTS					
Roasted, Edible Weights (no bone)					
Breast (¼):					
(from 17¼ oz. raw wt w/ bone)					
With skin, 12 oz.,					
(no bone)	**525**	**0**	**0**	**0**	**75**
Without skin, 10¾ oz.	**415**	**0**	**0**	**0**	**99.4**

	Calories	Total Carb	Fiber	Usable Carb	Protein
Leg (Thigh & Drumstick):					
(from 1lb raw wt w/ bone)					
With skin, 8½ oz.,					
(no bone)	*420*	*0*	*0*	*0*	*45.9*

TURKEY PRODUCTS

Louis Rich					
Fat Free Breast of Turkey					
Rotiss'd/Smoked/					
Roasted, 2 oz.	*60*	*1*	*0*	*1*	*8.1*
Turkey Ham & Chunks,					
cooked: Breast & White					
Turkey, 2 oz.	*60*	*2*	*0*	*2*	*11*
Turkey Ham/					
Pastrami, 2 oz.	*70*	*1*	*0*	*1*	*10*
Turkey Salami, 2 oz.	*100*	*0*	*0*	*0*	*7*
Franks:					
Medium, 1½ oz.	*80*	*2*	*0*	*2*	*4.5*
Large, 2 oz.	*110*	*3*	*0*	*3*	*.6*
Smoked Sausage/					
Kielbasa, 1 oz.	*45*	*2*	*0*	*2*	*4*
Turkey Nuggets,					
Cooked, each	*65*	*4*	*0*	*4*	*4*
Turkey Sticks,					
Cooked, each	*75*	*4*	*0*	*4*	*4*
Turkey Store					
Gobble Stix: Honey, each	*25*	*1*	*0*	*1*	*0*
Lean Burger Patties, 1 patty	180	5	0	5	22
Lean Italian Sausage,					
1 link	*190*	*2*	*0*	*2*	*27.5*

FISH, FRESH & CANNED

FRESH FISH

Low Oil (Less than 2.5% fat)					
White/pale colored flesh					
Per 4 oz. Edible Portion					
Raw, 4 oz. (no bones)	*90*	*0*	*0*	*0*	*20.4*
Steamed, Broiled,					
Baked	*130*	*0*	*0*	*0*	*26.1*
Medium Oil (2.5-5% fat)					
Pale colored flesh					
Raw, 4 oz. (no bones)	*140*	*0*	*0*	*0*	*17.6*

	Calories	Total Carb	Fiber	Usable Carb	Protein
Baked, Broiled, 4 oz.	*175*	*0*	*0*	*0*	*21*
Fried, 4 oz.	230	8	0	8	20.4
High Oil (Over 5% fat)					
Darker colored flesh					
Raw, 4 oz. (no bones)	*230*	*0*	*0*	*0*	*22.7*
CANNED FISH & SHELLFISH					
Edible Weights:					
(no bones/shell)					
Abalone: Raw, 4 oz.	120	7	0	7	19.3
Anchovy: Canned in oil,					
Drained, 5 only	*40*	*0*	*0*	*0*	*5.8*
Bass: Striped, raw,					
1 fillet, 5½ oz.	*150*	*0*	*0*	*0*	*27.8*
Blue Fish, raw,					
1 fillet, 5¼ oz.	*185*	*0*	*0*	*0*	*30*
Butterfish, raw, 4 oz.	*165*	*0*	*0*	*0*	*19.9*
Carp, raw, 4 oz.	*145*	*0*	*0*	*0*	*20.4*
Catfish: Raw, 4 oz.	*130*	*0*	*0*	*0*	*17.6*
Fried, breaded, 1 fillet, 3 oz.	200	7	0	7	15.3
Caviar: black/red,					
1 Tbsp, 16g	*40*	*0.5*	*0*	*0.5*	*3.9*
Clams:					
Raw, 3 oz., (4 lg/9 small)	*65*	*2*	*0*	*2*	*11.1*
Fried, breaded, ¾ cup, 4 oz.	450	39	0	39	15.9
Canned, 3 oz.	*125*	*4*	*0*	*4*	*21.3*
Minced, ¼ cup, 2 oz.	*25*	*0.5*	*0*	*0.5*	*4*
Cod, Atlantic/Pacific:					
Raw, 4 oz.	*95*	*0*	*0*	*0*	*20.4*
Canned, 3 oz.	*90*	*0*	*0*	*0*	*19.6*
Crab:					
Alaska King: Raw, 4 oz.	*95*	*0*	*0*	*0*	*20.8*
1 leg, cooked, 4¾ oz.	*130*	*0*	*0*	*0*	*25.9*
Blue: raw, 1 crab (⅓ lb					
whole crab, ¾ oz. flesh)	*18*	*0*	*0*	*0*	*3.8*
Canned, ½ cup, 2½ oz.	*65*	*0*	*0*	*0*	*13.8*
Dungeness, 1 crab,					
5¾ oz. edible (from					
1½ lb whole crab)	*140*	*2*	*0*	*2*	*28.3*
Imitation Crab Legs/					
Stix, 3 oz.	80	8.5	0	8.5	13
Crayfish, raw, 4 oz. (edible)	*100*	*0*	*0*	*0*	*18.2*

	Calories	Total Carb	Fiber	Usable Carb	Protein
Croaker, raw, 4 oz.	120	0	0	0	20.4
Cuttlefish, raw, 4 oz.	90	1	0	1	18.2
Dolphinfish, raw, 4 oz.	95	0	0	0	21
Eel: Raw, 4 oz.	210	0	0	0	21
Flounder/Sole, raw, 4 oz.	120	0	0	0	21.3
Grouper, raw, 4 oz.	105	0	0	0	22.2
Haddock: Raw, 4 oz.	100	0	0	0	21.6
Broiled, 1 fillet, 5¼ oz.	170	0	0	0	36
Smoked, 2 oz.	22	0	0	0	14.2
Halibut, raw, 4 oz.	125	0	0	0	23.9
Herring:					
Atlantic, raw, 4 oz.	180	0	0	0	20.4
Pickled, 2 pieces, 1 oz.	60	2	0	2	4
Rollmops, 1½ oz.	110	6	0	6	9.8
Smoked, kippered, 4 oz.	245	0	0	0	27.8
Ling, raw, 4 oz.	100	0	0	0	21.6
Lobster, Northern:					
Raw, 4 oz.	105	0.5	0	0.5	21.4
1 Lobster, 6¼ oz. (from					
1½ lb whole lobster)	135	0.5	0	0.5	28.2
Cooked, 1 cup, 5 oz.	140	2	0	2	29.7
Lox, Regular/Nova, 2 oz.	65	0	0	0	10.5
Mackerel: Atlantic,					
Raw, 4 oz.	235	0	0	0	21
Jack, can, ½ cup, 3⅓ oz.	150	0	0	0	21.6
King, raw, 4 oz.	120	0	0	0	23.3
Pacific/Jack, raw, 4 oz.	180	0	0	0	22.7
Spanish, raw, 4 oz.	160	0	0	0	22.2
Mahi-Mahi, raw, 4 oz.	140	0	0	0	23.9
Monkfish, raw, 4 oz.	75	0	0	0	16.5
Mullet, striped, raw	135	0	0	0	22.1
Mussels: Raw, 4 oz. (edible)	100	4	0	4	13.6
1 cup, 5¼ oz. (edible)	130	5	0	5	18
Cooked, moist heat, 3 oz.	150	6	0	6	20.4
Ocean Perch, raw, 4 oz.	90	0	0	0	21
Octopus, common,					
Raw, 4 oz.	95	2	0	2	17
Orange Roughy,					
Raw, 4 oz.	145	0	0	0	16.5
Oysters:					
Common, raw, 3 oz.	70	3.5	0	3.5	7.7

	Calories	Total Carb	Fiber	Usable Carb	Protein
Eastern raw:					
6 medium, 3 oz.	60	3	0	3	4.4
Fried/breaded,					
6 medium, 3 oz.	170	10	0	10	7.7
Pacific, raw,					
1 medium, 1¾ oz.	40	2	0	2	4.5
Perch, average,					
Raw, 4 oz.	105	0	0	0	22.2
Pollock, raw, 4 oz.	100	0	0	0	22.2
Pompano, Florida,					
Raw, 4 oz.	190	0	0	0	21
Rockfish, Pacific,					
raw, 4 oz.	110	0	0	0	21.6
Row, raw, 1 oz.	40	0.5	0	0.5	6.4
Salmon:					
Raw: Chinook, 4 oz.	205	0	0	0	22.7
Atlantic; Coho/Silver,					
4 oz.	160	0	0	0	24.4
Chum; Pink, 4 oz.	135	0	0	0	22.7
Red/Sockeye, 4 oz.	190	0	0	0	24.4
Smoked Salmon:					
Chinook, 3 oz.	100	0	0	0	15.7
Wild Oats, Pastrami					
Style, 2 oz.	130	0	0	0	5.5
Canned Salmon:					
Average All Brands					
Pink: 1 oz.	40	0	0	0	5.7
¼ cup, 63g (2.2 oz.)	90	0	0	0	12.5
3¾ oz. can, whole	155	0	0	0	21.3
7½ oz. can, whole	300	0	0	0	42.6
Red Sockeye: 1 oz.	50	0	0	0	5.8
¼ cup, 63g (2.2 oz.)	110	0	0	0	12.8
3¾ oz. can, whole	190	0	0	0	21.8
Atlantic, ½ cup, 3½ oz.	230	0	0	0	22
Chinook/King, ½ cup	210	0	0	0	25.3
Chum, ½ cup, 3½ oz.	140	0	0	0	26
Coho/Silver, ½ cup	155	0	0	0	24.5
Atlantic Steaks:					
Small, 8 oz.	320	0	0	0	48.1
Medium, 12 oz.	480	0	0	0	72.2
Large, 16 oz.	640	0	0	0	96.2

	Calories	Total Carb	Fiber	Usable Carb	Protein
Sardines (Canned):					
Average All Brands					
Drained of oil, 1 oz.	60	0	0	0	7
3¾ oz. can, drained,					
(3¼ oz.)	190	0	0	0	22.6
1 lg/2 medium 3"/					
5 small, 0.8 oz.	50	0	0	0	5.9
In Tom/Mustard Sce, 1 oz.	45	0	0	0	4.7
3¾ oz. can (8 sardines)	170	0	0	0	15.2
Scallop: Raw,					
6 lg/14 small, 3 oz.	75	2.5	0	2.5	14.5
Breaded/fried, 6 lg, 3 oz.	200	9	0	9	16.8
Seabass, raw, 4 oz.	110	0	0	0	26
Shark: Raw, 4 oz.	150	0	0	0	23.9
Batter-dipped, fried, 4 oz.	260	7	0	7	21
Shrimp: Raw,					
Shelled, 3 oz. (12 lg)	90	0.5	0	0.5	17.3
Breaded/fried, 3 oz.,					
(11 lg)	210	10	0.3	9.7	18.2
Canned, 2 oz.	60	0.5	0	0.5	13.1
Smelt, Rainbow, Raw, 4 oz.	115	0	0	0	19.9
Snapper, raw, 4 oz.	115	0	0	0	23.3
Sole, Lemon, raw, 4 oz.	90	0	0	0	19.4
Squid, raw, 4 oz.	105	3.5	0	3.5	18.2
Surimi (Imitation Crab), 4 oz.	110	7.5	0	7.5	17.4
Swordfish, raw, 4 oz.	140	0	0	0	22.7
Tilapia, Rain Forest					
Fillets, 3.5 oz.	95	0	0	0	20
Trout, Rainbow, Raw, 4 oz.	135	0	0	0	23.9
Tuna: Raw:					
Albacore, 4 oz.	190	0	0	0	16.7
Bluefin, 4 oz.	160	0	0	0	26.1
Skipjack, Yellowfin, 4 oz.	120	0	0	0	25
Tuna Canned:					
Average All Brands					
In Water, drained:					
Chunk/Solid, 2 oz. can	60	0	0	0	13.3
3 oz. can	90	0	0	0	20
In Oil, drained:					
Chunk Light, 2 oz.	110	0	0	0	16.5
6 oz. can, drained	275	0	0	0	49.4

	Calories	Total Carb	Fiber	Usable Carb	Protein
Solid White, 2 oz.	*90*	*0*	*0*	*0*	*13.3*
6 oz. can, drained	*225*	*0*	*0*	*0*	*40*
Tuna Salad: Deli Style,					
½ cup, 4 oz.	300	15	0	15	18.2
Whitefish: Raw, 4 oz.	*150*	*0*	*0*	*0*	*21.6*
Smoked, 3 oz.	*90*	*0*	*0*	*0*	*20*
Whiting, raw, 4 oz.	*100*	*0*	*0*	*0*	*21*

FROZEN MEALS

AMY'S (VEGETARIAN)

	Calories	Total Carb	Fiber	Usable Carb	Protein
Per Serving					
Pot Pies:					
Country Vege, 7½ oz.	370	47	4	43	12
Mexican Tamale, 8 oz.	150	27	4	23	5
Shepherd's Pie, 8 oz.	160	27	5	22	5
Vegetable (Non Dairy),					
7½ oz.	420	54	4	50	10
Bowls:					
Brown Rice & Veges, 10 oz.	240	46	5	41	9
Santa Fe Enchilada, 10 oz.	340	47	10	37	17
Teriyaki w/ Veges,					
Rice, 10 oz.	300	59	3	56	10
Entrees:					
Cheese Enchilada, 4.75 oz.	210	13	2	11	10
Black Bean Vege Enchilada,					
4.75 oz.	170	26	2	24	4
Cheese Lasagna, 10.25 oz.	330	36	6	30	19
Garden Vege/Tofu					
Lasagne, 9.5 oz.	300	41	6	35	13
Macaroni & Cheese, 9 oz.	410	47	3	44	16
Macaroni & Soy Cheeze,					
9 oz.	370	42	4	38	16
Pasta Primavera, 9 oz.	300	37	3	34	15
Ravioli w/ Sauce, 8 oz.	340	43	3	40	15
Vegetable Lasagne, 9.5 oz.	280	29	3	26	14
Burgers:					
Californian, 2½ oz.	100	17	5	12	6
Chicago Veggie,					
2½ oz. pattie	160	20	3	17	10
Classic All-American,					
1 burger	120	15	3	12	10

	Calories	Total Carb	Fiber	Usable Carb	Protein
Texas Veggie, 2½ oz.					
Pattie	120	14	3	11	12
Burritos:					
Bean & Rice, 6 oz.	280	49	5	44	9
w/ Cheddar Cheese, 6 oz.	270	48	6	42	10
Black Bean Vegetable, 6 oz.	320	54	4	50	9
Breakfast Burrito, 6 oz.	210	38	5	33	9
Burrito Especial, 6 oz.	260	45	3	42	8
Asian Meals:					
Thai Stir Fry, 9.5 oz.	270	36	5	31	8
Asian Noodle Stir Fry,					
10 oz.	240	41	4	37	7
Snacks:					
Cheese Pizza, 5-6 pc, 3 oz.	180	22	2	20	9
Spinach & Fetta Mini					
Pockets, 3 oz.	170	24	2	22	7
Whole Meals:					
Black Bean Enchilada, 10 oz.	320	55	9	46	7
Country Dinner, 11 oz.	380	60	8	52	11
Cheese Enchilada, 9 oz.	330	38	6	32	15
Chili & Cornbread, 10.5 oz	320	59	10	49	11
Veggie Loaf, 10 oz.	280	47	7	40	8
Pizza: Cheese; Spinach;					
Pesto, ⅓	300	38	2	36	12
Mushroom & Olive,					
⅓ pizza	250	33	2	31	10
Roasted Vegetable, ⅓, 4 oz.	260	43	2	41	6
Soy Cheese, ⅓ pizza	280	37	2	35	12
BANQUET					
Per Meal					
BBQ Chicken	330	37	0	37	13
Boneless Pork Rib	400	39	0	39	48.5
Chicken Fried Beef Steak	420	38	4	34	15
Chicken Nugget	410	38	0	38	13
Corn Dog	490	68	4	64	11
Meat Loaf	240	23	0	23	11
Mexican Style Enchilada					
Combo	370	55	9	46	10
Our Original Fried Chicken	470	35	0	35	0
Salisbury Steak Meal, 9.5 oz.	380	28	3.5	24.5	15.3
Sliced Beef, 9 oz.	270	17	4.1	12.9	26.4

	Calories	Total Carb	Fiber	Usable Carb	Protein
Spaghetti Meatballs	440	43	5	38	22
Swedish Meatballs	400	33	5	28	22
Turkey Mostly White Meat	270	30	0	30	16

BIRDS EYE—VOILA!

	Calories	Total Carb	Fiber	Usable Carb	Protein
Per Cup, Cooked (2 Cups frozen)					
Chicken Voila!:					
Garden Herb	310	28	2	26	16
Alfredo; 3-Cheese Chicken	230	26	2	24	15
Grilled Salsa Chicken					
w/ Rice	240	35	3	32	14
Italian Pesto; Teriyaki	240	24	1	23	15
Zesty Garlic Chicken	270	28	1	27	15
Steak Voila!:					
Beef Sirloin/Potato	240	26	3	23	13
Turkey Voila!:					
Turkey w/ Potato	200	24	3	21	12

BOCA (VEGETARIAN)

	Calories	Total Carb	Fiber	Usable Carb	Protein
Boca Burgers:					
Cheeseburger (1)	*130*	*6*	*4*	*2*	*13*
All American, 2.5 oz.	*110*	*6*	*4*	*2*	*14*
Garden Vegetable	120	9	4	5	15
Original	*90*	*6*	*4*	*2*	*13*
Roasted Garlic	*100*	*7*	*5*	*2*	*14*
Roasted Onion	140	11	4	7	15
Sausages:					
Italian (1), 2.5 oz.	*130*	*7*	*3*	*4*	*11*
Bratwurst	*130*	*3*	*2*	*1*	*11*
Smoked	130	7	2	5	12
Breakfast:					
Patties, (1), 1.4 oz.	*80*	*6*	*2*	*4*	*8*
Bkfst Links, (2), 1.5 oz.	*90*	*8*	*5*	*3*	*10*
Chik'n: Patties, (1), 2.5 oz.	150	12	2	10	13
Chik'n Nuggets: (4), 3 oz.	190	16	2	14	16

BUDGET GOURMET

	Calories	Total Carb	Fiber	Usable Carb	Protein
Classics: Per Serving					
Chinese Style Veg &					
White Chicken	250	40	3	37	8
Fettucini Alfredo w/					
Four Cheeses	480	40	0	40	30.5
Lasagna Mozzarella	360	40	0	40	25

	Calories	Total Carb	Fiber	Usable Carb	Protein
Macaroni & Cheese w/ Cheddar	310	45	0	45	16.8
Spaghetti Marinara	280	49	0	49	16
Spicy Szechuan Vege & Chicken	280	41	3	38	9
Stir Fry Rice & Vegetables	350	45	0	45	18
Ziti Parmesano	230	36	2	34	9
Dinner:					
Angel Hair Pasta w/ Tom Meat Sce, 8 oz.	240	39	0	39	8.2
Italian Style Meatballs & Vege	280	25	0	25	15

CASCADIAN FARM

	Calories	Total Carb	Fiber	Usable Carb	Protein
Per 9 oz. Bowl:					
Pasta Primavera	280	41	3	38	12
Country Herb Chicken w/ Veg Rice	250	38	2	36	15
Schechuan Rice Veggie	210	45	3	42	7
Teriyaki Rice Veggie	270	44	2	42	9
Per Tray:					
Chicken Fettuccine	380	43	2	41	23
Spinach Lasagna, 11 oz.	330	39	5	34	16

CELENTANO

	Calories	Total Carb	Fiber	Usable Carb	Protein
Eggplant:					
Parmigiana, 10 oz.	350	34	6	28	8
Great Choice Rollettes, 10 oz. pkg	290	24	5	19	7
Lasagne:					
Lasagne, ½ tray, 7 oz.	270	29	3.5	25.5	3.5
Lasagne Primavera, 10 oz. tray	260	39	6	33	10
Stuffed Shells:					
Broccoli, 10 oz. pkg	250	39	6	33	11

CROISSANT POCKETS

	Calories	Total Carb	Fiber	Usable Carb	Protein
Egg, Sausage & Cheese	350	38	2	36	11
Ham & Cheddar	340	36	2	34	13
Pepperoni Pizza	370	40	2	38	11
Philly Steak & Cheese	360	34	2	32	12

	Calories	Total Carb	Fiber	Usable Carb	Protein
EL MONTEREY					
Family Classics: Per Serving					
Burritos:					
Chicken Fajita, 5 oz.	250	40	2	38	10
Egg, Bacon, Cheese & Salsa, 4.5 oz.	270	33	1	32	12
Monterey Supreme, 5 oz.	290	37	1	36	13
Sausage Breakfast, 4.5 oz.	290	31	1	30	8
Steak Fajita, 5 oz.	250	40	2	38	10
Ultimate Chicken, 5 oz.	290	40	2	38	12
Chimichangas:					
Beef & Cheese, 5 oz.	310	35	1	34	14
Chicken & Cheese, 5 oz.	320	38	2	36	13
Taquitos:					
Beef & Cheese, 4.5 oz.	330	36	1	35	12
Chicken & Cheese, 4.5 oz.	310	36	1	35	11
Egg, Bacon, Cheese & Salsa, 4.5 oz.	290	38	1	37	12
Tacos:					
Soft Beef & Cheese, 5.5 oz.	440	42	3	39	19
Beef & Pork, 4 oz.	230	29	1	28	12
Spicy Chicken, 5.5 oz.	320	46	4	42	14
Spicy Beef & Chse, 5.5 oz.	420	40	2	38	19
Enchiladas:					
Beef w/ Sauce, 4.5 oz.	180	17	2	15	8
Cheese w/ Sauce, 4.5 oz.	210	15	1	14	10
Chicken w/ Sauce, 4.5 oz.	190	18	1	17	11
Tamales:					
Beef, 4.5 oz.	230	26	3	23	9
Chicken, 4.5 oz.	250	27	2	25	9
Regular: Per Serving					
Burritos: Beef & Bean (Reg/Green Chili/Spicy Red)					
5 oz. Size	370	42	4	38	10
8 oz. Size	580	68	6.4	61.6	16
10 oz. Size	730	85	8	77	20
Bean & Cheese, 8 oz. Size	470	70	6.4	63.6	16
Chicken, 4 oz.	210	32	1	31	5
EMPIRE KOSHER					
Express Meal:					
Chicken Fajita, 1	130	15	0	15	11.8

	Calories	Total Carb	Fiber	Usable Carb	Protein
Chicken w/ Pasta, 1 cup	140	17	0	17	13.5
Chicken Stir-Fry, 1 cup	160	20	0	20	14.3
Pierogies:					
Potato Cheese, 5.3 oz.	250	44	0	44	9.5
Potato Onion, 5.3 oz.	245	47	0	47	5.3
Pies:					
Chicken Pie, 8 oz.	440	41	0	41	21.8
Turkey Pie, 8 oz.	470	45	0	45	20.8
Blintzes:					
Cheese, 2	200	29	0	29	7.5
Blueberry, 2	190	36	0	36	2.5
Potato Pancakes:					
Mini, 12, 3 oz.	150	19	0	19	2.8
FORTUNE AVENUE					
Chicken Won Ton, 15 Pieces, 8 oz.	310	39	2	37	16
FOSTER FARMS					
Corn Dogs, 1 Dog, 2.6 oz.	200	24	0	24	0
GARDENBURGER (VEGETARIAN)					
Hamburger Style,					
Classic, 2.5 oz.	*90*	*8*	*6*	*2*	*12*
Savory Portabello, 1 piece	120	18	4	14	6
The Original, 2.5 oz.	110	16	4	12	6
Meatless:					
Meatballs, 6 balls, (25g)	110	8	0	8	9.5
Riblets w/ BBQ Sauce, 5 oz., (142g)	210	10	0	10	31.5
Flame Grilled:					
Hamburger Style	*120*	*7*	*4*	*3*	*14*
Chik'n Grill, 2.5 oz.	*100*	*5*	*3*	*2*	*13*
Gourmet Style:					
Santa Fe, 2.5 oz.	130	20	1	19	6
Fire Rsted Vege, 2.5 oz.	120	18	4	14	6
Veggie Medley, 2.5 oz.	90	18	3	15	5
GORTON'S					
Crunchy Fish Fillets: Breaded (Per Fillet)					
Lemon Pepper	135	9	0	9	4.5
Garlic & Herb; Hot & Spicy	125	10	0	10	5.6

	Calories	Total Carb	Fiber	Usable Carb	Protein
Grilled: Italian Herb;					
Lemon Pepper	*130*	*2*	*0*	*2*	*17*
Cajun Blackened;					
Lemon Butter	*120*	*1*	*0*	*1*	*17*
Bettered:					
Parmesan, 1 fillet	130	10	0	10	5.6
Plain; Garlic & Herb, 1 fillet	125	11	0	11	5.3
Lemon Pepper, 1 fillet	135	9	0	9	4.5
Homestyle Baked:					
Au Gratin, 4.6 oz.	230	14	0	14	16.5
Primavera, 1 fillet,					
4.6 oz.	*120*	*4*	*0*	*4*	*14.8*
Grilled Fillets:					
Garlic Butter (1)	*100*	*1*	*0*	*1*	*17*
Cajun Blackened (1),					
3.8 oz. fillet	*100*	*1*	*0*	*1*	*17*
Lemon Butter/Pepper (1),					
3.8 oz.	*100*	*0.5*	*0*	*0.5*	*16*
Shrimp Bowl:					
Alfredo, 1 bowl	290	49	1	48	14
Fried Rice, 1 bowl	320	65	2	63	11
Garlic Butter, 1 bowl	280	46	2	44	13
Primavera, 1 bowl	270	41	1	40	13
Teriyaki, 1 bowl	320	57	2	55	10
Fish Portions: 1 portion, 2½ oz.	170	12	0	12	5.8
Fish Sticks: Breaded, 6, 3 oz.	210	17	0	17	8.5
Popcorn Shrimp:					
20 shrimp, 3 oz.	240	26	0	26	7
Tenders:					
Extra Chunky, 3½ pcs	260	29	0	29	9
Original, 3½ pcs, 4 oz.	260	22	0	22	9.5
GREEN GIANT					
Create A Meal: Prepared with					
Meat & Oil (Prepared Weight—					
Approximately 10 oz.)					
Oven Roasted:					
Garlic Herb Chicken,					
1¾ cup	350	35	5	30	31
Lemon Pepper Chicken,					
1⅔ cup	310	30	5	25	29

	Calories	Total Carb	Fiber	Usable Carb	Protein
Parmesan Herb Chicken, 1¾ cup	340	29	5	24	31
Stir Fry:					
Beef & Broccoli Stir Fry, 1⅓ cup	290	15	2.2	12.8	15
Garlic & Ginger Stir Fry, 1½ cup	270	25	3.6	21.4	24.3
Lo Mein Stir Fry, 1¼ cup	320	33	3	30	30
Sweet & Sour Stir Fry, 1¼ cup	340	43	3	40	25
Szechuan Stir Fry, 1¼ cup	310	20	2.9	17.1	18.6
Teriyaki Stir Fry, 1¼ cup	230	18	4	14	27
Complete Skillet Meal!:					
Per 8 oz. (¼ Package)— Prepared					
Chicken Alfredo, 1¼ cup	270	37	2	35	15
Chicken & Cheesy Pasta, 1¼ cup	270	39	3	36	13
Chicken Lo Mein, 1¼ cup	250	30	3	27	16
Chicken Noodle, 1¼ cup	290	45	3	42	14
Chicken Teriyaki, 1¼ cup	250	45	3	42	15
Garlic Chicken Pasta, 1¼ cup	250	30	3	27	16
Sweet & Sour Chicken, 1¼ cup	320	62	3	59	14

HEALTH IS WEALTH

	Calories	Total Carb	Fiber	Usable Carb	Protein
Buffalo Wings, Meatless, 3, 2.2 oz.	100	11	3	8	10
Chicken:					
Nuggets, 4, 3 oz.	150	9	0	9	14
Chicken Free, 3, 2.25 oz.	90	11	2	9	10
Patties, 1, 3 oz.	150	9	0	9	13
Chicken Free, 1, 3 oz.	120	15	2	13	14
Tenders, 3, 3 oz.	130	11	0	11	13.8
Munchies, average, 2, 1 oz.	60	10	1	9	2
Egg Rolls:					
Oriental Veg, 1, 3 oz.	160	23	2	21	4
Oriental Chicken Free, 1	120	21	2	19	8
Spinach, 1, 3 oz.	180	20	3	17	7
Spring Rolls, 2 pces, 1.6 oz.	70	10	5	5	2

	Calories	Total Carb	Fiber	Usable Carb	Protein
HEALTHY CHOICE					
Bowl Creations:					
Beef Broccoli	300	41	1	40	17
Chicken Teriyaki w/ Rice	300	50	5	45	19
Duos:					
Grilled Chicken Breast & Pasta	240	26	4	22	20
Grilled Chicken Breast w/ Potato	190	19	4	15	19
Breaded Chicken & Macaroni Cheese	270	34	3	31	34
Sirloin Beef Tips & Mushroom Rice	270	35	4	31	20
Salisbury Steak & Mashed Potatoes	210	21	3	18	16
Turkey Breast w/ Mashed Potatoes	200	19	4	15	20
Solos:					
Beef Macaroni	220	34	5	29	19
Cheese Rice & Chicken	230	33	5	28	14
Chicken Enchilada	310	46	6	40	16
Dinners:					
Beef Pot Roast	320	39	6	33	19
Beef Tips Portabello	280	28	3	25	23
Blackened Chicken	300	36	5	31	20
Boneless Beef Ribs w/ BBQ Sauce	360	47	8	39	22
Chicken Broccoli Alfredo	300	34	2	32	25
Chicken Enchilada	360	59	6	53	16
Chicken Parmigiana	320	40	6	34	19
Chicken Teriyaki w/ Rice	270	37	6	31	16
Country Herb Chicken	280	37	5	32	18
Herb Baked Fish	360	55	5	50	16
Lemon Pepper Fish	320	50	5	45	11
Mesquite Beef w/ BBQ Sauce	340	40	8	32	22
Roasted Chicken Breast	280	32	7	25	18
Salisbury Steak	360	45	5	40	23
Stuffed Pasta Shells	370	41	9	32	15
Sweet & Sour Chicken	340	54	3	51	15
Traditional Meatloaf	300	36	6	30	18

	Calories	Total Carb	Fiber	Usable Carb	Protein
Mixed Grills:					
Chicken:					
w/ Ginger Dipping	450	59	5	54	31
w/ Barbecue Dipping Sauce	390	46	5	41	31
w/ Honey BBQ Dipping Sauce	390	46	5	41	31
w/ Roasted Garlic Tomato Sauce	420	45	5	40	34
w/ Roasted Red Pepper	390	39	7	32	36
Steak:					
w/ Teriyaki Dipping Sauce	450	62	6	56	26
w/ Zesty Dipping Sauce	340	37	6	31	24
Medleys:					
Beef Teriyaki	310	46	5	41	15
Chicken Breast w/ Veg & Pasta	230	29	6	23	18
Chicken Carbonara	310	39	2	37	23
Chicken Fettuccine Alfredo	280	28	3	25	25
Country Glazed Chicken	230	29	3	26	17
Mandarin Chicken	280	43	4	39	20
Oriental Style Chicken	240	28	7	21	21
Rigatoni w/ Broccoli & Chicken	280	34	3	31	19
Roast Turkey Breast	230	25	4	21	18
Sesame Chicken	260	34	4	30	13
HOT POCKETS					
Per Pocket (½ Pkg)					
Barbecue Sauce w/ Beef	340	47	2	45	10
Cheeseburger	340	46	2	44	14
Chicken Melt	360	39	3	36	10
Ham & Cheese	320	37	2	35	12
Italian Style Meat Trio	390	39	2	37	12
Pepperoni & Sausage Pizza	350	39	2	37	11
Pepperoni Pizza	360	41	2	39	11
Toaster Pizza Pepperoni	200	21	2	19	4
Turkey & Ham w/ Cheese	330	41	2	39	12
JOSÉ OLÉ					
Mexi Minis: Per Serving					
Beef & Cheese, 4 pce, 3 oz.	200	23	0	23	4.5
Beef & Cheese Mini Taco, 4 pce, 3 oz.	200	23	0	23	4.5

	Calories	Total Carb	Fiber	Usable Carb	Protein
Beef Steak Fajita Bowl, 12 oz.	330	37	0	37	21
Cheese Mini Burrito,					
3 pce, 3 oz.	200	27	0	27	5
Chicken & Cheese,					
4 pce, 3 oz.	140	20	0	20	5
Chicken & Cheese					
Rolled Tacos	270	33	0	33	12
Chicken Monterey,					
1 pce, 5 oz.	320	47	0	47	17.5
Grilled Chicken Quesadilla,					
3 pce, 3.4 oz.	220	27	0	27	10
Shredded Beef Taquitos,					
3 pce, 3 oz.	160	24	0	24	5
Chimichanga:					
Chicken, 5 oz. pce	330	45	0	45	10.5
Shredded Beef, 1 pce, 5 oz.	400	43	0	43	14.5
Wraps:					
Steak Fajita,1 pce, 4 oz.	340	46	0	46	16.5
Chicken Fajita, 1 pce, 5.3 oz.	330	46	0	46	14
Steak & Cheese,					
1 pce, 5.3 oz.	340	42	0	42	16
Chicken & Cheese,					
1 pce, 5.3 oz.	330	40	0	40	18
KROGER FISH PORTIONS					
Per 2 Pieces, 4 oz.					
Batter Dipt	260	22	0	22	11.5
Crispy Crunchy	270	18	0	18	9
LEAN CUISINE					
Bowls: Entrée					
Chicken Fried Rice	330	50	4	46	19
Chicken Teriyaki	330	59	3	56	16
Creamy Chicken & Veg.	390	57	3	54	22
Grilled Chicken Caesar	290	36	4	32	20
Teriyaki Steak	370	56	4	52	19
Three Cheese Stuffed					
Rigatoni	300	44	5	39	14
Everyday Favorites: Per Serving					
Angel Hair Pasta	240	43	3	40	9
Cheese Cannelloni	250	30	3	27	18
Cheese Ravioli	260	38	3	35	11
Chicken Chow Mein w/ Rice	240	37	2	35	12

	Calories	Total Carb	Fiber	Usable Carb	Protein
Chicken Enchilada					
Suiza w/ Rice	280	48	3	45	11
Chicken Fettuccini	270	33	2	31	20
Fettuccini Alfredo	280	40	2	38	13
Lasagna w/ Meat Sauce	300	41	3	38	19
Macaroni & Cheese	290	42	1	41	14
Roasted Potatoes w/ Broccoli	240	37	4	33	11
Rst Chicken w/					
Lemon Pepper Fettuccini	250	32	3	29	15
Santa Fe Style Rice & Beans	300	54	4	50	10
Spaghetti w/ Meat Sauce	300	51	5	46	13
Swedish Meatballs w/ Pasta	290	35	2	33	21
Café Classics: Per Serving					
Baked Chicken	240	33	3	30	17
Baked Fish, 9 oz.	290	40	2	38	20
Beef Portabello, 9 oz.	220	24	2	22	14
Chicken Breast in					
Wine Sauce	210	24	2	22	16
Chicken Carbonara	260	29	2	27	17
Chicken in Peanut Sauce	260	32	2	30	12
Chicken Parmesan	270	37	3	34	20
Chicken Piccata	270	40	2	38	12
Chicken & Vegetables	250	33	3	30	18
Chicken w/ Basil Cream					
Sauce	290	37	1	36	18
Fiesta Grilled Chicken	270	34	3	31	20
Glazed Chicken					
w/ Veg Rice	230	25	0	25	21
Herb Roasted Chicken	200	24	3	21	17
Honey Roasted Pork,					
9.5 oz.	240	31	3	28	17
Meatloaf w/ Whipped					
Potatoes	260	28	4	24	20
Roasted Garlic Chicken	230	29	1	28	18
Salisbury Steak	290	26	3	23	25
Shrimp & Angel Hair Pasta	280	44	3	41	15
Sweet & Sour Chicken	320	57	1	56	15
Teriyaki Chicken	320	51	0	51	19
Thai Style Chicken	270	39	1	38	18
Skillet Sensations:					
Beef Teriyaki & Rice, 8 oz.	290	31	9	22	9

	Calories	Total Carb	Fiber	Usable Carb	Protein
Chicken Alfredo	320	28	4	24	15
Chicken Teriyaki, Rice & Veg	300	37	9	28	14
Chicken Oriental, 6.8 oz.	290	23	5	18	12
Chicken Primavera	310	28	4	24	11
Garlic Chicken	350	32	4	28	10
Herb Chicken & Rst Potatoes	270	24	7	17	12
3 Cheese Chicken	340	26	7	19	13
Dinnertime Selections:					
Per Serving					
Chicken Fettuccine					
w/ Broccoli	410	55	5	50	29
Grilled Chicken					
w/ Penne Pasta	360	47	5	42	26
Grilled Chicken Tuscan	290	43	4	39	16
Jumbo Rigatoni	360	56	6	50	24
Roasted Chicken	370	57	4	53	23
Salisbury Steak Dinner	321	35	6	29	25
LEAN POCKETS					
BBQ Sauce w/ Beef	290	48	2	46	10
Chicken Fajita	260	38	2	36	11
Ham & Cheddar, 1 pce	280	40	2	38	13
Meatballs & Mozzarella	280	44	2	42	13
Pepperoni Pizza	290	42	2	40	13
Philly Steak & Cheese, 1 pce	280	42	2	40	12
Turkey/Broccoli/Cheese	270	39	2	37	10
LIGHTLIFE					
Vegetarian Meals: Per Serving					
Meatless 'Lightburgers,'					
2.5 oz.	120	12	5	7	15
Smart Deli Slices,					
3 slices, 1½ oz.	*50*	*2*	*0*	*2*	*9*
Smart Dogs, 1 link, 1½ oz.	*45*	*1*	*1*	*0*	*9*
Wonderdogs, 1½ oz.	*55*	*1*	*0*	*1*	*9*
LINDA MCCARTNEY					
Vegetarian Frozen Entrees					
Veg Burrito w/ Spanish Rice	450	51	1	50	16
Vegetable Lasagna	350	42	4	38	16
LOUIS KEMP					
Crab Delights, Surimi,					
½ cup, 2.5 oz.	80	10	0	10	10

	Calories	Total Carb	Fiber	Usable Carb	Protein
MARIE CALLENDER'S					
Meals & Dinners					
Beef Stroganoff	600	58.7	4.4	54.3	30.4
Breaded Fish w/ Mac & Cheese	550	53	3	50	22
Chunky Chicken & Noodle, 1 meal	520	47	5	42	21
Turkey w/ Gravy/dress, 1 dinner	504	51.8	0	51.8	31
MICHELINA'S					
Per Serving					
Black Bean & Chili w/ Rice, 8 oz.	300	58	8	50	10.4
Chicken a la King	280	39	2	37	13
Chili-Mac, 8 oz.	290	38	3	35	14
Fettucine Alfredo	390	45	3	42	14
Four Cheese Lasagna, 8 oz.	290	42	3	39	14
Lasagna Pollo	280	33	0	33	21.3
Lasagna Primavera	270	34	3	31	9
Lasagna w/ Meat Sauce, 8 oz.	240	29	2.5	26.5	12.3
Linguini w/ Clams & Sauce	290	52	2	50	11
Macaroni Cheese	260	40	2	38	12
Meatloaf, Gravy, Mashed Potato	340	20	2	18	12
Noodles Stroganoff w/ Beef, 8 oz.	340	38	2	36	17
Noodles w/ Chicken, 8 oz.	300	40	2	38	12
Penne Pasta w/ Mushroom Sauce	320	50	3	47	10
Penne Pollo	330	48	2	46	16
Pepper Steak & Rice	260	46	2	44	11
Rigatoni Pomodoro Italiano	260	49	3	46	8
Risotto Parmigiana	460	50	1	49	15
Salisbury Steak	330	21	2	19	13
Shells & Cheese w/ Jalapeno	360	45	2	43	14
Spaghetti & Meatballs	250	37	3	34	12
Spaghetti Marinara, 8 oz.	250	47	3	44	8
Spaghetti w/ Tomato Basil Sauce	250	46	3	43	9
Standard Wheels & Cheese	360	43	2	41	16

	Calories	Total Carb	Fiber	Usable Carb	Protein
Yu Sing:					
Chicken Fried Rice	360	58	2	56	14
Chicken Lo Mein	220	34	2	32	12
Roasted Garlic Chicken	240	43	2	41	8
Sweet & Sour Chicken					
w/ Rice	290	55	1	54	9
Teriyaki Beef	260	58	2	56	10
LOMA LINDA (VEGETARIAN)					
Chik Nuggets, 5 pieces, 3 oz.	240	13	4	9	14
Corn Dogs, 1 link	150	22	3	19	7
MRS PAUL'S					
Battered:					
Fish Sticks, 2	240	13	0	13	22.5
Fish Portions, 2	280	22	0	22	10
Batter Dipped:					
Fish Sticks, 2	330	28	0	28	16.3
Crispy Crunchy:					
Fish Sticks, 2	200	20	0	20	1
Fish Fillets, 2	250	11	0	11	22.3
Breaded Fish Portions, 2	240	20	0	20	13
Crunchy Batter:					
Fish Fillets, 2	280	23	0	23	17.5
Flounder Fillets, 2	260	24	0	24	9.5
Haddock Fillets, 2	250	25	0	25	10.5
Healthy Treasures:					
Fish Sticks, breaded,					
4 sticks	140	14	0	14	7.5
Fish Cakes, 2 cakes, 4 oz.	190	24	0	24	7.5
Light Seafood Entrees:					
Fish Dijon	200	17	0	17	21.8
Fish Florentine	220	10	0	10	27
Fish Mornay	230	12	0	12	23
NATURAL TOUCH (VEGETARIAN)					
Breakfast Pattie, 1	*80*	*4*	*1*	*3*	*8*
Corn Dogs, 1	170	22	3	19	8
Lentil Rice Loaf, 1" slice, 3 oz.	160	16	4	12	8
Nine Bean Loaf, 1" slice, 3 oz.	160	13	5	8	8
Okara Pattie, 1	*120*	*6*	*3*	*3*	*12*
Roasted Herb Chik'n, 1 fillet	110	9	2	7	13
Tex Mex Burger, 1	120	17	2	15	9

	Calories	Total Carb	Fiber	Usable Carb	Protein
Thai Burger, 1	*100*	*7*	*3*	*4*	*10*
Vegan Burger, 1	*70*	*6*	*3*	*3*	*11*
Veggie Medley, 1 Pattie	120	11	1	10	11
Vegetarian Chili, 1 cup, 8 oz.	170	21	11	10	18
ORTEGA					
Beef Taco Filling,					
⅓ cup, 2 oz.	*100*	*4*	*1*	*3*	*7.2*
Beef Enchilada	360	49	5	44	12
Cheese Enchilada	410	55	4	51	12
Chicken Enchilada	400	51	4	47	13
Skillet Fajitas:					
Steak, ½ cup, 2 oz.	*35*	*3*	*1*	*2*	*4*
Chicken, ¾ cup, 2½ oz.	*45*	*4*	*1*	*3*	*5*
Nachos Chicken Supreme,					
½ pkt, 11 oz.	380	49	8	41	20
Bowls:					
Chicken Santa Fe, 1	420	63	5	58	21
Pepper Jack Grilled					
Chicken, 1	480	60	4	56	23
Cheddar Rice & Grilled					
Chicken, 1	450	59	3	56	22
POPPERS					
Stuffed Jalapenos					
Cream Cheese (5), 5 oz.	304	27.1	2.5	24.6	5.9
ROSINA					
Turkey Meatballs,					
3 balls, 3 oz.	*170*	*7*	*3*	*4*	*15*
Italian Sausage Bites,					
4 bites, 1 oz.	*180*	*1*	*1*	*0*	*8.7*
Swedish Meatballs,					
6 balls, 3 oz.	*260*	*5*	*3*	*2*	*12*
SAFEWAY SELECT					
Gourmet Club Meals: Per Serving					
Bacon Wrapped					
Sirloin Tip Fillets	*350*	*0*	*0*	*0*	*23*
Beef Meatloaf	180	9	0	9	12
Beef Sirloin Tip Fillets:					
w/ Black Pepper Glaze	*210*	*5*	*1*	*4*	*29*
w/ Teriyaki Glaze	*250*	*3*	*0*	*3*	*29*
Beef Tamales w/ Sauce	472	44	6	38	20

	Calories	Total Carb	Fiber	Usable Carb	Protein
Beer Battered Cod Fillets	160	13	2	11	10
Boneless Pork Shoulder Ribs	180	9	0	9	14
Cheese & Broccoli Potatoes	260	34	3	31	8
Cheese Enchiladas w/ Mole Sauce	200	22	2	20	6
Chicken Breasts	230	13	0	13	17
Chicken Enchiladas	180	13	1	12	5
Chicken Fried Steak w/ Gravy	330	27	0	27	27
Chicken Nuggets	210	10	0	10	17
Chicken Stew w/ Dumplings	400	38	2	36	27
Chicken Strips	230	11	0	11	19
Chile Belleno w/ Polenta, Cheese	510	46	15	31	22
Chili Pot Roast	160	8	2	6	20
Deluxe Beef Shepherd's Pie	360	17	4	13	28
Deluxe Chicken Pot Pie	480	36	4	32	21
Extra Lean Steakhouse Beef Patties	*130*	*1*	*0*	*1*	*19*
Fillet of Sole	190	18	1	17	8
Gorditas	410	35	7	28	21
Italian Six Cheese Lasagna	310	34	5	29	18
Italian Style Penne Pasta	190	30	1	29	9
Jumbo Chicken Wings: BBQ Style	200	6	0	6	11.9
Hot Buffalo Style	*160*	*1*	*0*	*1*	*15.8*
Low Fat Chicken Fillets, Average	50	6	0	6	2
Low Fat Turkey Lasagna	300	48	5	43	19
Macaroni & Cheese	350	30	0	30	13
Meat Lasagna	290	30	5	25	18
Mexican Style Lasagna	390	26	3	23	20
Mozzarella & Bacon Beef Steak Patties	*300*	*0*	*0*	*0*	*18*
Peppercorn Glazed Beef Kabobs	*120*	*4*	*0*	*4*	*22*
Pork Carnitas, Rice & Salsa	714	79.5	21	58.5	31.5
Pot Roast & Vegetables	210	15	2	13	22
Roasted Garlic Mashed Potatoes	285	33	3	30	4.5

	Calories	Total Carb	Fiber	Usable Carb	Protein
Salisbury Steak w/ Gravy	380	9	0.5	8.5	23
Seasoned Boneless					
Beef Strips	120	13	1	12	11
Southwestern Quesadilla	280	21	3	18	16
Southwestern Wraps	260	26	2	24	12
Stuffed Baked Potatoes,					
1 potato	280	35	3	32	10
St Louis Style Pork Spareribs	370	17	0.5	16.5	22
Tamale Bake	400	32	2	30	16
Three Cheese & Bacon					
Stuffed Baked Potatoes	210	22	2	20	6
Vegetable Lasagna,					
1 lasagna	310	27	3	24	13
Vegetable Quesadilla	330	33	2	31	15
Stir Fry:					
Chicken & Vegetables	180	26	4.6	21.4	16
Chicken Fajita	130	14	3.4	10.6	13.7
Shrimp & Vegetable	140	24	4.6	19.4	10.3
Teriyaki Beef	190	28	3.4	24.6	16
Beef & Broccoli	260	19	2	17	15
Chicken & Pork Potstickers	330	54	3	51	9
Ginger Beef	310	22	12	10	15
Orange Chicken	390	35	0	35	27
Pepper Beef	270	16	0.5	15.5	14
Pork Fried Rice	330	32	0.5	31.5	11
Sesame Pork	410	28	0.5	27.5	28
Shrimp Fried Rice	300	33	0.5	32.5	11
Sweet & Sour Pork	250	42	2	40	12
Szechuan Chicken	250	28	2	26	14
Vegetable Potstickers	250	36	6	30	9
SEAPAK					
Crunchy Clam Strips,					
1 packet, 5 oz.	410	41	0	41	56
Popcorn Fish, 7 pces, 3 oz.	240	23	0	23	12.5
Popcorn Shrimp,					
15 pieces, 3 oz.	210	18	0	18	7.5
SEEDS OF CHANGE					
Per 11 oz. Bowl					
Bowtie Primavera	380	51	8	43	18
Creamy Spinach Lasagna	370	36	7	29	19
Macaroni & Cheese	420	52	4	48	20

	Calories	Total Carb	Fiber	Usable Carb	Protein
Mushroom Wild Pilaf	350	40	5	35	13
Penne Marinara	290	44	5	39	13
Seven Grain Pilaf	390	52	10	42	15
Spicy Peanut Noodles	370	53	4	49	15
Teriyaki Stir-Fried Rice	340	56	6	50	10
SKYLINE CHILI					
Original Chili, 1 cup	*310*	*5*	*2*	*2*	*24*
Chili & Beans, 1 cup	350	63	5	12	23
Chili & Spaghetti, 1 cup	340	37	4	40	25
Coney Calzonies, 1 piece, 5 oz.	340	33	1	22	13
STOUFFER'S					
Entrees: Per Meal					
Beef, Roast Potato & Peppers	300	44	0	44	20.5
Cheesy Spaghetti Bake	460	47	4	43	21
Chicken a la King	370	47	2	45	21
Chicken Pie, 10 oz.	730	61	4	57	23
Creamed Chipped Beef	435	24.9	0	24.9	31.1
Fettuccini Alfredo	520	51	4	47	19
Fish Fillet w/ Mac & Cheese	410	44	2	42	23
Five Cheese Lasagna	340	39	6	33	20
Lasagna w/ Meat Sauce, 10 ½ oz.	370	35	4	31	27
Macaroni & Beef w/ Tomatoes	350	41	3	38	20
Macaroni & Cheese w/ Broccoli	350	38	4	34	16
Macaroni & Cheese, 1 cup	330	32	3	29	15
Maxaroni, Macaroni & Cheese	390	44	2	42	16
Roasted Garlic Chicken	320	39	0	39	11.8
Spaghetti w/ Meat Sauce	350	56	5	51	20
Spaghetti w/ Meatballs	390	49	5	44	19
Stuffed Pepper, 10 oz.	240	24	2	22	10
Swedish Meatballs w/ Pasta	520	48	4	44	25
Tuna Noodle Casserole	360	36	2	34	18
Turkey Tetrazzini	400	36	2	34	20
Veg & Chicken Pasta Bake	410	40	4	36	24
Yankee Pot Roast	320	40	0	40	23.3

	Calories	Total Carb	Fiber	Usable Carb	Protein
Homestyle:					
Beef Pot Roast	270	43	8	35	21
Baked Chicken in Gravy w/ Potato	260	18	0	18	22.5
Beef Stroganoff	350	37	2	35	17
Breaded Boneless Pork Cutlet	370	34	4	30	13
Fried Chicken & Mashed Potatoes	350	34	3	31	16
Meatloaf w/ Whipped Potatoes	580	38	5	33	29
Roast Chicken w/ Mushrooms	380	31	2	29	26
Roast Chicken w/ Stuffing Bake	510	37	4	33	24
Roast Pork w/ Sweet Potatoes, Stuffing	400	46	3	43	14
Salisbury Steak in Gravy w/ Onions	550	49	5	44	28
Veal Parmigiana	530	66	7	59	27
Family Style Recipes:					
Per Serving					
Chicken & Broccoli Pasta Bake, 1/5 Pkt	340	28	2	26	19
Chicken Cordon Bleu Pasta, 1/4	360	35	2	33	21
Grandma's Chicken & Veg Rice Bake	360	36	2	34	19
Lasagna w/ Meat Sauce, 1/2 pkg	330	28	3	25	16
Macaroni & Cheese, 1 cup	370	37	2	35	16
Meatloaf in Gravy, 1 loaf, 5.5 oz.	222	10	1	9	16
Hearty Portion:					
Fried Chicken Breast, 15⅛ oz.	520	66	0	66	28
Pork w/ Roast Potatoes, 15⅜ oz.	570	75	0	75	34
Side Dishes:					
Corn Souffle	170	21	2	19	5
Cheddar Potato Bake, 1/2 cup	250	21	2	19	7

	Calories	Total Carb	Fiber	Usable Carb	Protein
Harvest Apples	210	43	3	40	1
Spinach Souffle	130	10	1	9	5
Welsh Rarebit	120	6	0	6	5
Whipped Potato & Gravy	320	31	3	28	5
Pot Pies:					
Chicken, 10 oz.	730	61	4	57	23
Turkey, 10 oz.	590	53	4	49	25
Skillet Sensations: Per ½ Pkg					
Broccoli & Beef	300	46	6	40	17
Chicken & Dumplings	280	33	0	33	19.8
Chicken Alfredo	470	52	3	49	30
Grilled Chicken & Vegetable	400	42	2	40	25
Homestyle Beef	370	37	6	31	22
Homestyle Chicken	370	43	6	37	29
Teriyaki Chicken	340	40	5	35	22
SWANSON					
Standard Meal:					
Boneless White Meat Fried Chicken	450	50	5	45	23
Chicken Teriyaki (Original)	430	71	4	67	20
Classic Fried Chicken, 11½ oz.	640	41	5	53	24
Fish 'N Chips	470	52	0	52	18.5
Grilled Glazed Turkey Medallions	380	45	4	41	25
Grilled White Meat Chicken w/ Penne	310	31	3	28	21
Mexican Style Fiesta, 13.25 oz.	470	63	0	63	18
Salisbury Steak	470	33	0	33	16.5
Turkey Breast w/ Stuffing & Gravy	420	39	0	50	19
Hungry Man Dinners:					
Mexican	690	87	0	87	25
Boneless Pork Rib	770	78	0	78	29
Boneless White Meat Fried Chicken	430	72	8	64	34
Buffalo Chicken Strips	870	106	8	98	50
Classic Fried Chicken, 16½ oz.	790	75	6	69	33

	Calories	Total Carb	Fiber	Usable Carb	Protein
Mexican Style Fiesta	710	87	0	87	25
Salisbury Steak	610	46	0	46	32.5
Turkey Breast	630	82	5	77	30
TGI FRIDAY'S					
Chicken Quesadilla Rolls	250	26	2	24	10
Honey BBQ Wings	180	7	0	7	12
Potato Skins, 3 pc, 2.8 oz.	210	19	3	13	7
UNCLE BEN'S					
Breakfast Bowls: Per Bowl					
Egg, Cheese & Salsa, 7.5 oz.	310	16	4	12	14
French Toast & Sausage, 6 oz.	420	45	3	42	11
Pancakes:					
Apple Cinnamon, 6 oz.	330	59	3	56	5
Peach & Pecan, 6 oz.	300	54	4	50	5
Sausage, Egg & Biscuit, 7.5 oz.	350	31	5	26	13
Mini Bowls, 8 oz.:					
Pepperoni Pizzeria	330	34	1	33	19
Noodle Bowls:					
Honey Ginger Chicken	430	69	3	66	25
Spicy Thai Style Chicken	432	60	6	54	21
Pasta Bowls: Per 12 oz.					
Garden Vegetable Lasagna	320	44	6	38	19
Parmesan Shrimp Penne	380	58	2	56	24
3 Cheese Ravioli	380	61	6	55	21
4 Cheese Lasagna	330	41	7	34	24
Rice Bowls: Per 12 oz.					
Chicken Fried Rice	400	67	3	64	24
Chicken & Vegetable	360	56	3	53	21
Spicy Beef & Broccoli	370	62	1	61	21
Sweet & Sour Chicken	360	65	2	63	20
Teriyaki Chicken	380	66	3	63	20
Teriyaki Stir Fry Vegetable	360	74	4	70	8
VAN DE KAMP'S					
Fish Sticks, Breaded, 6 sticks, 4 oz.	290	23	0	23	11.3
Battered Fillets, 1 fillet, 2.6 oz.	180	12	0	12	8.3
Crisp & Healthy:					
Breaded, 1 fillet, 1.8 oz.	85	12	0	12	5.8

	Calories	Total Carb	Fiber	Usable Carb	Protein
Grilled: Italian Herb, 1, 4 oz.	**130**	**2**	**0**	**2**	**17**
Breaded Butterfly Shrimp, 7, 4 oz.	300	32	0	32	11.4
Lemon Pepper, 1, 3.6 oz.	**130**	**0**	**0**	**0**	**19**
Salmon, Creamy Dill, 1	**90**	**1**	**0**	**1**	**15.8**
Tuna, Barbecue, 1, 1.8 oz.	100	5	0	5	18.8
Tuna, Sesame Teriyaki, 1	**110**	**4**	**0**	**4**	**20**
WEIGHT WATCHERS					
Main Street Bistro Selections: Per Meal					
Basil Chicken, 9 oz.	270	34	2	32	20
Fajita Chicken Supreme, 9.25 oz.	280	33	2	31	19
Fire-Grilled Chicken & Vegetables, 10 oz.	280	40	2	38	18
Golden Baked Garlic Chicken, 10 oz.	280	40	3	37	19
Peppercorn Beef Fillet	230	24	0	24	15.5
Rst Chicken w/ Sour Cream & Chives	190	23	0	23	16.5
Slow Roast Turkey Breast, 10 oz.	220	20	2	18	18
Smart Ones: Per Meal					
Chicken Enchiladas Suiza, 9 oz.	280	38	2	36	14
Chicken Oriental	230	34	0	34	13.5
Fettuccini Alfredo w/ Broccoli, 9.25 oz.	270	39	3	36	14
Fiesta Chicken, 8.5 oz.	210	35	3	30	13
Grilled Salisbury Steak	260	25	0	25	26.5
Lasagna Florentine, 10.5 oz.	290	36	5	31	15
Lemon Herb Chicken Piccata	250	36	0	36	15.5
Mac & Cheese; Lasagna Bolognese	240	45	0	45	9.5
Ravioli Florentine, 8.5 oz.	220	43	4	39	9
Santa Fe Style Rice & Beans, 10 oz.	300	49	6	43	12
Teriyaki Chicken & Veg Bowl	280	48	0	48	15.5
Southwestern Style Chicken Bowl	230	35	0	35	17
Spaghetti Marinara, 9 oz.	280	46	4	42	9

	Calories	Total Carb	Fiber	Usable Carb	Protein
Spicy Penne Mediterranean	260	40	0	40	11.5
Spicy Szechuan Vegetables & Chicken	230	34	0	34	12.5
Swedish Meatballs, 9 oz.	280	34	3	31	20.5
Smartwiches:					
Ham & Cheddar	260	36	2	34	9
Average other varieties	270	38	2	36	12
WORTHINGTON (VEGETARIAN)					
Bolono, 3 slices, 2 oz.	*80*	*2*	*2*	*0*	*10*
Chicken Roll, 1 slice, 2 oz.	*90*	*2*	*0.5*	*1.5*	*9*
Chicken Diced, ¼ cup, 2 oz.	*60*	*3*	*0.5*	*2.5*	*11*
Chic-Ketts, 2 slices	*120*	*2*	*2*	*0*	*13*
ChikStiks, 1 piece	*110*	*3*	*2*	*1*	*10*
Choplets, 2 slices	*90*	*3*	*2*	*1*	*17*
FriChik, 2 pieces	*140*	*3*	*1*	*2*	*12*
Low Fat FriChik, 2 pieces	*80*	*4*	*1*	*3*	*12*
FriPats, 1 pattie	*130*	*4*	*3*	*1*	*14*
Veja-Links, 1 link	*40*	*1*	*0*	*1*	*5*

FROZEN PIZZAS

AMY'S
Per ⅓ Pizza:					
Cheese, Spinach, & Pesto	300	38	2	36	12
Roasted Vegetable, 4 oz.	270	43	2	41	6
Soy Cheese & Veggie					
Combo, Average	280	37	1	36	10
Mushroom & Olive	250	33	2	31	10

CELESTE
Pizza For One:					
Cheese, 1 pizza	390	42	6	36	13
Deluxe	440	42	6	36	14
Sausage & Pepperoni;					
Suprema	500	44	6	38	17
Zesty Chicken Supreme	360	40	6	34	14

DI GIORNO
Rising Crust (Large):					
Per ⅙ pizza					
Four Cheese	320	40	3	37	16
Sausage & Pepperoni	360	40	2	38	17

	Calories	Total Carb	Fiber	Usable Carb	Protein
Rising Crust (Small):					
Per ⅓ Pizza					
Four Cheese	270	34	2	32	14
Pepperoni	310	35	2	33	15
Sausage & Pepperoni	320	35	2	33	15
Spicy Chicken Supreme	280	35	2	33	16
Spinach, Mushroom & Garlic	260	36	3	33	12
Supreme	330	35	2	33	15
ELLIO'S (MCCAIN)					
Cheese, 1 slice	160	22	2	20	7
FRESCHETTA					
Sauces Stuffed Crust:					
Supreme, ⅕ pizza	360	42	2	40	12
HEALTHY CHOICE: FRENCH BREAD PIZZA					
Solos:					
Cheese & Pepperoni, 6 oz.	360	57	5	52	20
Supreme, 6.35 oz.	360	58	6	52	21
Vegetable, 6 oz.	320	50	4	46	18
HOME RUN INN					
Large: Cheese, ⅛ pizza	290	27	1	26	10
Sausage, ⅛ pizza	310	27	1	26	14
Small: Cheese, ⅙ pizza	260	26	1	25	9
Sausage, ⅙ pizza	280	26	1	25	12
JACK'S (KRAFT)					
Original: Cheese, ⅓ pizza	330	38	3	35	16
Sausage & Pepperoni, ¼ pizza	310	29	0	29	14
JEWEL					
Cheese, ⅓ pizza	310	40	2	38	14
Pepperoni, ¼ pizza	290	32	2	30	12
Supreme, ¼ pizza	320	32	2	30	14
LEAN CUISINE: FRENCH BREAD PIZZA					
Cheese, 6 oz.	340	46	3	43	18
Deluxe, 6⅛ oz.	330	44	3	41	18
Pepperoni, 5¼ oz.	300	44	2	42	16
MR. P'S PIZZA					
Cheese Pizza, 6.5 oz.	410	58	5	53	20.9
Combination (Saus/Pepp), 1	460	58	5	53	19

	Calories	Total Carb	Fiber	Usable Carb	Protein
MYSTIC					
Cheese, ⅓ pizza	360	36	1	35	19
House Special, ⅓ pizza	375	36	2	34	14
Pepperoni, ⅓ pizza	380	36	1	35	18
OLD ITALIAN					
Microwaveable Little Pizza:					
Per 1 Pizza					
Pepperoni, 4.2 oz.	350	41	4	37	11
Party, 4.2 oz.	340	40	4	36	10.5
RALPH'S					
Large (Self-Rising Crust):					
Four Cheese, ⅙	330	48	2	46	15
Pepperoni, ⅙	390	49	2	47	16
Supreme, ⅙	390	49	2	47	12
Small:					
Cheese, 1	440	62	6	56	22
Combination, 1	520	61	6	55	22
Pepperoni, 1	510	62	5	57	21
RED BARON					
Classic (Large):					
4 Cheese, ¼ pizza	420	36	1	35	18
Pepperoni, ¼ pizza	440	36	1	35	17
Sausage & Pepperoni, ⅕	360	29	1	28	14
Supreme, Special Deluxe, ⅕	350	30	2	28	12
Bake To Rise:					
4 Cheese, ⅙ pizza	330	39	2	37	16
Pepperoni, Special					
Deluxe, ⅙ pizza	360	40	2	38	16
Deep Dish Pan Style:					
4 Cheese, ⅓ pizza	370	39	2	37	14
Supreme, ⅓ pizza	410	40	2	38	15
Deep Dish Singles:					
Cheese, 1 pizza	430	41	2	39	17
Pepperoni, 1 pizza	460	41	2	39	17
Supreme, 1 pizza	470	40	2	38	16
Deep Dish Mini Pizzas:					
Cheese, 4 pizzas	380	44	2	42	17.5
Pepperoni, 4 pizzas	400	41	2	39	16
Supreme, 4 pizzas	430	43	1.3	41.7	14.7

	Calories	Total Carb	Fiber	Usable Carb	Protein
REGGIO'S					
Family Size:					
Cheese, ⅙ pizza	320	38	2	36	15
Sausage, ⅙ pizza	330	38	3	35	18
Dinner Size:					
Cheese, ¼ pizza	330	41	2	39	14
Pepperoni & Sausage, ¼ pizza	400	41	2	39	18
Sausage, ¼ pizza	380	41	2	39	17
STOP & SHOP					
Single Serving:					
Cheese, 1	390	42	6	36	13
9 Slices:					
Cheese, 2 slices	350	49	2	47	15
STOUFFERS: FRENCH BREAD PIZZA					
Cheese, 1 piece, (½ pkg)	370	43	3	40	14
Deluxe, 1 piece	420	50	5	45	11
Extra Cheese, 1 piece	400	49	4	45	16
Pepperoni, 1 piece	410	47	3	44	11
Sausage, 1 piece	420	49	4	45	11
Three Meat, 1 piece	460	50	6	44	15
White Cheese/Garlic/Herbs, 1 piece	460	45	3	42	17
THE OLD CITY CAFÉ					
Mushroom Pizza, ¼	165	28	1	27	8
Pizza DeDeluxe, ¼	195	29	1	28	8
TOMBSTONE					
Original (Large):					
Deluxe, ⅕ pizza	300	31	3	28	15
Extra Cheese, ¼ pizza	340	37	3	34	18
Sausage & Mushroom, ⅕ pizza	300	30	3	27	15
Mexican Style (Large):					
Cheese Quesadilla, ⅓ pizza	360	37	3	34	16
Chicken Fajita, ¼ pizza	300	29	2	27	15
Nacho Grande, ¼ pizza	380	37	3	34	15
Original (Small 9"):					
Extra Cheese, ½ pizza	370	42	3	39	19
Classic Sausage, ⅓ pizza	270	28	2	26	14

	Calories	Total Carb	Fiber	Usable Carb	Protein
Oven Rising:					
Pepperoni, 1/6 pizza	330	35	2	33	17
Thin Crust:					
3 Cheese, 1/4 pizza	350	27	2	25	19
Italian, 1/4 pizza	380	27	2	25	18
Pepperoni, 1/4 pizza	400	27	2	25	18
TONY'S					
Original:					
Cheese, 1/3 pizza	390	33	1	32	15
Sausage, 1/3 pizza	440	34	2	32	15
Supreme, 1/3 pizza	420	39	1	38	12
Thin Crust:					
Cheese, 1/3 pizza	290	31	1	30	14
Sausage, 1/3 pizza	330	32	2	30	14
Supreme, 1/3 pizza	340	33	2	31	14
Super Rise:					
4 Cheese, 1/4 pizza	340	40	2	38	14
Sausage, 1/4 pizza	380	41	2	39	15
TOTINO'S					
Crisp Crust Party Pizza:					
Per 1/2 Pizza, Cheese	320	34	2	32	15
VERDI (SAFEWAY SELECT)					
Self-Rising Crust (Large):					
Meat Magnifico, 1/6 pizza	370	41	1	40	17
Primo Pepperoni, 1/6 pizza	370	42	1	41	16
Quatro Formaggio, 1/6 pizza	300	41	1	40	14
Supremo Classico, 1/6 pizza	368	43	1	42	13
Self-Rising Crust (Small):					
Rstd Mushroom & Garlic, 1/3 pizza	230	33	2	31	10
Primo Pepperoni, 1/3 pizza	300	32	1	31	13
Roasted Vegetable Speciale, 1/3 pizza	240	33	2	31	11
Supremo Classico, 1/3 pizza	300	33	2	31	13
WEIGHT WATCHER'S (SMART ONES)					
Per Whole Pizza					
BBQ-Style Chicken Pizza	400	69	3	66	19
Four Cheese Pizza	400	58	3	55	20
Pepperoni Pizza	400	65	4	61	22
Veggie Ultimate Pizza	400	65	5	60	18

	Calories	Total Carb	Fiber	Usable Carb	Protein
WOLFGANG PUCK					
Large:					
4 Cheese & Pesto, ¼ pizza	440	38	1	37	20
Barbecue Style Chicken,					
⅕ pizza	310	30	3	27	18
Italian Sausage &					
Pepperoni, ¼ pizza	410	36	4	32	20
Small:					
BBQ Chicken, ½ pizza	330	32	3	29	19
Primavera Vegetable,					
½ pizza	300	30	4	26	14
Spicy Grilled Chicken,					
½ pizza	380	35	1	34	19
Thai Style Chicken, ½ pizza	390	36	1	35	20

CANNED & PACKAGED MEALS

	Calories	Total Carb	Fiber	Usable Carb	Protein
BANQUET					
Homestyle Bake:					
Prepared Per Serving					
Creamy Turkey & Stuffing	260	29	4	25	12
Cheesy Ham & Hashbrowns	240	31	3	28	6
Country Chicken					
Potato Biscuit	380	55	3	52	11
BETTY CROCKER					
Chicken Helper:					
Per Cup, Prepared					
Homestyle Chicken					
& Biscuit	440	35	0	35	22
Homestyle Chicken					
& Dumplings	290	27	0	27	23
Southwestern Chicken	240	29	0	29	23
Average other flavors	300	28	0	28	0
Hamburger Helper:					
Per Cup, Prepared					
Cheddar & Broccoli	350	33	0	33	22
Cheesy Enchilada	380	27	0	27	32
Nacho Cheese	350	30	0	30	21.5
Philly Cheesesteak	330	25	0	25	21
Potato:					
Average, ⅓ cup dry mix	80	18	1	19	2

	Calories	Total Carb	Fiber	Usable Carb	Protein
Suddenly Salad: Prepared					
Caesar, 1 cup	170	34	1	33	6
Classic, ¾ cup	250	38	2	36	7
Ranch & Bacon, ¾ cup	330	30	1	29	7
Roasted Garlic & Parmesan,					
¾ cup	260	33	0	33	7
Tuna Helper:					
Fettuccine Alfredo,					
¾ cup dry mix	170	30	1	29	5
Supper Bakes:					
Per ⅙ Box, Prepared					
Lemon Chicken w/ Herb Rice	340	43	2	41	26
Herb Chicken w/ Rice	330	40	1	39	27
Garlic Chicken w/ Pasta	370	44	2	42	33
Savory Pork Chops	380	31	2	29	24
CEDARLANE (VEGETARIAN)					
Bruschetta, Pesto, Mozzarella,					
Tomato, (1)	100	10	0.5	9.5	3
Burrito, Beans, Rice, &					
Cheese, (1) 6 oz.	260	48	7	41	13
Eggplant Parmesan,					
½ pkg, 5 oz.	190	16	3	13	7
Enchilada: Garden Veg,					
(1) 4.8 oz.	140	20	3	17	9
Three-Layer Pie, ½ pkg,					
5.5 oz.	215	27	3	24	13
Focaccia:					
Tomato & Basil, ⅓ loaf	275	33	2	31	14
Mediterranean Stuff, ⅓ loaf	296	37	1	36	13
Lasagne: Cheese, ½ carton,					
5 oz.	190	22	1.5	20.5	12.5
Garden Veg, ½ ctn, 5 oz.	180	26	2	24	10
Pizza, Mini Bistro, (3), 4 oz.	280	27	2	25	10
Wrap: Veggie "Ham" &					
Cheese, 6 oz.	350	36	1	35	29
CHEF BOYARDEE					
Beefaroni, all types, 1 cup	260	35	0	35	10
Homestyle, 15 oz. Can:					
Per Cup, 9 oz.					
Cannelloni	240	36	2	34	9
Chicken Alfredo w/ Pasta	250	24	1	23	10

	Calories	Total Carb	Fiber	Usable Carb	Protein
Rigatoni	250	31	0	31	9
Mini Bites, 14.75 oz. Can:					
Per Cup					
Mini Beef Ravioli					
w/ Meatballs	300	36	0	36	10
Mini Pasta Shells					
w/ Meatballs	270	32	0	32	8
Mini Spaghetti					
w/ Meatballs	280	31	0	31	9
Pepperoni Pizza Roli	320	46	0	46	10
Chef Jr: Micro Ravioli, 1 cup	220	36	0	36	7
Dinosaurs w/ M'Balls					
in Tomato Sauce	290	39	0	39	8
Other varieties, 1 cup, 9 oz.	200	43	0	43	5
Jumbo (14.75 oz. Can):					
Per Cup					
99% Fat Free:					
Beef Ravioli	190	37	0	37	7
Cheese Ravioli	240	45	0	45	7
Lasagna	270	36	0	36	9
Spaghetti w/ Jumbo					
Meatballs	280	30	0	30	11
Overstuffed Italian					
Sausage Ravioli	280	50	0	50	10

DENNISON'S CHILI

	Calories	Total Carb	Fiber	Usable Carb	Protein
Per 1 Cup Serving (15 oz. Can)					
Chili Con Carne w/ Beans:					
Original; Hot	350	36	0	36	18
Chunky; Hot & Chunky	320	32	0	32	21
Micro Cup, 7.5 oz. Bowl	290	26	0	26	17.5
99% Fat Free:					
Beef Chili w/ Beans	220	27	0	27	23.5
Turkey Chili w/ Beans	210	29	0	29	17
Vegetarian w/ Beans	180	35	0	35	8
Mild Green w/ Beans	370	32	0	32	22.5
No Bean Chili Con Carne	330	21	0	21	21

DINTY MOORE (HORMEL FOODS)

	Calories	Total Carb	Fiber	Usable Carb	Protein
Noodles & Chicken	200	21	0	21	7
Micro Cup:					
Beef Stew, 1 cup	160	16	0	16	6
Corned Beef Hash, 1 cup	350	19	0	19	19

	Calories	Total Carb	Fiber	Usable Carb	Protein
Chili Con Carne, 1 bowl	290	26	0	26	15.5
Mac & Cheese	190	28	0	28	6
Chicken & Noodles	270	28	0	28	21.5
Chicken Breast/Roast Beef & Gravy w/ Potato	240	24	0	24	25
Hearty Lasagna	340	28	0	28	21
Salisbury Steak w/ Potato	300	24	0	24	22
Turkey & Dressing w/ Gravy	290	32	0	32	22.5
DON MIGUEL XLNT					
Flautas:					
Garlic Chicken, (2) 4 oz.	250	40	2	38	12
Shredded Beef, (2) 4 oz.	230	39	2	37	12
Tamales: Beef, (1) 3 oz.	200	17	3	14	5
Chimichangas:					
Beef, (1) 4.8 oz.	260	35	2	33	1
Chicken, (1) 4.8 oz.	280	36	2	34	11
DR. MCDOUGALL'S					
Per Cup					
Pasta w/ Beans, Mediterranean	180	29	7	22	8
Pinto Beans & Rice, Southwestern	190	38	7	31	9
Rice & Pasta Pilaf	210	36	2	34	6
EDEN					
Per ½ Cup, 4½ oz.					
Baked Beans w/ Sorghum & Mustard	150	27	7	20	7
Chili Beans w/ Jalapeno & Peppers	130	21	7	14	9
Ginger Blacks w/ Ginger & Lemon	120	21	7	14	7
FANTASTIC					
Per Packet					
Cha-Cha Chili	250	44	13	31	17
Noodles, average	140	27	4	23	8
FRANCO AMERICAN					
Spaghetti O's:					
w/ Tomato Sauce & Cheese					
A to Z's, 1 cup	180	36	0	36	6
Garfield, 1 cup	210	39	0	39	6

	Calories	Total Carb	Fiber	Usable Carb	Protein
Where's Waldo, 1 cup	200	38	0	38	7
Meatballs in Tomato Sauce:					
A to Z's, 1 cup	260	33	0	33	11
Knights & Castles, 1 cup	270	33	0	33	10
GREEN GIANT					
Per Cup					
Pork & Beans w/					
Tomato Sauce	240	46	8	38	10
Spicy Chili Beans	220	40	10	30	12
HEALTH VALLEY (VEGETARIAN)					
Fat-Free Beans & Chili:					
Chili Burrito/Enchilada, ½ cup	80	15	7	8	7
Chili in a Cup, All Types,					
¾ cup	120	21	6	15	10
Chili, Fajita flavored, ½ cup	80	15	7	8	7
Mild/Spicy Vegetarian Chili:					
All flavors, ½ cup	80	15	7	8	7
HORMEL					
Per Cup					
Kid's Kitchen:					
Beans 'N Wieners	310	37	0	37	11.5
Beefy Macaroni	190	23	0	23	11
Cheezy Mac 'N Cheese	260	30	0	30	10.5
Cheezy Mac 'N Franks	300	26	0	26	12
Mini Beef Ravioli	240	34	0	34	10.5
Spaghetti & Mini Meatballs	230	26	0	26	12
Spaghetti Rings & Franks	240	32	0	32	9
Noodle Rings & Chicken	150	16	0	16	10.5
Spaghetti Rings w/					
Meatballs	230	35	0	35	7
Microwave Cup:					
Chili w/ Beans	220	27	0	27	14.5
Chili no Beans	190	15	0	15	14.5
Lasagna w/ Meat Sauce	210	29	0	29	10
Scalloped Potatoes & Ham	240	20	0	20	8.5
Spaghetti w/ Meat Sauce	220	31	0	31	8.5
Chili, 15 oz. Can: Per Cup					
With Beans:					
Reg/Hot/Chunky	270	34	0	34	18
Homestyle Chili	330	24	0	24	16

	Calories	Total Carb	Fiber	Usable Carb	Protein
Turkey (99% Fat Free)	200	26	0	26	17.5
Vegetarian (99% Fat Free)	200	38	0	38	10
No Beans, 1 cup	210	17	0	17	15.5

HUNGRY JACK POTATOES

	Calories	Total Carb	Fiber	Usable Carb	Protein
Casseroles: ½ cup, average	150	24	2	22	2
Idaho Mashed: ½ cup, avg	155	21	1	20	3
Instant Potato Flakes: ⅓ cup	80	18	0.9	17.1	1.8
Potato Pancake Mix,					
2 T, made up	90	16	1	15	2

KRAFT PASTA DINNERS

	Calories	Total Carb	Fiber	Usable Carb	Protein
Per Cup, Prepared					
Macaroni & Cheese:	320	44	0	44	13.5
Light	290	48	0	48	14.5
Easy Mac, 1 pouch	250	38	0	38	8
Velveeta: All varieties	360	46	0	46	15
Oven Classic Chicken Bake:					
⅙ Pkt, Prepared					
Au Gratin; Traditional Roast	340	33	0	33	27
Herb & Garlic	320	34	0	34	26
Homestyle BBQ	360	43	0	43	27
Honey Mustard	380	43	0	43	28
Lemon	370	48	0	48	26
Roasted Garlic	310	28	0	28	25

LIPTON PACKET MEALS

	Calories	Total Carb	Fiber	Usable Carb	Protein
Per Cup, Prepared					
Rice & Sauce:					
Spanish	270	47	0	47	3.5
Cheddar Broccoli;					
Chicken	280	46	0	46	4
Noodles & Sauce:					
Butter & Herb	310	42	0	42	4
Chicken Flavor;					
Chicken Broccoli	300	42	0	42	8.5
Recipe Secrets:					
Golden Onion	50	9	1	8	1
Onion	*20*	*4*	*0*	*4*	*1*
Onion & Mushroom;					
Savory Herb	30	6	0.3	5.7	0.8
Vegetable	30	9	1	8	0.8

	Calories	Total Carb	Fiber	Usable Carb	Protein
Sizzle & Stir: ⅙ Pkt, Prepared					
3 Cheese Alfredo Chicken & Penne	410	29	0	29	7
Savory Herbed Chicken & Pasta	340	28	0	28	5
Spanish Chicken; Teriyaki Stir Fry	360	34	0	34	5
LOMA LINDA (VEGETARIAN)					
Big Franks, 1 link, 1.8 oz.	*110*	*2*	*2*	*0*	*10*
Chicken Supreme Mix,					
⅓ cup mix	*90*	*6*	*3.6*	*2.4*	*13.5*
Dinner Cuts, 2 slices, 1.4 oz.	*90*	*3*	*2*	*1*	*17*
Fried Chik'n w/ Gravy,					
2 pieces, 3 oz.	*150*	*5*	*2*	*3*	*12*
Linketts, 1 link, 1¼ oz.	*70*	*1*	*1*	*0*	*7*
Little Links, 2 links, 1.6 oz.	*90*	*2*	*2*	*0*	*8*
Nuteena, ⅜" slice, 2 oz.	*160*	*6*	*2*	*4*	*6*
Ocean Platter, ⅓ cup					
dry mix, 1 oz.	*90*	*8*	*4*	*4*	*14*
Redi-Burger, ⅝" slice, 3 oz.	*120*	*7*	*4*	*3*	*18*
Savory Dinner Loaf,					
⅓ cup dry mix	*90*	*7*	*5*	*2*	*14*
Swiss Steak, 1 piece, 3¼ oz.	*120*	*8*	*4*	*4*	*9*
Tender Bits, 6 pieces, 3 oz.	*110*	*7*	*3*	*4*	*11*
Tender Rounds, 6 pieces,					
2¾ oz.	120	6	1	5	14
Vege-Burger, ¼ cup, 2 oz.	*70*	*2*	*2*	*0*	*11*
Vita-Burger Granules,					
3 T, ¾ oz.	*70*	*6*	*3*	*3*	*10*
MIDLAND HARVEST					
Fat Free & Lowfat Dry Mix:					
Taco Filling & Dip, 2.7 oz.	50	7	2	5	8
Chili Fixins, 8 oz.	160	24	8	16	15
Sloppy Joe Fixins, 3.6 oz.	70	11	3	8	8
Burger Loaf Dry Mix:					
Per 3.2 oz.	*120*	*8*	*5*	*3*	*17*
Frozen Patties:					
Sausage, 2 oz.	*80*	*5*	*3*	*2*	*10*
Other varieties, 3.2 oz.	*120*	*8*	*5*	*3*	*18*

	Calories	Total Carb	Fiber	Usable Carb	Protein
MORNINGSTAR FARMS (VEGETARIAN)					
Better'n Burger,					
1 pattie, 3 oz.	**80**	**6**	**3**	**3**	**14.5**
Better'n Eggs, ¼ cup, 2 oz.	**20**	**0**	**0**	**0**	**5**
Breakfast Links,					
2 links, 1½ oz.	**80**	**3**	**1.9**	**1.1**	**10**
Breakfast Patties:					
Frozen 1 pattie, 1⅓ oz.	**80**	**3**	**2**	**1**	**10**
Breakfast Strips, 2 strips	**60**	**2**	**0**	**2**	**2**
Buffalo Wings,					
5 nuggets, 3 oz.	200	18	3	15	14
Burger-Style Recipe					
Crumbles, ⅔ cup	**80**	**4**	**2**	**2**	**10.4**
Chik Nuggets, 4 nuggets	180	17	5	12	14.5
Chik Patties, 1 pattie	150	16	2	14	9
Corn Dog (Meat Free):					
1 link	150	22	3	19	6.5
Mini, 4 pieces, 2.7 oz.	170	21	1	20	11
Garden Veg Patties (1),					
2⅓ oz.	100	9	4	5	10
Grillers:					
Original, 1 pattie, 2¼ oz.	**140**	**5**	**3**	**2**	**16.5**
Prime, 1 pattie, 2½ oz.	**170**	**5**	**2**	**3**	**17.5**
Ground Meatless					
Crumbles, ½ cup, 2 oz.	**60**	**4**	**2.1**	**1.9**	**10.3**
Harvest Burgers, 1 pattie,					
3.2 oz.	**140**	**8**	**5**	**3**	**18**
Mushroom & Pepper					
Burger, 1	120	9	3	6	12
Pot Pie:					
Hearty Chik'n, 269 g	350	45	9	36	11
Homestyle Chili Pie, 255 g	330	49	7	42	13.5
Sausage Recipe Crumbles,					
⅔ cup, 2 oz.	**90**	**5**	**3.1**	**1.9**	**11.2**
Scramblers, ¼ cup, 2 oz.	**35**	**2**	**0**	**2**	**6**
Spicy Black Bean Burger,					
1 pattie	110	16	5	11	11
Supreme Pizza, ½ pizza	300	38	2	36	15
Tomato & Basil Pizza					
Burger, 2.3 oz.	**130**	**7**	**3**	**4**	**11**
Veggie Dog, 1 link, 2 oz.	80	6	1	5	13

	Calories	Total Carb	Fiber	Usable Carb	Protein
Breakfast Sandwiches:					
Muffin/Scramblers/Pattie/					
Cheese	280	35	5	30	28
Muffin/Scramblers/Pattie	240	32	5	27	22
NATURAL TOUCH (VEGETARIAN)					
Canned & Dry Products					
Roasted Soy Butter,					
2 tbsp, 1.1 oz.	170	10	1	9	6
Vegetarian Chili,					
1 cup, 8 oz.	170	21	11	10	18
NEAR EAST					
Prepared As Directed, Per Cup					
Couscous:					
Original Plain	230	46	0	46	7
Chicken & Herbs	200	42	3	39	7
Rice Pilaf	190	42	0	42	4.5
NEW MENU (VITASOY) VEGETARIAN					
VegiBurgers, 3 oz.	110	12	1	11	13
VegiDogs, 1 link, 1.5 oz.	*45*	*1*	*0*	*1*	*9*
Tofumate (Seasoning Mixes):					
¼ Pkt	*25*	*4*	*0*	*4*	*1*
NILE SPICE					
Per Cup, Couscous:					
Minestrone	180	34	0	34	7.5
Parmesan	200	34	0	34	9.5
NISSIN					
Cup Noodles,					
All types, average	300	38	0	38	5.6
OLD EL PASO: PER SERVING					
One Skillet Mexican					
(Prepared):					
Rice Burrito (1)	190	35	0	35	15
Salsa; Taco, average (2)	460	56	0	56	23
Dinner Kits (Prepared):					
Soft Taco	390	33	0	33	22
Burrito (1)	270	27	0	27	14
Hard & Soft Taco (2)	360	32	0	32	19
Fajita (2)	330	35	0	35	24
Taco Dinner (2)	300	19	0	19	17

	Calories	Total Carb	Fiber	Usable Carb	Protein
Side Dishes: Per Serving					
Canned:					
Chili w/ Beans, 1 cup	240	19	0	19	17
Spanish Rice, 1 cup	140	30	0	30	3
Tamales in Chili Gravy (1)	320	31	0	31	7
Boxed:					
Chsy Mexican Rice, ⅓ Pkt	250	55	0	55	4
Spanish Rice, ⅓ Pkt	280	55	0	55	5
Refried Beans:					
Reg, Black, ½ cup	100	17	6	11	6
w/ Green Chilies, ½ cup	100	19	6	13	6
w/ Cheese, ½ cup	130	18	6	12	7
w/ Sausage, ½ cup	200	14	4	10	7
Fat Free Varieties, ½ cup	100	18	6	12	6
Mex/Pinto Beans, ½ cup	110	19	7	12	7
Black/Garbanzo Beans,					
½ cup	100	17	4	13	6
PASTA-RONI					
Per Cup, Prepared					
Angel Hair Pasta Primavera	330	39	2	37	9
Butter & Garlic	260	40	2	38	8
PRITIKIN: VEGETARIAN					
Chili, 1 cup	160	27	0	27	11
RICE-A-RONI					
Per Cup, Prepared					
Beef; Herb & Butter	310	52	0	52	5.5
Chicken & Broccoli	230	41	0	41	3
Chicken & Garlic;					
Chicken Teriyaki	260	41	1	40	6
Fried Rice	320	51	0	51	4.5
Long Grain & Wild Rice	240	43	0	43	3.5
Rice Pilaf; Risotto	310	51	0	51	6.5
STAGG CHILI					
15 oz. Can: Per Cup (8.7 oz.)					
Chili w/ Beans:					
Classic/Dynamite	330	28	0	28	16.5
Country/Laredo	320	29	0	29	15
Fiesta Grille	240	25	0	25	15
Rancho House Chicken	290	32	0	32	20.5

	Calories	Total Carb	Fiber	Usable Carb	Protein
No Beans:					
Steakhouse/Double	330	16	0	16	19.5
99% Fat Free:					
Veg Garden/4 Bean	200	37	0	37	11
Turkey Ranchers/					
Silvarado Beef	240	31	0	31	22.5

SWEET SUE

	Calories	Total Carb	Fiber	Usable Carb	Protein
Chicken & Dumplings, 1 cup	218	22.8	0	22.8	15.6
Whole Chicken;					
w/out giblets, 2 oz.	*80*	*0*	*0*	*0*	*9*

WESTBRAE

	Calories	Total Carb	Fiber	Usable Carb	Protein
Ramen Noodles:					
Per ½ Container					
Average all varieties	140	30	3	27	5

WHITE WAVE (VEGETARIAN)

	Calories	Total Carb	Fiber	Usable Carb	Protein
Tempeh:					
Five Grain, ⅓ pkg	140	15	4	11	11
Original, ⅓ pkg	*150*	*10*	*6*	*4*	*14*
Sea Veggie, ⅓ pkg	*120*	*11*	*8*	*3*	*12*
Wild/Soy Rice, ⅓ pkg	140	13	5	8	13
Seitan:					
Chicken w/ Broth, 5 oz.	130	12	5	7	13
Traditional, 4 oz.	*140*	*4*	*1*	*3*	*31*
Tofu:					
Baked: all flavors, 2 oz.	*120*	*3*	*1*	*2*	*13*
Organic: Soft/Firm,					
⅛ pkg, 3.2 oz.	*90*	*1*	*1*	*0*	*10*
Fat-Reduced, ⅛ pkg, 3.2 oz.	90	4	2	2	10
Extra Firm, ¼ pkg, 3 oz.	*80*	*1*	*1*	*0*	*10*

WORTHINGTON (VEGETARIAN)

	Calories	Total Carb	Fiber	Usable Carb	Protein
Canned & Dry Products:					
Chili, 1 cup, 8 oz.	290	21	9	12	19
Low Fat Chili, 1 cup, 8 oz.	170	21	11	10	18
Corned Beef, 4 slices, 2 oz.	140	5	0	5	10
Country Stew, 1 cup, 8½ oz.	210	20	5	15	13
Crispy Chic Patties, 1 pattie	150	16	2	14	9
Diced Chic, ¼ cup, 2 oz.	*50*	*2*	*1*	*1*	*9.3*
Dinner Roast, ¾" slice,					
3 oz.	*180*	*5*	*3*	*2*	*12*
Fillets, 2 pces, 3 oz.	*180*	*8*	*4*	*4*	*16*

	Calories	Total Carb	Fiber	Usable Carb	Protein
Golden Croquettes, 4 pieces, 3 oz.	210	14	2	12	15
Leanies, 1 link	*100*	*2*	*1*	*1*	*7*
Multigrain Cutlets, 2 slices, 3¼ oz.	*100*	*5*	*4*	*1*	*15*
Numete, ⅜" slice, 2 oz.	*130*	*5*	*3*	*2*	*6*
Salami, 3 slices, 2 oz.	*130*	*2*	*2*	*0*	*12*
Smoked Beef, 6 slices, 2 oz.	130	7	0.5	6.5	11
Smoked Turkey, 3 slices, 2 oz.	*140*	*3*	*0*	*3*	*10*
Wham, 2 slices, 1½ oz.	*90*	*2*	*0*	*2*	*8*

YVES VEGGIE CUISINE (VEGETARIAN)

	Calories	Total Carb	Fiber	Usable Carb	Protein
Breakfast:					
Breakfast Links, (2), 1.8 oz.	*60*	*3*	*2*	*1*	*11*
Breakfast Patties, (1), 2 oz.	*70*	*4*	*2.3*	*1.7*	*11*
Canadian Veg Bacon, 3 slices, 2 oz.	*80*	*1*	*1*	*0*	*16.4*
Burgers:					
Veggie Burger, (1), 3 oz.	120	9	3	6	9
Garden Vegetable Patties, (1), 3 oz.	*90*	*11*	*7*	*4*	*11.5*
Black Bean & Mushroom, (1), 3 oz.	100	13	7	6	12
Veggie Chick 'N Burger, (1), 3 oz.	*120*	*6*	*2.3*	*3.7*	*15*
Dogs:					
Good Dog, (1)	*80*	*2*	*1*	*1*	*13*
Hot & Spicy Veggie Chili, (1)	*70*	*3*	*2*	*1*	*13*
Veggie Dog, (1)	*60*	*1*	*1*	*0*	*11*
Jumbo Veggie Dog, (1)	100	7	2	5	16
Tofu Dog, (1)	*45*	*2*	*0*	*2*	*9*
Veggie Ground Round:					
⅓ cup, 1.93 oz.	60	4	3	1	10
Slices:					
Bologna, 2 oz.	*80*	*4*	*1*	*3*	*15*
Pizza Pepperoni, 1.7 oz.	*70*	*4*	*3*	*1*	*14*
Veggie Ham, 2 oz.	80	6	1	5	14
Veggie Turkey, 2 oz.	*90*	*4*	*2*	*2*	*15*

	Calories	Total Carb	Fiber	Usable Carb	Protein
Veggie Entrees:					
Per 300g Tray, 10.5 oz.					
Country Stew	170	24	7	17	18.5
Chili; Macaroni; Penne,					
Average	230	38	14	24	21
Lasagne	300	51	4	47	17

SOY & TOFU

SOYBEAN PRODUCTS

	Calories	Total Carb	Fiber	Usable Carb	Protein
Miso, ½ cup, 5 oz.	280	39	7.4	31.6	16.2
Tempeh, 1 pc, 3 oz.	170	14	0	14	15.8

TOFU

	Calories	Total Carb	Fiber	Usable Carb	Protein
Azumaya Tofu:					
Soft (Silken), 3 oz.	*45*	*4*	*0*	*4*	*3*
Firm, 3 oz.	*60*	*3*	*0*	*3*	*6*
Extra Firm, 3 oz.	*80*	*2*	*0*	*2*	*10*
Age (Tofu Puff), ½ oz.	*40*	*2*	*0*	*2*	*4*
Nama-Age (Fried Tofu), 3 oz.	130	8	0	8	15
Mori-Nu Tofu (Silken):					
Soft, 4 oz.	*60*	*3*	*0.1*	*2.9*	*5.5*
Firm, 4 oz.	*70*	*3*	*0.1*	*2.9*	*8*
Extra Firm, 4 oz.	*70*	*3*	*0.1*	*2.9*	*8.4*
Nasoya Tofu:					
Soft, 3 oz.	*60*	*2*	*0.2*	*1.8*	*7*
Silken, 3 oz.	*50*	*2*	*0.2*	*1.8*	*6*
Firm, 3 oz.	*80*	*2*	*0.2*	*1.8*	*9*
Extra Firm, 3 oz.	*90*	*1*	*0.2*	*0.8*	*10.5*
Chinese 5 Spice Tofu, 3 oz.	*80*	*2*	*0.5*	*1.5*	*9*

SOUPS

HOMEMADE & RESTAURANT

	Calories	Total Carb	Fiber	Usable Carb	Protein
Restaurant & Take-Out					
Per 8 fl. oz.					
Bean Medley	200	34	8	26	7
Beef Consomme	*30*	*2*	*0*	*2*	*5.3*
Bouillabaisse	400	10	0	10	56
Chicken & Corn	290	20	2.2	17.8	17.4
Chicken & Wild Rice	80	9	0	9	5
Chicken Noodle	80	12	1	11	6
Chicken Soup	80	6	1	5	3.6

	Calories	Total Carb	Fiber	Usable Carb	Protein
Chili w/ Bean	250	25	8	17	20
Clam Chowder	240	17	1	16	8
Corn Chowder	150	16	2	14	7
Cream of Broccoli	200	20	1	19	15
Cream of Potato	220	25	3	22	5
Cream of Mushroom	290	20	1	19	3
French Onion	420	25	1	24	2
Gazpacho	60	13	0	13	0
Lentil Soup	250	28	14	14	11
Lobster Bisque	320	10	1	9	6
Matzo (w/ one large ball)	180	24	0	24	5
Minestrone	140	14	3	11	3
Pea & Ham	240	25	0	25	5
Potato & Bacon	170	19	2	17	6
Shark Fin Soup	*220*	*21*	*0*	*4*	*6.9*
Split Pea Soup	150	18	8	10	10
Vegetable (Fat Free)	75	18	4	14	3
Vegetable Beef	80	10	2	8	4
Vichyssoise	200	15	0	15	14.8
BOUILLON CUBES & POWDERS					
Average all types					
Regular, 1 cube	*8*	*1*	*0*	*1*	*1*
Powders: Average, 1 Tsp	*8*	*1*	*0*	*1*	*0.6*
Soup Oyster Crackers					
40 small/20 large, ½ oz.	60	8	0	8	0
AMY'S					
Per Cup (½ Can)					
Black Bean Vegetable	110	22	5	17	6
Cream of Mushroom, ¾ cup	120	10	2	8	3
Cream of Tomato	100	17	4	13	2
Lentil	130	19	9	10	8
No Chicken Noodle	90	12	2	10	5
Organic Vegetable Broth	35	8	0	8	1
Split Pea	100	19	4	15	7
Vegetable Barley	50	10	0	10	0.5
BETTY CROCKER					
Bowl Appetit! Per 2.7 oz. Serving					
3-Cheese Rotini	370	52	0	52	13.5
Cheddar Broccoli Rice	300	52	0	52	5
Herb Chicken Veg Rice	260	50	0	50	6

	Calories	Total Carb	Fiber	Usable Carb	Protein
Homestyle Chicken Flavor					
& Pasta	260	42	0	42	9.5
Pasta Alfredo	360	51	0	51	14.5
Tomato Parmesan Penne	350	57	0	57	12.5
BIRDS EYE					
Hearty Spoonfuls Soup Bowls					
(Frozen)					
Cheesy Cream of Broccoli	230	25	6	19	9
Chicken Noodle	140	19	2	17	11
Chicken, Rice & Vegetables	160	26	2	24	10
Italian Minestrone	240	37	7	30	11
CAMPBELL'S					
Red & White Label					
Per 1 Cup Prepared					
(from ½ Cup Condensed)					
Bean & Bacon	180	25	0	25	8.8
Beef Broth	*15*	*1*	*0*	*1*	*3*
Broccoli Cheese	110	9	0	9	3
Californian Veg;					
Chicken Gumbo	60	10	2	8	2
Cheddar Cheese	130	11	0	11	3.5
Chicken Alphabet	80	11	0	11	4.5
Chicken Broth	*30*	*1*	*0*	*1*	*2*
Chicken Noodle w/ Stars	70	9	0	9	3
Chicken Vegetable	80	12	2	10	3
Chicken w/ White &					
Wild Rice	60	10	0	10	1.5
Clam Chowder, Manhattan	60	12	1	11	2
Clam Chowder,					
New England	100	15	1	14	4
Cream of Asparagus; Celery	110	9	0	9	3
Cream of Broccoli; Shrimp	100	9	0	9	2.5
Cream of Mushroom	110	9	0	9	3
Cream of Mushroom w/					
Roasted Garlic	70	10	0	10	2
Cream of Potato	90	14	0	14	2
Curly Noodle	80	12	1	11	3
Double Noodle in					
Chicken Broth	100	15	0	15	4.5
French Onion	45	6	1	5	2
Golden Mushroom	80	10	0	10	3.5

	Calories	Total Carb	Fiber	Usable Carb	Protein
Goldfish Pasta Chicken	70	8	1	7	3
Goldfish Pasta Tomato	110	25	2	23	3
Mega Noodle	70	10	0.9	9.1	2
Minestrone	100	16	3	13	4
Split Pea w/ Ham; Green Pea	180	28	0	28	9
Tomato	80	18	1	17	2
Tomato Bisque	130	24	0	24	2
Tomato Rice (Old Fashioned)	120	23	0	23	2.5
Vegetable	90	16	2	14	3
Vegetable & Beef;					
Turkey Noodle	80	10	1	9	4
Simply Home:					
Per Cup					
Chicken & Pasta;					
Chicken Noodle	90	14	0	14	6
Chicken w/ Rice	100	19	1	18	5
Country Vegetable	110	23	3	20	3
Minestrone	140	27	3	24	5
Soup At Hand:					
Per 10 ¾ oz. Ctn					
Blended Vege Medley	110	21	0	21	2
Classic Tomato	120	26	0	26	4
Cream of Broccoli	160	17	0	17	3
Creamy Chicken	170	17	0	17	5.5
Soup & Recipe Mixes (Dry):					
Per 1 Tbsp					
Chicken Noodle w/ Broth	30	5	0	5	1.5
Onion	20	5	0	5	0
Chunky (Red Can):					
19 oz. Can: Per ½ Can Serving					
Baked Potato w/					
Cheddar & Bacon	180	23	2	21	5
Beef w/ White & Wild Rice	140	23	2	21	8
Cheese Tortellini	110	18	0	18	4
Chicken Broccoli Cheese	200	14	0	14	5
Chicken Corn Chowder	250	18	0	18	10.8
Classic Chicken Noodle	130	16	0	16	9.8
Grilled Chicken Veg & Pasta	110	17	0	17	6
Grilled Sirloin Steak & Vegies	120	19	4	15	8
Hearty Bean & Ham	180	30	0	30	8.5
Hearty Chicken & Vegetables	90	12	0	12	6

	Calories	Total Carb	Fiber	Usable Carb	Protein
Herb Rst Chicken w/					
Potatoes & Garlic	110	17	0	17	6
Honey Rst Ham w/ Potatoes	130	20	0	20	8
New England Clam Chowder	300	26	0	26	11
Potato & Ham Chowder	220	16	0	16	7.5
Savory Chicken & Rice	140	18	0	18	10.2
Sirloin Burger	180	20	0	20	9.3
Slow Rst Beef w/ Mushrooms	110	14	0	14	9
Vegetable	160	15	0	15	16
Select: Per Cup					
Beef w/ Roasted Barley	130	21	0	21	8
Beef w/ Portabello					
Mushrooms	120	14	0	14	9.5
Chicken & Pasta w/ Garlic	110	17	0	17	6
Chicken Rice w/ Vegetables	100	18	0	18	4
Chicken w/ Long Grain Rice	110	19	0	19	7.5
Creamy Potato w/ Garlic	180	21	0	21	7.5
Fiesta Vegetable	120	24	0	24	5
Grilled Chicken w/					
Tomato & Veg	100	17	0	17	4.6
Honey Roasted Chicken w/					
Golden Potato	110	17	1	16	7
Herbed Chicken w/ Rst Veg	90	14	0	14	7.5
Italian Style Wedding	120	16	0	16	11
Minestrone	120	21	0	21	3.3
New England Clam Chowder	190	14	0	14	27
Fat Free	110	17	0	17	10.5
Roast Chicken w/					
Rotini & Penne	110	17	1	16	6
Rosemary Chicken w/					
Roasted Vegetable	110	18	0	18	0
Tomato Garden	100	22	0	22	1.8
Vegetable	110	20	0	20	5.2
CUP-A-RAMEN					
Beef; Cajun Chicken, 1 cup	310	36	0	36	5.5
Chicken; Shrimp, 1 cup	320	36	0	36	5.8
DR. MCDOUGALL'S					
Per Container Cup (Mix)					
Minestrone & Pasta	180	31	5	26	9
Split Pea w/ Barley	200	36	9	27	12
Tortilla Soup w/ Baked Chips	190	37	5	32	7

	Calories	Total Carb	Fiber	Usable Carb	Protein
FANTASTIC CUP SOUPS					
Per Container Cup (Mix)					
Split Pea	220	38	9	29	15
Cha-Cha Chili	250	44	13	31	17
Corn & Potato Chowder	170	34	3	31	6
Creamy Soups: Average	150	27	2	25	7
Big Soup Noodle Bowls:					
Per Cup, ½ Pkg					
Hot & Sour	140	25	1	24	4
Miso w/ Tofu	110	21	0	21	5
Sesame Miso	100	19	0	19	4
HEALTH VALLEY					
Per Cup					
Bean Vegetable	140	32	13	19	10
Beef Broth	*20*	*0*	*0*	*0*	*5*
Carotene varieties, Average	70	17	6	11	7
Chicken Broth	*45*	*0*	*0*	*0*	*7*
Chicken Noodle/Rice	130	20	2	18	9
Country Corn & Veg;					
Super Broccoli	70	17	7	10	5
Garden/Tomato Vegetable	80	17	4	13	6
Italian Minestrone	90	21	11	10	8
Lentil & Carrots	90	25	14	11	10
Real Minestrone; Italian Plus	80	20	6	14	7
Rotini & Vegetables	100	20	4	16	4
Split Pea & Carrots	110	17	8	9	10
Pasta Soups:					
Pasta Fagioli	120	25	4	21	6
Other varieties	110	23	3	20	3
Organic: Black Bean;					
Split Pea	110	25	12	13	11
Mushroom Barley;					
Potato Leek	60	15	8	7	5
Lentil; Tomato; Minestrone	90	20	9	11	9
Vegetable	80	18	6	12	5
Dry Soups: ⅓ cup, average	120	24	3	21	3
HEALTHY CHOICE					
Per Cup					
Bean & Pasta	100	18	3	15	6
Chicken & Dumplings	140	19	4	15	11

	Calories	Total Carb	Fiber	Usable Carb	Protein
Rst Chicken & Garlic	130	21	2	19	8
Chicken w/ Pasta	120	18	2	16	6
Chicken w/ Rice	100	12	2	10	7
Classic Italian Bean & Pasta	100	17	3	14	6
Creamy Tomato	100	21	2	19	3
Garden Vegetable	120	27	4	23	6
New England Clam Chowder	120	22	3	19	4
Roasted Italian Style Chicken	130	22	4	18	9
Split Pea & Ham	170	28	4	24	11
Zesty Gumbo	100	15	3	12	6

HORMEL

Microwave Cup Hearty Soups:
1 Cup, 7½ oz.

	Calories	Total Carb	Fiber	Usable Carb	Protein
Chicken Noodle	110	13	0	13	14

IMAGINE

Per Cup
Organic Creamy:

	Calories	Total Carb	Fiber	Usable Carb	Protein
Broccoli	70	10	2	8	3
Butternut Squash	120	23	2	21	2
Portabello Mushroom	80	10	2	8	4
Potato Leek	90	14	2	12	3
Sweet Corn	100	15	1	14	5
Tomato	90	17	2	15	2
Vegetable Broth	*30*	*5*	*1*	*4*	*1*
Free Range Chicken Broth	*20*	*2*	*0.5*	*1.5*	*1*

JUANITA'S

Per Cup

Menudo Blanco/	Calories	Total Carb	Fiber	Usable Carb	Protein
Mas picoso	170	12	3	9	15
Menudo Sin Maiz	*170*	*1*	*1*	*0*	*20*
Pozole	170	22	5	17	8

LIPTON

Cup-a-Soup:
Per Envelope

	Calories	Total Carb	Fiber	Usable Carb	Protein
Broccoli & Cheese	70	9	1	8	2
Cream of Chicken	70	12	0.5	11.5	1
Creamy Chicken Vegetable	80	10	0	10	0
Chicken Noodle	65	10.5	0.4	10.1	2.7

	Calories	Total Carb	Fiber	Usable Carb	Protein
Recipe Secrets Mixes:					
Per Serving					
Beefy Onion	25	5	0	5	0
Chicken Noodle	80	11	0	11	4.5
Onion	*20*	*4*	*0*	*4*	*1*
Onion Mushroom	*30*	*5*	*0.3*	*4.7*	*0.8*
Savory Herb w/ Garlic;					
Vegetable	30	6	0.3	5.7	0.9
PACIFIC FOODS					
Heat & Serve:					
Per Cup (8 fl. oz.)					
All Natural Chicken Broth	*4*	*0*	*0*	*0*	*1*
French Onion	28	6	0	6	1
Organic Vegetable Broth	*0*	*0*	*0*	*0*	*0*
Creamy: Tomato	100	17	1	16	5
PROGRESSO					
Per 1 Cup Serving					
Beef Barley	130	13	3	10	10
Chickarina	130	12	0	12	8
Chicken w/ Wild Rice	100	15	2	13	7
Chicken Barley	110	16	3	13	8
Chicken Broth	*20*	*1*	*0*	*1*	*1*
Chicken Noodle	90	9	0	9	9
Chicken Rice w/ Vegetable	90	13	1	12	6
Escarole in Chicken Broth	*25*	*3*	*1*	*2*	*1*
French Onion	50	9	1	8	0.9
Green Split Pea	170	25	5	20	10
Hearty Black Bean	170	30	10	20	8
Hearty Chicken & Rotini	90	12	0	12	8
Hearty Penne in					
Chicken Broth	80	14	0	14	4
Home Style Chicken					
w/ Vegetables	90	11	0	11	7
Lentil	140	22	7	15	9
Macaroni & Bean	160	23	6	17	7
Manhattan Clam Chowder	110	11	3	8	12
Minestrone	120	21	5	16	5
New England Clam Chowder	190	21	7	14	5
Rsted Chicken Garden Herb	70	9	0	9	6
Roasted Chicken Italiano	80	10	0	10	6

	Calories	Total Carb	Fiber	Usable Carb	Protein
Southwestern Style					
Corn Chowder	200	29	3	26	4
Split Pea w/ Ham	150	20	5	15	9
Steak & Baked Potato	130	18	1	17	8
Steak & Mushrooms					
w/ Vegetables	100	12	1	11	8
Tomato; Tomato Basil	100	19	1	18	2
Tomato Vegetable Italiano	90	15	4	11	3
Tortellini in Chicken Broth	70	10	2	8	3
Turkey Noodle	90	11	0	11	7
Turkey & Rice w/ Veg	110	18	1	17	7
Vegetable	90	17	2	15	3
99% Fat Free:					
Per 1 Cup Serving					
Beef Barley	130	20	4	16	9
Chicken Noodle	90	13	1	12	7
Lentil; Minestrone	130	20	6	14	8
New England					
Clam Chowder	110	18	2	16	5
White Cheddar Potato	100	20	2	18	2
PUCK					
Canned: Per Cup					
Chicken & Egg Noodles	150	16	0.9	15.1	8
Chicken & Vegetables	140	17	2	15	8
Chicken w/ Sweet Corn	200	20	1	19	9
Creamy Chicken	210	15	0	15	10
Hearty Vegetable Beef	140	13	2	11	8
New England					
Clam Chowder	240	18	1	17	11
Old World Minestrone	180	24	3	21	6
Roast Chicken w/ Wild Rice	150	18	0.9	17.1	8
Spicy 7 Bean w/					
Italian Sausage	230	22	5	17	11
Thick Country Vegetable	170	23	3	20	4
SWANSON					
Per Cup					
Canned:					
Beef Broth	*20*	*1*	*0*	*1*	*2*
Chicken Broth	*30*	*1*	*0*	*1*	*2*
100% Fat Free	*15*	*1*	*0*	*1*	*3*
Vegetable Broth	*20*	*3*	*0*	*3*	*0*

	Calories	Total Carb	Fiber	Usable Carb	Protein
WALNUT ACRES					
Per Cup, 250g					
Autumn Harvest	100	19	2	17	3
Classic Minestrone	100	22	3	19	3
Country Corn Chowder	150	28	2	26	4
Cuban Black Bean	150	30	8	22	7
Four Bean Chili	140	28	4	24	6
Ginger Carrot	100	22	3	19	2
Mediterranean Lentil	130	26	8	18	7
Savory Tomato	120	23	2	21	4
WESTBRAE					
Canned: Per Cup					
240g, Unless Indicated					
Alabama Black Bean Gumbo	140	26	6	20	8
California Unchicken Broth	*20*	*2.7*	*0*	*2.7*	*1.3*
Great Plains Savory Bean	120	23	7	16	8
Hearty Milano Minestrone	120	24	6	18	7
Instant Miso Soup,					
1 packet	*35*	*3*	*0*	*3*	*2*
Louisiana Bean Stew	130	25	7	18	8
Mediterranean Lentil	140	24	10	14	10
Monte Carlo Creamy					
Mushroom	93	13.3	0	13.3	1.3
New York Unchicken Noodle	60	10	0.5	9.5	2
Old World Split Pea	150	28	6	22	10
Santa Fe Vegetable	160	31	8	23	9
Spicy Southwest Vegetable	130	25	6	19	7
Tuscany Tomato,					
¾ cup, 180g	70	16	0	16	2.7

HERBS & SPICES, CONDIMENTS

HERBS & SPICES					
Per Teaspoon:					
Allspice, ground	*5*	*1*	*0.4*	*0.6*	*0.1*
Chili Powder	*8*	*1*	*0.9*	*0.1*	*0.3*
Cinnamon, ground	*6*	*2*	*1.2*	*0.8*	*0.1*
Curry Powder	*6*	*1*	*0.7*	*0.3*	*0.3*
Garlic Powder	*9*	*2*	*0.3*	*1.7*	*0.5*
Nutmeg, ground	*12*	*1*	*0.5*	*0.5*	*0.1*
Onion Powder	*7*	*2*	*0.1*	*1.9*	*0.2*

	Calories	Total Carb	Fiber	Usable Carb	Protein
Parsley, dried	1	0.2	0.1	0.1	0.1
Pepper, black/red/					
white, average	6	1	0.6	0.4	0.2
Saffron	2	0	0	0	0.1
Tumeric, ground	8	1	0.5	0.5	0.2
Seeds:					
Fenugreek	12	2	0.9	1.1	0.9
Mustard, Poppyseed	15	1	0.5	0.5	0.8
Other types, average	7	1	0.4	0.6	0.3
SEASONINGS & FLAVORINGS					
Angostura Bitters, 1 tsp	12	3	0	3	0
Bacon Bits, average, 1 Tbsp	30	0	0	0	5.3
Bacon Chips (Durkee),					
1 Tbsp	45	2	0	2	7
Butter Buds	8	2	0	2	0
Molly McButter, 1 tsp	10	0	0	0	0
Salt: Regular, Sea Salt,					
Lite Salt	0	0	0	0	0
Taco Seasoning,					
Average, ¼ pkg	30	4	0.8	3.2	0
Old El Paso:					
Cheesy Taco Seasoning					
Mix, 1 Tbsp	15	3	0	3	0
Taco/Burrito Seasoning					
Mix, 2 tsp	15	4	0	4	0
Enchilada Seasoning					
Mix, 2 tsp	10	2	0	2	0
Fajita Seasoning					
Mix, 1 tsp	10	3	0	3	0
CONDIMENTS, SAUCES					
Average of Brands					
& Homemade					
Barbecue: avg, 1 Tbsp	11	1.9	0.2	1.7	0.3
Cheese, homemade,					
¼ cup, 2½ oz.	110	4.3	0.3	4	4.2
Chili Sauce:					
Heinz, 1 Tbsp	15	4	0.2	3.8	0.3
Del Monte, 1 Tbsp	20	5	0	5	0
Cocktail Sauce: ¼ cup	100	24	0	24	1
Cranberry Sauce, all types,					
¼ cup, 2½ oz.	110	27	0.5	26.5	1.5

	Calories	Total Carb	Fiber	Usable Carb	Protein
Honey Mustard (French's):					
1 tsp	*5*	*1*	*0*	*1*	*0*
Horseradish, 1 tsp	*2*	*0*	*0*	*0*	*0*
Ketchup: Regular, 1 Tbsp	*16*	*4*	*0*	*4*	*0*
Heinz Kick'rs, 1 Tbsp	*16*	*4*	*0*	*4*	*0*
Mustard, average, 1 tsp	*5*	*0.5*	*0.2*	*0.3*	*0.2*
Pesto, ¼ cup, 2 oz.	*35*	*4*	*1*	*3*	*1*
Pizza Sauce, canned,					
¼ cup, 2 oz.	*20*	*4*	*1*	*3*	*0*
Seafood Cocktail Sauce,					
¼ cup	100	24	0	24	1
Soy Sauce, all types,					
average, 1 Tbsp	*10*	*0*	*0*	*0*	*0*
Sour Cream Sauce, ½ cup	180	17	0	17	5.5
Spaghetti Sauce,					
½ cup, 4½ oz.	*61*	*11*	*9*	*2*	*1.5*
Steak Sauce: Heinz/A1,					
1 Tbsp	*15*	*3*	*0.2*	*2.8*	*0.3*
Tabasco Sauce, 1 Tbsp	*2*	*0*	*0*	*0*	*0*
Taco Sauce, average,					
2 Tbsp	*10*	*1*	*0*	*1*	*0*
Tartar Sauce: Heinz,					
2 Tbsp, 30g	*140*	*4*	*1*	*3*	*0.1*
Vinegar: White or Wine,					
1 fl. oz.	*4*	*1*	*0*	*1*	*0*
White Sauce, ½ cup, 5 oz.	130	12	0.3	12	4.8
Worcestershire Sauce,					
1 tsp	*5*	*1*	*0*	*1*	*0.1*

PICKLES & GRAVY

PICKLES & RELISH

Average All Brands					
Bread & Butter Pickles,					
4 slices, 1 oz.	24	6	0	6	0
Chutney, 2 Tbsp, 1¼ oz.	40	12	0	12	0
Dill Pickle:					
Slices, 4 slices, 1 oz.	*5*	*1.2*	*0*	*1.2*	*0.1*
1 large, 2¼ oz.	24	5.6	0	5.6	0.7
Extra large, 5 oz.	30	6	0	6	0.7
Halves: small, 1 oz.	*5*	*1.2*	*0*	*1.2*	*0.1*
Large, 2½ oz.	*13*	*2.9*	*0*	*2.9*	*0.4*

	Calories	Total Carb	Fiber	Usable Carb	Protein
Sweet, small, ½ oz.	17	4.5	0	4.5	0.1
Gherkins, sweet, 1 med, 1 oz.	41	10	0	10	0
Green Chilies, chopped,					
2 Tbsp	10	3	0	3	0
Horseradish, 1 Tbsp	7	2	0.5	1.5	0.2
Jalapenos, pickled,					
2 whole	10	1	0	1	0
Jalapeno Relish,					
1 Tbsp, ½ oz.	5	1	0	1	0
Mustard,					
average all brands, 1 tsp	5	0.5	0.2	0.3	0.2
Peppers: Hot/Mild, 1 oz.	6	1.4	0	1.4	0.3
Pickled: Beets, ½ cup, 4 oz.	75	19	3	16	0.9
Pickles:					
Sweet, 2 Tbsp, 1 oz.	35	9	0	9	0.1
Large, 1¼ oz.	24	5.6	0	5.6	0.7
Relishes:					
Sandwich Spread, 1 Tsp	29	5	0	5	0
Cranberry-Orange, 1 Tbsp	51	13	0	13	0.1
Hot Dog (Heinz), 1 Tbsp	17	28	0	28	0
Sweet Pickle, 1 Tbsp	20	5	0	5	0
Sauerkraut, ½ cup, 3½ oz.	25	5	0	5	1
Sweet Cauliflower	35	8	0	8	0.8
SALSA					
Average All Types					
Regular, no oil, 1 Tbsp	15	3.5	0	3.5	0
w/ Oil, homemade, 1 Tbsp	59	8	0	8	0
Del Monte, all flavors,					
2 Tbsp	10	2	0	2	0
Wild Oats, 2 Tbsp, 1 oz.	8	2	0	2	0
GRAVY					
Homemade Gravy:					
Thin, little fat, 2 Tbsp,					
1 oz.	20	3	0	3	0
Thick, 2 Tbsp, 1¼ oz.	50	9	0	9	0
Franco-American (Canned):					
Beef/Mushroom; Turkey					
Gravy, 2 oz.	25	3	0	3	0
Chicken Gravy, ¼ cup, 2 oz.	40	3	0.5	2.5	0
98% Fat Free, ¼ cup, 2 oz.	25	3	0	3	1

	Calories	Total Carb	Fiber	Usable Carb	Protein
GRAVY-IN-JARS—HOMESTYLE					
Boston Market, all types,					
¼ cup, 2 oz.	30	4	0	4	0
Heinz, regular, all types,					
¼ cup, 2 oz.	25	3	0	3	1
Fat Free Rst Turkey,					
¼ cup, 2 oz.	10	2	0	2	1
Vons, all types, ¼ cup, 2 oz.	20	3	0	3	1

SAUCES—PASTA, COOKING

	Calories	Total Carb	Fiber	Usable Carb	Protein
AMY'S					
Per ½ Cup					
Family Marinara	50	8	3	5	1
Garlic Mushroom	120	10	3	7	3
Puttanesca	*40*	*5*	*1*	*4*	*1*
Tomato Basil	80	11	3	8	2
BARILLA					
Per ½ Cup					
Marinara; Sweet Peppers					
& Garlic	70	11	2	9	2
Roasted Garlic & Onion	80	13	1	12	2
Tomato & Basil	70	12	3	9	2
BULLSEYE					
BBQ, 1 Tbsp	88	6.5	0	6.5	0
CONTADINA					
Pasta Sauces					
Marinara Sauce, ½ cup	80	9	1.5	7.5	1.5
Pizza Squeeze Sauce,					
¼ cup	*35*	*6*	*1.3*	*4.7*	*1.4*
DEL MONTE					
Pasta Sauces: Per ½ Cup					
Chunky Sauce, average					
all varieties	60	11	0	11	2
Spaghetti Sauce:					
Traditional	60	15	3	12	2
Garlic & Onion	80	16	2	14	2
w/ Mushroom & Meat	60	14	3	11	3
Sloppy Joe Sauce, ¼ cup	70	16	0	16	1

	Calories	Total Carb	Fiber	Usable Carb	Protein
FRENCH'S GRILL & GLAZE					
Honey Mustard, 2 Tbsp	90	18	1	17	1
Teriyaki, 2 Tbsp	60	13	0	13	0.9
GREEN GIANT					
Sloppy Joe S'wich Sauce,					
¼ cup, 2.5 oz.	50	11	2	9	2
Sloppy Joe Sauce & Meat	200	11	2	9	14
HEALTHY CHOICE					
Per ½ Cup					
Four Cheese Creamy Alfredo	94	6	0	6	4
Garlic Lovers	96	26	6	20	4
Traditional Pasta Sauce	50	13	3	10	3
Super Chunky:					
Vege Primavera	60	13	3	10	2
Tomato, Mushroom Garlic	48	10	3	7	2
HEINZ					
Per 1 Tbsp, Approx ½ oz.					
Barbecue Sauces, All flavors	35	9	0	9	0.3
Chili Sauce, 1 Tbsp	*15*	*4*	*0.2*	*3.8*	*0.3*
Horseradish Sauce	*70*	*2*	*1.2*	*0.8*	*0.2*
Mustard:					
Pourable/Mild	*8*	*0.5*	*0*	*0.5*	*0*
Spicy Brown	*13*	*1*	*0.5*	*0.5*	*0.7*
Seafood Cocktail Sauce	*20*	*3*	*0.1*	*2.9*	*0.2*
Steak Sauce 57	*15*	*4*	*0.2*	*3.8*	*0.3*
Tartar Sauce	*70*	*2*	*1*	*1*	*0.1*
Tomato Ketchup	*16*	*4*	*0.2*	*3.8*	*0.2*
Worcestershire Sauce	*8*	*1*	*0*	*1*	*0.1*
KC MASTERPIECE					
Per 1 Tbsp					
Marinades:					
Garlic & Herb	*30*	*4*	*0*	*4*	*0*
Honey Teriyaki	35	7	0	7	1
Original BBQ	40	7	0	7	0
KRAFT BARBECUE SAUCES					
Average, 2 Tbsp	39	9	0.3	8.7	0.2
LAWRY'S 30 MINUTE MARINADE					
Per 1 Tbsp					
Caribbean Jerk; Teriyaki	25	6	0	6	0

	Calories	Total Carb	Fiber	Usable Carb	Protein
Hawaiian; Dijon & Honey	20	3.5	0	3.5	0
Mediterranean;					
Lemon Pepper	10	2	0	2	0
Mesquite	5	1	0	1	0
Thai Ginger; Herb &					
Garlic	10	2	0	2	0
MR. YOSHIDA'S					
Original Gourmet, 2 Tbsp	90	20	0	20	2
Hawaiian Sweet & Sour,					
2 Tbsp	70	18	0	18	0
MUIR GLEN					
Per ½ Cup					
Organic Pasta Sauce:					
Mushroom Marinara;					
Portabello Mushroom	50	11	0	11	2
Other varieties, Average	50	11	0	11	2
NEWMAN'S OWN					
Per ½ Cup					
Bombolina (Tomato & Basil)	100	15	7	5	2
OLD EL PASO					
Salsa:					
Thick 'n Chunky,					
2 Tbsp, 1 oz.	8	2	0	2	0
Homestyle; Green					
Chili; Verde, 2 Tbsp	10	2	0	2	0
Enchilada Sauce,					
all types, ¼ cup, 2 oz.	20	3	0	3	0
Tomato & Green Chiles/					
Jalapenos, ¼ cup, 2 oz.	10	2	0	2	0
PACE					
Per 2 Tbsp, 1oz.					
Picante Sauce	10	2	0	2	0
Chunky Salsa, average,					
all types	10	2	0	2	0
Salsa Con Queso	45	4	0	4	0.5
PREGO					
Pasta Bake: Per ⅛ Jar					
3-Cheese Marinara	100	11	2	9	3
Hearty Meat Sauce	102	12	2	10	4

	Calories	Total Carb	Fiber	Usable Carb	Protein
Tomato, Garlic & Basil	80	11	2	9	1
Mushroom w/ Garlic & Onion	90	13	2	11	2
Regular: Per ½ Cup					
Hamburger	120	17	3	14	3
Italian Sausage & Garlic	120	16	3	13	3
Mini Meatball	160	20	3	17	4
Mushroom & Garlic	110	20	3	17	2
Pepperoni	120	18	3	15	3
Roast Red Pepper/ Herb & Garlic	110	18	3	15	2
Roast Garlic Parmesan	120	23	3	20	3
Savory Chicken	130	17	3	14	4

RAGU

	Calories	Total Carb	Fiber	Usable Carb	Protein
Cheese Creations Per ½ Cup:					
Roasted Garlic Parmesan	240	6	0	6	4

WALNUT ACRES

	Calories	Total Carb	Fiber	Usable Carb	Protein
Per ½ Cup					
Organic Pasta Sauce, avg	55	10	1	9	2

WILD OATS

	Calories	Total Carb	Fiber	Usable Carb	Protein
Per 2 Tbsp, 1 oz.					
Wasabi; Seafood Marinade & Grill	*30*	*4*	*0*	*4*	*0*
Korean Sesame Marinade & Grill	30	8	0	8	0

MAYONNAISE

AVERAGE ALL BRANDS

	Calories	Total Carb	Fiber	Usable Carb	Protein
Regular, 1 Tbsp	*100*	*0*	*0*	*0*	*0*
Light/Reduced Fat					
Kraft; Best Foods, 1 Tbsp	*50*	*1*	*0*	*1*	*0.1*
Hellman's; Estee, 1 Tbsp	*25*	*2*	*0*	*2*	*0*
Smart Balance, 1 Tbsp	*50*	*2*	*0*	*2*	*0*
Wild Oats, 1 Tbsp	*35*	*1*	*0*	*1*	*0*
Fat Free					
Kraft; Weight Watchers, 1 Tbsp	*10*	*2.1*	*0.3*	*1.8*	*0*
Mayonnaise Type Dressing					
Gour Mayo (French's), 1 Tbsp, 0.5 oz.	*50*	*1*	*0*	*1*	*0*

	Calories	Total Carb	Fiber	Usable Carb	Protein
Miracle Whip Salad Dressing:					
Light, 1 Tbsp, 0.5 oz.	40	3	0	3	0
Free, 1 Tbsp, 0.5 oz.	15	3	0.3	2.7	0
Nayonaise (Nasoya)					
(Tofu Base/Dairy Free/Eggless)					
Regular, 1 Tbsp	35	1	0	1	0.5
Fat-Free, 1 Tbsp	10	2	0	2	0.5

SALAD DRESSINGS

AVERAGE ALL BRANDS

Per 2 Tbsp, approx 1 fl. oz.					
Blue Cheese: Regular	150	2	0	2	0
Light/Reduced Fat	80	1	0	1	1
Caesar: Regular	140	2	0	2	1.5
Light/Reduced Fat	50	0.5	0	0.5	0.8
French: Regular	130	5	0	5	2.8
Light/Reduced Fat	50	4	0	4	1.8
Fat/Oil-Free	40	4	0	4	6
Italian: Regular	130	3	0	3	4.8
Light/Reduced Fat	70	2	0	2	0
Fat/Oil-Free	10	2	0	2	0.5
Ranch: Regular	180	3	0	3	1.5
Light/Reduced Fat	90	3	0	3	0
Fat-Free	50	2	0	2	10.5
Russian: Regular	130	3	0	3	3.3
Light/Reduced Fat	50	2	0	2	0
Fat-Free	30	2	0	2	5.5
Thousand Island: Regular	130	5	0	5	0.5
Light/Reduced Fat	63	3	0	3	0
Fat-Free	35	3	0	3	2

ANNIE'S NATURALS

Per 2 Tbsp, approx 1 fl. oz.					
Caesar	120	1	0	1	1
Cowgirl Ranch	120	3	0	3	1
French	90	3	0	3	0
Goddess	90	3	0	3	0.5
Organic:					
Buttermilk	70	1	0	1	0.5
Green Garlic	90	2	0	2	0.5
No Fat Yogurt	20	3	0	3	1

	Calories	Total Carb	Fiber	Usable Carb	Protein
Thousand Island	90	5	0	5	0.5
Tuscany Italian	80	5	0	5	0
Vinaigrette:					
Balsamic	*100*	*3*	*0*	*3*	*0*
Basil & Garlic	*130*	*0.5*	*0*	*0.5*	*0*
Black Olives & Truffle	*110*	*1*	*0*	*1*	*0*
Cilantro & Lime	*100*	*2*	*0*	*2*	*0*
Low Fat:					
Honey Mustard	45	6	0	6	0
Gingerly	*40*	*4*	*0*	*4*	*1*
Raspberry	35	5	0	5	0
Roasted Red Pepper	*70*	*3*	*0*	*3*	*0*
Sea Veggie & Sesame	*110*	*1*	*0*	*1*	*1*
Shitake & Sesame	*120*	*1*	*0*	*1*	*0*
Yellow Pepper & Tomato	*70*	*2*	*0*	*2*	*0*
BERNSTEIN'S					
Per 2 Tbsp, approx 1 fl. oz.					
Balsamic Italian	*110*	*2*	*0*	*2*	*1*
Cheese: Garlic Italian;					
Fantastico	*110*	*2*	*0*	*2*	*1*
Creamy Caesar	*120*	*1*	*0*	*1*	*3.5*
Fat Free Cheese &					
Garlic Italian	*10*	*2*	*0*	*2*	*0.5*
Italian	*110*	*1*	*0*	*1*	*0*
Olive Oil Vinaigrette	*90*	*3*	*0*	*3*	*0*
Red Wine & Garlic Italian	*110*	*2*	*0*	*2*	*1*
Restaurant Recipe Italian	*130*	*1*	*0*	*1*	*2.5*
Light Fantastic:					
Cheese Fantastico	*25*	*3*	*0*	*3*	*0*
Roasted Garlic Balsamic	*45*	*3*	*0*	*3*	*0.5*
CARDINI'S					
Per 2 Tbsp, approx 1 fl. oz.					
Caesar	*160*	*1*	*0*	*1*	*1*
Fat-Free Caesar	40	9	0	9	1
Light Caesar	80	5	0	5	0
Extra Virgin Olive					
Oil Italian	*120*	*1*	*0*	*1*	*0*
Honey Mustard	140	5	0	5	1
Kalamata Olive w/					
Romano Cheese	*120*	*2*	*0*	*2*	*0*
Lemon Herb	*120*	*1*	*0*	*1*	*0*

	Calories	Total Carb	Fiber	Usable Carb	Protein
Parmesan Ranch	*150*	*2*	*0*	*2*	*1*
Poppyseed w/ Shallots	160	8	0	8	0
Vintage White Wine	*110*	*1*	*0*	*1*	*0*
Zesty Garlic	*120*	*2*	*0*	*2*	*0*
GIRARDS					
Per 2 Tbsp, approx 1 fl. oz.					
Balsamic Basil	*90*	*3*	*0*	*3*	*0*
Shitake Chardonnay	*100*	*4*	*0*	*4*	*0*
HIDDEN VALLEY					
Per 2 Tbsp, approx 1 fl. oz.					
Regular Range:					
Caesar w/ Garlic	*120*	*4*	*0*	*4*	*1.5*
Cole Slaw	150	5	0	5	0
French w/ Honey & Bacon	150	10	0	10	0.5
Original Ranch:					
w/ Garlic	*130*	*2*	*0*	*2*	*1.5*
w/ Sundried Tomato	*140*	*2*	*0*	*2*	*1.5*
Light Range:					
Original Ranch w/					
Sour Cream	145	6	0	6	14
Fat Free:					
French Honey & Bacon	50	11	0	11	0
Original Ranch	30	6	0	6	1.5
KNOTT'S BERRY FARM					
Per 2 Tbsp, approx 1 fl. oz.					
Honey Dijon	*130*	*4*	*0*	*4*	*0.5*
Honey Poppyseed	120	10	0	10	0
Oriental Chicken Salad	130	5	0	5	0.5
Parmesan & Peppercorn	*160*	*1*	*0*	*1*	*1*
Roasted Garlic Caesar	140	10	0	10	0
Sun Dried Tomato	*100*	*3*	*0*	*3*	*0.5*
Low Fat:					
Raspberry	50	8	0	8	0
Tropical Fruit	45	9	0	9	0
KRAFT					
Per 2 Tbsp, approx 1 fl. oz.					
Regular Dressings:					
3 Cheese Ranch	*170*	*1*	*0*	*1*	*0.5*
Buttermilk Ranch	*150*	*2*	*0*	*2*	*0*
Caesar w/ Bacon	*150*	*1*	*0*	*1*	*3*

	Calories	Total Carb	Fiber	Usable Carb	Protein
Catalina	90	8	0	8	0
Classic Caesar	*110*	*0.5*	*0*	*0.5*	*0*
Coleslaw	150	8	0	8	0
Cucumber Ranch	*140*	*2*	*0*	*2*	*0*
Creamy Italian	*110*	*3*	*0*	*3*	*0*
French	*120*	*4*	*0*	*4*	*0*
Ranch w/ Bacon	*150*	*1*	*0*	*1*	*0.5*
Roka Brand Blue Cheese	90	5	0	5	2
Thousand Island	110	5	0	5	0
Thousand Island w/ Bacon	120	5	0	5	0
Zesty Italian	*110*	*2*	*0*	*2*	*1*
Kraft Free (Fat Free):					
Italian	*10*	*2*	*0.1*	*1.9*	*0.2*
Blue Cheese, Catalina,					
French	50	12	1	11	0
Classic Caesar; Ranch	50	11	0	11	1.5
Thousand Island; Sour					
Cream & Onion	45	11	1	10	0
Light Done Right!:					
Classic Caesar	*70*	*3*	*0*	*3*	*1*
Catalina	60	11	0	11	0
Ranch	*77*	*3.1*	*0.2*	*2.9*	*0.3*
Roka Blue Cheese	*70*	*3*	*0*	*3*	*1*
Thousand Island	70	8.5	0	8.5	0
3 Cheese Ranch	*80*	*2*	*0*	*2*	*0.5*
Special Collection:					
Balsamic Vinaigrette	*90*	*4*	*0*	*4*	*0.5*
Classic Italian					
Vinaigrette	*50*	*4*	*0*	*4*	*0*
Sun Dried Tomato	*60*	*4*	*0*	*4*	*0*
Sweet Honey Catalina	130	8	0	8	0
Seven Seas:					
Viva Italian	*110*	*2*	*0*	*2*	*0*
Red Wine Vinaigrette	*90*	*2*	*0*	*2*	*0.5*
NEWMAN'S OWN					
Per 2 Tbsp, approx 1 fl. oz.					
Balsamic Vinaigrette	*90*	*3*	*0*	*3*	*0*
Caesar; Olive Oil &					
Vinegar	*150*	*1*	*0*	*1*	*0*
Creamy Caesar	*170*	*1*	*0*	*1*	*0*
Family Recipe Italian	*120*	*1*	*0*	*1*	*1*

	Calories	Total Carb	Fiber	Usable Carb	Protein
Parmesan & Rstd Garlic	110	2	0	2	1
Ranch	180	2	0	2	1

SEEDS OF CHANGE

Per 2 Tbsp, approx 1 fl. oz.

	Calories	Total Carb	Fiber	Usable Carb	Protein
Balsamic/Greek Feta					
Vinaigrette	60	4	0.5	3.5	0
Italian Herb Vinaigrette	50	4	2	2	0

SPECTRUM

Per 2 Tbsp, approx 1 fl. oz.

Fat Free:

	Calories	Total Carb	Fiber	Usable Carb	Protein
Creamy Dill	25	4	0	4	2.5
Creamy Garlic	20	4	0	4	1
Sweet Onion & Garlic;					
Toasted Sesame	15	3	0	3	1
Lowfat:					
Blue Cheese Style	35	3	0	3	1.5
Creamy Roasted Pepper	45	5	0	5	2
Honey Dijon	35	4	0	4	0.5
Mango Madness	50	7	0	7	1
Southwestern Caesar	40	3	0	3	2.5

T. MARZETTI'S

Per 2 Tbsp, approx 1 fl. oz.

Regular:

	Calories	Total Carb	Fiber	Usable Carb	Protein
Balsamic Vinaigrette	100	4	0	4	0
Caesar Lite	70	2	0	2	1
Italian	100	3	0	3	0
Ranch	160	2	0	2	1
Roasted Garlic Vinaigrette	130	8	0	8	0
Sesame Oriental	110	8	0	8	0
Sun Dried Tomato					
Vinaigrette	130	6	0	6	0
Wild Berry Vinaigrette	100	4	0	4	0

WALDEN FARMS

Fat Free, Calorie Free Range

	Calories	Total Carb	Fiber	Usable Carb	Protein
Average all types, 2 Tbsp	0	1	0	1	0

WILD OATS

Per 2 Tbsp, approx 1 fl. oz.

	Calories	Total Carb	Fiber	Usable Carb	Protein
Caesar Style	116	1	0	1	1
Creamy Peppercorn	100	1	0	1	1
Honey Toasted Sesame					

	Calories	Total Carb	Fiber	Usable Carb	Protein
Ginger	*100*	*3*	*0*	*3*	*0.5*
Italian Balsamic Vinaigrette	80	5	0	5	0
Ranch	*115*	*3*	*0*	*3*	*1*
Thousand Island	90	5	0	5	0.5

WISHBONE

Per 2 Tbsp, approx 1 fl. oz.
Regular:

	Calories	Total Carb	Fiber	Usable Carb	Protein
Chunky Blue Cheese	*170*	*2*	*0*	*2*	*2.5*
Classic Caesar	*110*	*2*	*0*	*2*	*3*
Creamy Caesar	*180*	*1*	*0*	*1*	*3.5*
French: Deluxe French	120	5	0	5	0.5
Sweet 'N Spicy	140	6	0	6	2
Italian: Regular	*80*	*3*	*0*	*3*	*0*
House Italian	*110*	*3*	*0*	*3*	*2*
Robusto Italian	*90*	*4*	*0*	*4*	*0.5*
Ranch:					
Original	*160*	*1*	*0*	*1*	*1*
w/ Garlic/Spring Onion	*150*	*2*	*0*	*2*	*2*
Russian: Regular	110	15	0	15	0
Thousand Island	130	7	0	7	0
Vinaigrette:					
Red Wine; Balsamic	*60*	*3*	*0*	*3*	*0*
Fat Free:					
Chunky Blue Cheese	35	7	0	7	2
Italian	*15*	*2*	*0*	*2*	*2*
Ranch	40	9	0	9	1
Dressing & Marinades:					
Asian	45	6	0	6	0
Balsamic Olive Oil & Herbs	*35*	*4*	*0*	*4*	*0*
Lemon Garlic & Herb	45	5	0	5	0
Tangy Honey Mustard	70	9	0	9	0
Just 2 Good!:					
Blue Cheese	45	6	0	6	1
Classic/Creamy Caesar; Ranch	40	5	0	5	1
Country Italian	*30*	*3*	*0*	*3*	*0*
Italian	35	5	0	5	0
Parmesan Peppercorn Ranch	45	6	0	6	1
Thousand Island	60	9	0	9	0

	Calories	Total Carb	Fiber	Usable Carb	Protein

BREAKFAST CEREALS

COOKED CEREALS

	Calories	Total Carb	Fiber	Usable Carb	Protein
Corn/Hominy Grits:					
Dry, ¼ cup, 1.4 oz.	145	33	0.6	32.4	3.5
Cooked, ¾ cup, 6½ oz.	110	25	0.4	24.6	2.7
Farina:					
Cooked, ¾ cup, 6 oz.	85	18	2.4	15.6	2.6
Oatmeal:					
Dry, ⅓ cup, 1 oz.	110	19	2.8	16.2	4.3
Regular, cooked,					
¾ cup, 6 oz.	110	19	3	16	4.4
Instant: Regular,					
Average, 1 oz.	100	18	3.1	14.9	4.3

COLD CEREALS

	Calories	Total Carb	Fiber	Usable Carb	Protein
Corn Flakes, 1 cup, 1 oz.	110	24	0.3	23.7	2.1
Granola, ¼ cup, 1 oz.	130	14.9	2.9	12	4.1
Puffed Rice, 1 cup, ½ oz.	55	12	0.2	11.8	0.9
Puffed Wheat, 1 cup, ½ oz.	55	12	0.7	11.3	2.2
Rice Crisps, 1 cup, 1 oz.	110	25	0.4	24.6	1.5

GRAINS & FLOURS

GRAINS & FLOURS

Per ½ Cup (8 level Tbsp)	Calories	Total Carb	Fiber	Usable Carb	Protein
Amaranth	350	60	14.8	45.2	14
Arrowroot	230	57	2.2	54.8	0.3
Barley: Regular	325	56	9.4	46.6	7.8
Pearled, raw	350	78	15.5	62.5	9.8
Buckwheat: Regular	290	61	8.5	52.5	11.2
Groats, roasted, dry	285	60	8.8	51.2	10
Roasted, cooked	90	19	2.7	16.3	3.4
Flour, whole-groat	200	42	6	36	7.6
Bulgur: Dry	240	54	2.8	51.2	8.6
Cooked	75	17	4.1	12.9	2.8
Corn Bran	*85*	*32*	*32*	*0*	*3.2*
Corn Flour/Masa	210	44	5.5	38.5	5.3
Cornmeal: Average					
All types, 1 oz.	100	22	2.1	19.9	2.3
Cornstarch: 1 Tbsp	30	7	0.1	6.9	0
Couscous: Dry, 3¼ oz.	345	72	4.6	67.4	11.7
Cooked, 4.1 oz.	60	12	1.6	10.4	4.4

	Calories	Total Carb	Fiber	Usable Carb	Protein
Farina: Dry, 3 oz.	325	70	1.7	68.3	8.9
Cooked, 4.1 oz.	60	13	1.6	11.4	1.7
Flax Seeds, 2 oz.	280	22	15.8	6.2	11.1
Garbanzo, ½ cup, 2 oz.	170	26.6	5	21.6	10.3
Kuzu Root Starch, 1 Tbsp	35	8	0	8	0
Millet: Raw, ½ cup, 3½ oz.	375	72.8	8.5	64.3	11
Cooked, ½ cup, 4¼ oz.	104	20.5	1.1	19.4	3
Oat Bran:					
Raw, ½ cup, 1.7 oz.	115	31	7.2	23.8	8.1
Cooked, ½ cup, 4 oz.	44	12.5	2.8	9.7	3.5
Oats, rolled/oatmeal:					
Dry/Groats, ½ cup, 1.5 oz.	195	34.5	6	28.5	7.5
Cooked, ½ cup, 4.2 oz.	75	13	2	11	2.9
Quinoa, dry, ½ cup, 3 oz.	320	58.6	5.1	53.5	11
Cooked, ½ cup	105	17	1.5	15.5	6
Rice Bran, ⅓ cup, 1 oz.	123	19.4	8.2	11.2	5.3
Rice Flour, ½ cup, 2¾ oz.	290	63	3.6	59.4	5.5
Rye Flour:					
Dark, 1 cup, 4½ oz.	415	88	28.4	59.6	17.9
Medium, 1 cup, 3½ oz.	360	79	14.9	64.1	9.6
Light, 1 cup, 3½ oz.	375	82	14.9	67.1	8.6
Rye Grain: ½ cup, 3 oz.	280	59	12.3	46.7	12.4
Semolina, ½ cup, 3 oz.	305	61	3.3	57.7	10.6
Soy Bean Flour:					
Defatted, 1 cup	330	34	4.3	29.7	47
Low-Fat, 1 cup	325	30	3.7	26.3	40.9
Full-Fat, 1 cup	370	27	4	23	29.4
Tapioca, pearl, Dry:					
½ cup, 2.7 oz.	260	67	0.8	66.2	0.2
Triticale: Flour, whole-grain,					
½ cup	220	47	9.5	37.5	8.5
Wheat Bran, unprocessed,					
½ cup, 1 oz.	65	20	12.5	7.5	4.5
Wheat Germ: ¼ cup, 1 oz.	105	15	3.7	11.3	6.6
Toasted, ¼ cup, 1 oz.	108	14	3.7	10.3	8.2
Wheat Flour: White,					
All Purpose/Self-Rising					
1 level Tbsp, 0.6 oz.	61	13	0.5	12.5	1.8
½ cup, 2.1 oz.	225	47	1.7	45.3	6.5
Whole Wheat,					
1 cup, 4.2 oz.	410	87	14.4	72.6	16.4

	Calories	Total Carb	Fiber	Usable Carb	Protein
RICE					
BROWN RICE					
Average Short or Long Grain					
Raw/ Dry: ½ cup, 3½ oz.	350	72	3.2	68.8	7.4
Cooked: Hot, ½ cup, 3½ oz.	110	23	1.8	21.2	2.4
WHITE RICE					
Raw:					
Short/Med Grain, 1 cup, 7 oz.	720	156	5.6	150.4	13
Long Grain, 1 cup, 6½ oz.	670	144	2.4	141.6	13.1
Glutinous, 1 cup, 6½ oz.	680	150	5.2	144.8	12.6
Cooked (Boiled/Steamed):					
Short/Medium Grain:					
Hot, ½ cup, 3¼ oz.	103	22.2	0.3	21.7	2.1
Long Grain:					
Hot, ½ cup, 2¾ oz.	100	22	0.3	21.7	2.1
Glutinous/Sticky, Cooked, 1 cup, 6 oz.	170	36	1.7	34.3	3.5
Precooked/Instant:					
Dry, ½ cup, 3½ oz.	180	40	0.8	39.2	3.6
Cooked, Hot, ½ cup, 3 oz.	90	20	0.5	19.5	1.6
Wild Rice:					
Raw, 1 cup, 5½ oz.	570	120	9.9	110.1	23.5
Cooked, hot, 1 cup, 5¾ oz.	165	35	3	32	6.6
PASTA, SPAGHETTI & NOODLES					
DRY SPAGHETTI/MACARONI					
1 oz.	105	21	0.7	20.3	3.6
1 lb box/pkg, 16 oz.	1680	336	10.9	325.1	57.7
Elbows, 1 cup, 3¾ oz.	395	77	2.5	74.5	13.3
Shells, small, 1 cup, 3¼ oz.	340	66	2.2	63.8	11.8
Spirals, 1 cup, 3 oz.	315	61	2	59	10.7
COOKED SPAGHETTI/MACARONI					
Spaghetti, ½ cup, 2½ oz.	90	18	0.9	17.1	3.3
Elbows/Spirals, 1 cup, 5 oz.	197	38	1.8	36.2	6.6
Small shells, 1 cup, 4 oz.	150	31	1.5	29.5	5.4
Whole-wheat:					
Dry, 1 oz.	100	21	2.4	18.6	4.2
Cooked, 1 cup, 5 oz.	175	37	3.9	33.1	7.4

	Calories	Total Carb	Fiber	Usable Carb	Protein
NOODLES					
Plain/Egg:					
Dry, 1 oz.	108	20	0.8	19.2	4
1 cup, 1⅓ oz.	145	28	1	27	5.3
Cooked, 1 oz.	38	7	0.3	6.7	1.3
½ cup, 2¾ oz.	105	20	0.9	19.1	3.8
1 cup, 5½ oz.	210	40	1.8	38.2	7.5
Chinese: Cellophane/					
Rice, dry, 1 oz.	100	25	0.1	24.9	0
Chow Mein/hard, dry, 1 oz.	150	17	1.1	15.9	2.4
Japanese: Somen, dry, 1 oz.	100	22	1.2	20.8	3.2
EGG ROLL SKINS/WON TON					
Per 2.1 oz.					
Won Ton Wrappers:					
(Dynasty) 10 wrappers	170	36	1	35	5
Egg Roll/Spring Roll Wrapper:					
(Dynasty) 3 wrappers	170	36	1	35	5
BREAD					
AVERAGE ALL VARIETIES					
Thin slice (¼"), 1 oz.	70	13	0	13	2
Extra thin slice, ¾ oz.	55	10	0.7	9.3	1.3
Thick slice (⅜"), 1.5 oz.	69	12	0	12	3
BREADS					
Boule, ½" thick, 2 oz.	130	29	0.6	28.4	5
Challah, 1 oz. slice	85	14	0.2	13.8	3
Cracked Wheat Sourdough,					
1½ oz.	130	27	2	25	5
Croutons, 2 Tbsp	35	6	0.5	5.5	1.2
11-Grain, 1¾ oz. slice	90	17	3	14	4
French Stick/Baguette,					
1 oz. slice	70	15	0.5	14.5	3
French Toast, Sticks					
(Aunt Jemima), 1 pce, 1 oz.	75	12	0.3	11.7	1.3
Italian Bread, 1 oz.	75	15	0.3	14.7	2.5
MultiGrain:					
1 slice, 1 oz.	75	14	3	11	4
Fat Free, 1 oz.	70	15	1.5	13.5	2
Oatmeal/Oatbran Bread,					
1 oz. slice	70	13	2	11	4

	Calories	Total Carb	Fiber	Usable Carb	Protein
Pita Bread, average all types, 2 oz.	150	30	1.1	28.9	5.1
Mini/Pocket, 1 oz.	75	15	0.5	14.5	2
Pumpernickel, 1 oz.	75	15	0.7	14.3	2.2
Raisin Bread, 1 oz.	80	14	1.1	12.9	2
Raisin Walnut, 2 oz.	160	29	1.8	27.2	4.6
Roman Meal, 1 oz.	70	14	0.7	13.3	2.6
Country Potato & Oat, 1½ oz.	110	20	1	19	4
Rye: average, 1 thin slice, 1 oz.	53	9	1	8	2
Sourdough, 1 oz. slice	70	12	0.5	11.5	2.5
Sprouted 7-Grain, 1.5 oz. slice	80	16	3	13	4

BREAD ROLLS & BUNS

	Calories	Total Carb	Fiber	Usable Carb	Protein
Dinner Rolls:					
1 small, 1 oz.	85	15	0.8	14.2	2.4
1 medium, 1½ oz.	130	23	1.3	21.7	3.6
English Muffins, average, 2 oz.	140	27	1.5	25.5	4.4
Frankfurter/Hot Dog:					
1½ oz. size	120	23	1.2	21.8	3.7
Hamburger:					
Regular, 1½ oz.	120	23	1.2	21.8	3.7
Large, 3 oz.	240	46	2.3	43.7	7.3
Sourdough Roll, 1¼ oz.	100	18	0.5	17.5	3.4

BAGELS & BREAD PRODUCTS

BAGELS

	Calories	Total Carb	Fiber	Usable Carb	Protein
Average All Brands					
Plain/Onion:					
1 mini/bagelette, 1 oz.	80	15	0.6	14.4	2.2
1 small bagel, 2 oz.	160	30	1.3	28.7	6
1 medium bagel, 3 oz.	240	45	2	43	8.9
1 large bagel, 4 oz.	320	60	2.6	57.4	11.9
Bagel Bites (Ore-Ida), 4 pieces	190	25	2	23	8
Bagel Crisps (Burns Ricker), 1 oz.	133	20	1	19	3

BAGEL SPREADS

	Calories	Total Carb	Fiber	Usable Carb	Protein
Cream Cheese:					
Plain, 1 oz.	*80*	*2*	*0*	*2*	*0*
Reduced Fat, 1 oz.	*60*	*2*	*0*	*2*	*2*

	Calories	Total Carb	Fiber	Usable Carb	Protein
Flavors:					
Lox, 1 oz.	*75*	*1*	*0*	*1*	*4.5*
Raisin Walnut, 1 oz.	90	8	0	8	1
Strawberry, 1 oz.	60	7	0	7	1.5
Sundried Tomato, 1 oz.	*80*	*2*	*0*	*2*	*2.5*
Vegetable, 1 oz.	*60*	*1*	*0*	*1*	*0.5*
BREAD PRODUCTS					
Bread Crumbs, dry:					
Plain or seasoned, 1 oz.	110	20	0.7	19.3	3.5
1 cup, 3½ oz.	390	73	2.4	70.6	12.3
Corn Flake Crumbs, 1 oz.	104	24	1	23	2
Croutons: Average all brands,					
1 oz.	116	20.9	1.4	19.5	3.4
Stuffing: Average,					
Dry mix, 1 oz.	110	21.6	0.9	20.7	3.1
Made-up, ½ cup, 4 oz.	202	24.6	3.4	21.2	3.4
CRISPBREADS					
Ak-Mak: Sesame,					
5 crackers, 1 oz.	116	19	3.5	15.5	4.6
BAKING INGREDIENTS					
ALMOND PASTE					
Marzipan, 1 oz.	125	12	0	12	3.5
BAKING POWDER					
Regular, 1 tsp	*3*	*0.5*	*0.1*	*0.4*	*0*
CREAM OF TARTAR					
1 tsp	*2*	*0.5*	*0*	*0.5*	*0*
BUTTER/MARGARINE					
½ cup, 4 oz.	*820*	*0*	*0*	*0*	*0*
CAROB FLOUR					
½ cup	90	26	20.5	5.5	2.4
CHOCOLATE BAKING BARS					
Average All Brands					
Unsweetened, 1 oz.	*150*	*8*	*4.4*	*3.6*	*3*
Grated, 1 cup	680	36	20.3	15.7	13.9
Semi-sweet, 1 oz.	160	18	0	18	1
Bitter-sweet/White Baking,					
1 oz.	160	17	0	17	1

	Calories	Total Carb	Fiber	Usable Carb	Protein
CHOCOLATE BAKING CHIPS					
Average All Brands					
Milk Choc/Semi-sweet, 1 oz.	160	20	0	20	2
¼ cup, 1½ oz.	240	30	0	30	3
COCOA POWDER, BAKING					
Nestle, 1 Tbsp	*15*	*3*	*1.8*	*1.2*	*1.1*
⅓ cup, 1 oz.	65	15.4	9.4	6	5.6
CORNSTARCH					
1 Tbsp	54	13	0.1	12.9	0.1
FLOUR					
White					
1 Tbsp, 0.6 oz.	55	12	0.5	11.5	1.8
1 cup, 4.4 oz.	450	95	3.4	91.6	12.9
Whole Wheat, 1 cup, 4.2 oz.	410	87	14.4	72.6	16.4
FLAVOR EXTRACTS					
Average All Brands					
Imitation, 1 tsp	*15*	*3.5*	*0*	*3.5*	*0*
Pure Extract, 1 tsp	*20*	*4*	*0*	*4*	*0*
Almond Vanilla, 1 tsp	*10*	*3*	*0*	*3*	*0*
GELATIN					
Dry, ¼ oz. pkg	30	6.4	0	6.4	0.6
LEMON/ORANGE PEEL					
¼ cup	*30*	*9.1*	*6*	*3.1*	*0.9*
RENNIN					
1 pkg, 11g	40	10	0.6	9.4	0.3
SPRINKLES					
All types, 1 Tbsp, ½ oz.	70	10	0.3	9.7	0.7
VINEGAR					
Average all types, 1 oz.	*4*	*2*	*0*	*2*	*0*
YEAST					
Fleischmann's, 0.6 oz. pkg	*15*	*2*	*0*	*2*	*3*

SUGAR, SYRUP, JAM, HONEY

	Calories	Total Carb	Fiber	Usable Carb	Protein
SUGAR					
White Sugar, granulated:					
1 level tsp	*15*	*4*	*0*	*4*	*0*
1 heaping tsp	25	6.5	0	6.5	0

	Calories	Total Carb	Fiber	Usable Carb	Protein
2 cubes	19	5	0	5	0
Single portion, 1 pkt	23	6	0	6	0
1 Tbsp	48	12	0	12	0
1 oz.	110	27	0	27	0
1 cup, 7 oz.	770	189	0	189	0
1 lb.	1760	432	0	432	0
Brown Sugar:					
1 Tbsp	50	13	0	13	0
1 oz.	109	28	0	28	0
1 cup, not packed, 5 oz.	540	140	0	140	0
1 cup, packed, 7¾ oz.	845	218	0	218	0
Powdered/Confectioners:					
Unsifted, 1 cup, 4¼ oz.	460	117	0	117	0
Other Sugars:					
Glucose, 1 oz.	110	27	0	27	0
Barley/Wheat/Rye Malt,					
1 Tbsp; ¾ oz.	60	14	0	14	1
Cinnamon Sugar, 1 tsp	*15*	*4*	*0*	*4*	*0*
Dextrose, 1 oz.	110	27	0	27	0
Fructose, 3 Tbsp, 1 oz.	110	27	0	27	0
Sorbitol, 1 oz.	110	27	0	27	0
Turbinado Sugar,					
2 Tbsp, 1 oz.	110	27	0	27	0
Unrefined Cane Sugar, 1 oz.	110	27	0	27	0

SUGAR SUBSTITUTES

DiabetiSweet, 1 tsp	*9*	*4*	*0*	*4*	*0*
Equal: Granulated, 1 pkg	*0*	*1*	*0*	*1*	*0*
Nutra Taste, 1 pkt	*0*	*0*	*0*	*0*	*0*
Sweet 'N Low, 1 pkt	*0*	*0*	*0*	*0*	*0*
Sweet One, 1 pkt	*0*	*0*	*0*	*0*	*0*

HONEY, JAM, PRESERVES

Average All Brands					
Honey:					
- 1 tsp, ¼ oz.	22	5.5	0	5.5	0
1 Tbsp, ¾ oz.	65	17	0	17	0.1
1 cup, 12 oz.	1030	269	0.7	268.3	1.7
Single Portion, ½ oz. pkg	43	11	0	11	0.1
Jams/Jellies/Marmalade/					
Preserves					
Regular, 1 tsp, ¼ oz.	*18*	*5*	*0.1*	*4.9*	*0*
1 Tbsp, ¾ oz.	55	16	0.2	15.8	0.1

	Calories	Total Carb	Fiber	Usable Carb	Protein
Single Portion, ½ oz. pkg	38	9.6	0.1	9.5	0.1
Apple/Fruit Butters, 1 Tbsp, 0.6 oz.	29	7.3	0.3	7	0.1

SYRUPS, MOLASSES

	Calories	Total Carb	Fiber	Usable Carb	Protein
Syrups:					
Average All Types & Brands					
Regular/Dark/Light Color:					
1 Tbsp, ½ fl. oz.	55	14	0	14	0
¼ cup (4 Tbsp)	220	55	0	55	0
Lite: 1 Tbsp	25	6	0	6	0
¼ cup (4 Tbsp)	100	25	0	25	0
Sugar-Free:					
Cary's, 2 Tbsp, 1 oz.	*30*	*1.2*	*0*	*1.2*	*0*
Cozy Cottage, 2 Tbsp, 1 oz.	*10*	*3*	*0*	*3*	*0*
Molasses: Dark/Light:					
1 Tbsp, ¾ oz.	55	14	0	14	0
1 cup, 11½ oz.	880	224	0	224	0
Blackstrap:					
1 Tbsp, ¾ oz.	47	13	0	13	0
1 cup, 11½ oz.	750	208	0	208	0

ICE CREAM TOPPINGS

	Calories	Total Carb	Fiber	Usable Carb	Protein
Average All Types & Brands					
Butterscotch, Caramel, 2 Tbsp	140	30	0.4	29.6	0.6
Chocolate, Hot Fudge, 2 Tbsp	140	22	1	21	2
Fat Free (Hershey's), 2 Tbsp	100	23	0	23	1
Pineapple, Strawberry, 2 Tbsp	110	28	0.4	27.6	0
Smuckers:					
Guilt Free, All flavors	100	24	1	23	1
Magic Shell, 2 Tbsp	220	16	0	16	1
Milky Way, 2 Tbsp	130	24	0	24	1
Lite Hot Fudge, 2 Tbsp	90	23	2	21	2

POPCORN

HOME-POPPED POPCORN

	Calories	Total Carb	Fiber	Usable Carb	Protein
Air-popped (no oil),					
Plain, 1 oz.	108	22	4.3	17.7	3.4
1 cup	31	6.2	1.2	5	1

	Calories	Total Carb	Fiber	Usable Carb	Protein
Oil-popped, plain, 1 oz.	140	16.2	2.8	13.4	2.6
1 cup	55	6.3	1.1	5.2	1
MICROWAVE POPCORN					
Average All Brands (Popped)					
Butter:					
Regular, 1 cup	*35*	*4*	*0.5*	*3.5*	*0.5*
Light, 1 cup	*25*	*4*	*0.5*	*3.5*	*0.5*
Act II Popcorn:					
Butter, 1 cup, 0.3 oz.	*35*	*4*	*0.5*	*3.5*	*0.5*
Light Butter, 1 cup, 0.2 oz.	*25*	*4*	*0.5*	*3.5*	*0.5*
Butter Lovers, 1 cup, 0.3 oz.	*45*	*4*	*1*	*3*	*1*
Healthy Choice					
Butter, 6 cups	92	19.2	3.8	15.4	3.1
Natural, 6 cups	90	19.4	3.7	15.7	3
Newman's Own					
Butter, 1 oz.	161	15.1	2.8	12.3	1.9
Orville Redenbacher's:					
Per Cup Popped					
Corn on the Cob	*35*	*3*	*0.5*	*2.5*	*0*
BAGGED POPCORN					
Boston's					
Lite, 2 cups, 1 oz.	140	19	3	16	3
Gourmet Super Premium,					
2 cups, 1 oz.	160	13	3	10	2
40% Less Fat, 2¾ cup, 1 oz.	140	17	3	14	3
Cracker Jack					
Original, ½ cup, 1 oz.	120	23	1	22	2
Fat Free varieties, ¾ cup, 1 oz.	110	26	1	25	0
Crunch 'N Munch					
Buttery Toffee, ⅔ cup, 1 oz.	150	22	0.5	21.5	2
Fiddle Faddle					
Skippy, ¾ cup, 1 oz.	130	23	1	22	2
W/Real Planters Peanuts,					
⅔ cup	130	24	0.5	23.5	1
Wild Oats					
All types, 2½ cups, 1 oz.	160	15	1.9	13.1	2.8
MOVIE THEATER POPCORN					
Small (7 cups):					
Plain	400	30	8.5	21.5	9
w/ Butter	580	30	8.5	21.5	9

	Calories	Total Carb	Fiber	Usable Carb	Protein
Medium (16 cups):					
Plain	900	70	20	50	20
w/ Butter	1170	70	20	50	20
Large (20 cups):					
Plain	1150	90	24	66	26.5
w/ Butter	1500	90	24	66	26.5

SNACKS

BEEF JERKY

	Calories	Total Carb	Fiber	Usable Carb	Protein
Average, 1 oz.	*116*	*3*	*0.5*	*2.5*	*9.4*

PORK SKINS/RIND

	Calories	Total Carb	Fiber	Usable Carb	Protein
Baken-ets, 1 oz.	*160*	*0*	*0*	*0*	*14.2*
Lance, 1 package	*158*	*2*	*0*	*2*	*15*

SOY NUTS

	Calories	Total Carb	Fiber	Usable Carb	Protein
Dry Roasted, 1 oz.	130	9	2	7	10
Choc-coated, 12-15 pcs, ½ oz.	70	7	0.5	6.5	2

GRANOLA, SPORTS & DIET BARS
(PER BAR)

ARBONNE BALANCED

	Calories	Total Carb	Fiber	Usable Carb	Protein
Nutrition	190	24	0	24	14

ATKINS ADVANTAGE

	Calories	Total Carb	Fiber	Usable Carb	Protein
Almond Brownie, 2.11 oz.	220	21	7	14	21
Other flavors, average, 2.11 oz.	230	23	9	14	19

BALANCE BAR

	Calories	Total Carb	Fiber	Usable Carb	Protein
High Protein, avg, 1.76 oz.	200	23	1	22	14
Gold, avg, 1.76 oz.	210	22	0.5	21.5	15

BARBARA'S BAKERY

	Calories	Total Carb	Fiber	Usable Carb	Protein
Granola Bars, average, ¾ oz.	80	15	2	13	2

BIOCHEM

	Calories	Total Carb	Fiber	Usable Carb	Protein
Ultimate Lo Carb, 2.1 oz.	*155*	*3*	*0*	*3*	*20*

BODY SMARTS

	Calories	Total Carb	Fiber	Usable Carb	Protein
Choc P'nut Crunch	210	34	2	32	5
Yogurt Berry Crunch	200	35	2	33	5

CARB SOLUTIONS TASTE SENSATIONS

	Calories	Total Carb	Fiber	Usable Carb	Protein
Choc Peanut Butter, 2.1 oz.	250	14	1	13	26
Choc Toffee Hazelnut, 2.1 oz.	260	15	1	14	25
Other flavors, 2.1 oz, avg	240	16	0.5	15.5	26

	Calories	Total Carb	Fiber	Usable Carb	Protein
CARBOLITE					
Choc Almond, 1.75 oz.	230	25	1	24	4
Milk/Dairy Chocolate,					
Average, 1.75 oz.	250	28	1	27	4
CHOICE					
All types, 1.23 oz. bar	140	19	3	16	6
CLIF BAR					
Luna Bar, average	180	27	2	25	8
Ice Series (w/ caffeine), 2.4 oz.	250	43	5	38	10
Mojo Bar, average	210	29	2	27	9
Nutrition Sustained					
Energy, 68g:					
Apricot; Cranberry; Apple;					
Cherry	220	44	5	39	8
Other varieties, average	250	44	5	39	8
COACH'S ICED ENERGY BARS					
2 oz. bar	240	38	3	35	7
DETOUR					
2.8 oz. bar	310	25	3	22	30
DR SOY					
Protein Bar					
Lemon, 1.76 oz.	180	28	0	28	11
Chocolate/Peanut, 1.76 oz.	185	27	1	26	11
EXTREME BODY					
3 oz. bar	340	24	2	22	34
FIT! (MEDIFAST)					
1.5 oz. bar	160	21	2	19	10
GENERAL MILLS					
Milk 'n Cereal					
Chex; Cheerios;					
Cocoa Puffs, 1.4 oz.	160	26	1	25	6
Cinnamon Toast Crunch,					
1.6 oz.	180	31	1	30	6
GENISOY					
Average all bars, 2.2 oz.	230	41	3	38	11
HANSEN'S					
Natural Bars, 50g	195	25	1	24	14
Active Nutrition Bars, Avg, 40g	140	20	1	19	7

	Calories	Total Carb	Fiber	Usable Carb	Protein
IRON-TEK					
Vanilla Fudge, 2.73 oz.	290	21	2	19	28
JENNY CRAIG					
Meal Bars, 1.97 oz					
Milk Choc; Lemon Meringue	210	32	0	32	10
Choc Peanut; Yogurt Peanut	220	33	1	32	10
Oatmeal Raisin	210	35	3	32	10
KASHI GOLEAN BARS					
Average, 78g	290	45	6	39	13
KID SPORT BARS					
Average, 1.76 oz.	200	29	20	9	10
KUDOS					
Granola; M&M's; Snickers	105	16	0	16	1
MLO BIO PROTEIN					
2.85 oz. bar	300	39	1	38	21
NATROL PROLAB					
1.76 oz.	190	12	0.5	11.5	19
NATURE VALLEY GRANOLA					
Average	145	24	1	23	2
NATURE'S PLUS					
Energy Bar, 1.45 oz.	140	24	5	19	7
Chi Chinese Herbal, 1.5 oz.	150	20	4.9	15.1	5.9
Calcium Almond Blitz, 1.5 oz.	150	29	2	27	2
Spiru-tein, all flavors, 1.4 oz.	150	20	3	17	10
NEXT PROTEINS					
Designer Whey, 78g	*260*	*6*	*1*	*5*	*30*
U-Turn Protein, 2.8 oz	300	26	2	24	30
ODWALLA ENERGY BARS					
Carrot	225	45	4	41	4
Chocolate	240	40	4	36	6
Chocolate Chip Peanut	245	39	4	35	7
Cranberry C Monster	225	47	4	43	4
Peanut Crunch	255	40	3	37	8
Super Protein	235	31	3	28	16
Superfood	225	41	5	36	4
POWER BAR					
Harvest, average, 2.3 oz.	240	45	4	41	7

	Calories	Total Carb	Fiber	Usable Carb	Protein
PREMIER					
Protein Eight, 2.4 oz.	260	23	1	22	30
Protein Meal Replacement, 2.5 oz.	280	20	2	18	31
Complete Nutrition, 48g	190	28	1	27	10
Odyssey Protein, 80g	310	29	3	26	30
PROMAX					
Average, 2.7 oz. bar	290	40	2	38	20
PURE FIT					
Average, 2 oz. bar	230	27	16	11	18
QUAKER					
Chewy Dipps Granola Bars:					
Caramel Nut	145	21	1	20	2
Chocolate Fudge	165	21	1	20	2
Peanut Butter	155	19	1	18	2
Chewy Granola Bars:					
Low Fat	110	23	1	22	1
Baby Ruth; Butterfinger	120	22	0.5	21.5	2
Choc Chip; Nestle Crunch	120	21	1	20	2
Peanut Butter	110	18	1	17	2
Peanut Butter & Choc Chunk	120	20	1	19	2
Fruit & Oatmeal Bars:					
Apple Crisp	***90***	***15***	***15***	***0***	***1***
Average other flavors	140	26	1	25	1
Fruit & Oatmeal Bites, 3 pieces	140	27	1	26	2
Fruit & Oatmeal Breakfast Bar	130	24	1	23	1
REVIVAL SOY BARS (DIRECT)					
Cook Krispy Protein:					
Choc Temptation	220	30	0.5	29.5	15
Apple Cinnamon; Marsh Krunch	220	33	0.5	32.5	17
Peanut Butter/Choc Pal, average	240	32	1	31	16
SLIM-FAST BARS					
Meal Options, 1.97 oz.	220	36	2	34	8
Snack Options, 1 oz.	130	22	0	22	0.5
Solid Protein Meal, 2.75 oz.	270	14	0.5	13.5	34
Think Protein Bar, 2.3 oz.	280	18	0	18	21

	Calories	Total Carb	Fiber	Usable Carb	Protein
WHOLE FOODS					
Everyday Bars, 1.76 oz.					
Choc Fudge/Raspberry	172	17	1	16	17
Honey Peanut Yogurt	200	18	2	16	18
Zone Perfect, avg, 1.76 oz.	210	24	1	23	14

NUTS & SEEDS

NUTS					
Acorns, raw, 1 oz.	105	12	0.7	11.3	1.8
Almonds, Dried/Dry Roasted:					
Whole, 24-28 med, 1 oz.	*170*	*7*	*3.4*	*3.6*	*6.2*
Chopped, ½ cup	380	16	8.1	7.9	15.2
Oil Rstd (Blue Diamond), 1 oz.	*175*	*5*	*3*	*2*	*6*
Honey Roasted, 1 oz.	*170*	*8*	*3.9*	*4.1*	*5.1*
Brazil Nuts,					
8 medium, 1 oz.	*185*	*3.5*	*1.5*	*2*	*4.1*
Cashews, Dry or Oil Roasted:					
14 large/18 med/26 small, 1 oz.	165	10	0.9	9.1	4.3
Honey Roasted, 1 oz.	160	9	1	8	1
Chestnuts:					
Dried, 1 oz.	105	22	1.4	20.6	1.4
Raw/ Fresh, 1 oz.	60	13	0.3	12.7	0.5
Coconut:					
Flesh (no shell), 1 oz.	*100*	*4*	*2.6*	*1.4*	*0.9*
Raw: 1 piece, 1.6 oz.	*160*	*7*	*4.1*	*2.9*	*1.5*
Dried (Desiccated):					
Unsweetened, 1 oz.	*187*	*6.9*	*4.6*	*2.3*	*1.9*
Sweetened, shredded, 1 oz	140	13	1.3	11.7	0.8
Cream (can), ½ cup, 5.2 oz.	285	12	3.3	8.7	4
Water (center liquid), ½ cup, 4¼ oz.	*23*	*4.5*	*1.3*	*3.2*	*0.8*
Filberts or Hazelnuts:					
Shelled, 18-20 nuts	*180*	*4.5*	*2.6*	*1.9*	*4*
Chopped, ¼ cup	*180*	*4.5*	*2.8*	*1.7*	*4.3*
Ground, ¼ cup	*120*	*3*	*1.8*	*1.2*	*2.8*
Ginko Nuts, can:					
14 med, 1 oz.	*32*	*6*	*2.6*	*3.4*	*0.7*
Hickory, 30 sm nuts	*190*	*5*	*1.8*	*3.2*	*3.6*

	Calories	Total Carb	Fiber	Usable Carb	Protein
Macadamia Nuts, shelled:					
Raw, 7 med/14 small,					
1 oz.	*200*	*4*	*2.4*	*1.6*	*2.3*
Oil roasted, 1 oz.	*205*	*3.5*	*2.3*	*1.2*	*2.2*
Mixed Nuts:					
18-22 nuts, 1 oz.	*175*	*7*	*2.6*	*4.4*	*4.9*
Planters:					
Dry Roasted/Honey	151	9	1.9	7.1	1.9
Sweet Roasts, 26 pces,1 oz	160	10	1.9	8.1	4.7
Peanuts: Raw/ Dried:					
In shell, 1 oz.	*117*	*3*	*1.2*	*1.8*	*5.3*
Shelled, 1 oz.	*160*	*4.5*	*2.4*	*2.1*	*7.3*
Roasted, 30 large/					
60 small, 1 oz.	*165*	*6*	*2.3*	*3.7*	*6.7*
1 cup, 5.1 oz.	840	31	11.7	19.3	34.5
Planters:					
Beer Nuts, 1 oz. pkg	170	7	2	5	7
Cocktail, oil roasted,					
1 oz.	*170*	*6*	*2*	*4*	*5*
Dry Roasted, 1 oz.	*160*	*6*	*2*	*4*	*5.3*
Honey Roasted, 1 oz.	150	10	2	8	6
Honey/Dry Roasted, 1 oz.	160	7	2	5	6
Spanish Oil Roasted, 1 oz	*180*	*5*	*2*	*3*	*8.5*
Pecans:					
Kernel halves (20 jumbo					
or 31 large halves), 1 oz.	*190*	*5*	*2.7*	*2.3*	*2.6*
1 cup halves, 3.8 oz.	720	20	10.4	9.6	9.8
Chopped, ½ cup, 2 oz.	*380*	*10*	*5.7*	*4.3*	*5.4*
Oil Roasted, 1 oz.	*195*	*4.5*	*2.7*	*1.8*	*2.6*
Honey Roasted, 1 oz.	*200*	*5*	*2.7*	*2.3*	*2.7*
Pinenuts, dried:					
1 Tbsp	*50*	*1.5*	*0.4*	*1.1*	*2.1*
Pistachios:					
Lance, 1⅛ oz. pkg	*95*	*4*	*2*	*2*	*4*
Planters:					
Dry Roasted, 1 oz.	*170*	*6*	*2*	*4*	*5.3*
Trail Mix, 3 Tbsp, 1 oz.	140	13.8	1.7	12.1	3.4
Soy Nuts:					
Dry Roasted, 1 oz.	130	9	2	7	10
½ cup, 3 oz.	390	28	6	22	30

	Calories	Total Carb	Fiber	Usable Carb	Protein
Dr Soy:					
Choc coated, 1 oz. pkg	130	18	2	16	5
Honey Roasted, 1 oz.	140	11	4	7	6
Flavors, average, 1oz.	*150*	*8*	*4*	*4*	*13*
Walnuts:					
Black: 15-20 halves, 1 oz.	*175*	*3.5*	*1.4*	*2.1*	*6.9*
Chopped, ¼ cup	*190*	*4*	*1.6*	*2.4*	*7.6*
English Persian:					
14 halves, 1 oz.	*185*	*5*	*1.9*	*3.1*	*4.3*
Chopped, ¼ cup	*195*	*5*	*2*	*3*	*4.6*
SEEDS					
Alfalfa Seeds, sprout,					
½ cup, ½ oz.	*5*	*1*	*0.4*	*0.6*	*0.7*
Caraway, Fennell, 1 tsp	*10*	*1*	*0.8*	*0.2*	*0.4*
Cottonseed Kernels,					
Roasted, 1 Tbsp	*50*	*2*	*0.6*	*1.4*	*3.3*
Flax Seeds, 3 Tbsp, 1 oz.	*150*	*11*	*7.9*	*3.1*	*5.5*
Pumpkin & Squash Seeds,					
Whole: Dried, 1 oz.	*155*	*5*	*1.1*	*3.9*	*7*
Sesame Seeds:					
Dried, 1 Tbsp	*50*	*1*	*0.9*	*0.1*	*2.1*
Roasted/Toasted, 1 oz.	*160*	*7*	*4.8*	*2.2*	*4.8*
Sunflower Kernels/Seed:					
Dry Roasted, 1 Tbsp	*45*	*1.5*	*0.9*	*0.6*	*1.5*
¼ cup, 1 oz.	*160*	*6*	*3.2*	*2.8*	*5.5*
Oil Roasted, ¼ cup, 1 oz.	*208*	*5*	*2.3*	*2.7*	*7.2*
NUT & SEED BUTTERS					
Almond Butter:					
1 Tbsp, ½ oz.	*89*	*3*	*0.5*	*2.5*	*2.1*
Cashew Butter: 1 Tbsp	*92*	*4.5*	*0.3*	*4.2*	*2.8*
Peanut Butter:					
Average All Brands					
1 tsp, 6g	*35*	*1.5*	*0.3*	*1.2*	*1.1*
1 Tbsp, 0.6 oz.	*105*	*3.5*	*1*	*2.5*	*3.5*
1 oz. quantity, 28g	*170*	*6*	*1.8*	*4.2*	*6.2*
½ cup, 5 oz.	850	30	8.9	21.1	31.1
Natural Peanut Butter,					
1 Tbsp	*100*	*3.5*	*1*	*2.5*	*3.5*
Sesame Butter/Tahini,					
1 Tbsp, ½ oz.	*90*	*3.9*	*1.4*	*2.5*	*2.7*

	Calories	Total Carb	Fiber	Usable Carb	Protein
COUGH & PHARMACEUTICAL					
COUGH/COLD SYRUPS					
Regular, 1 Tbsp:					
w/ sugar	35	9	0	9	0
w/ alcohol	46	9	0	9	0
Sugar-Free (Diabetic Tussin),					
1 Tbsp	*0*	*0*	*0*	*0*	*0*
COUGH DROPS					
Halls Defense Vit C, 1 drop	*15*	*4*	*0*	*4*	*0*
Halls Fruit Breezers,					
1 drop	*14*	*4*	*0*	*4*	*0*
Halls Menthol Drops,					
1 drop	*15*	*4*	*0*	*4*	*0*
Sugar Free, 1 drop	*6*	*1.5*	*0*	*1.5*	*0*
Halls Plus, 1 drop	18	5	0	5	0
Listerine Lozenge	*9*	*2*	*0*	*2*	*0.5*
Luden's Throat Drops,					
all flavors	*10*	*2*	*0*	*2*	*0.5*
Rolaids/Sodium Free, 1	*4*	*1*	*0*	*1*	*0*
Sather's Peppermint					
Lozenges, 1	*13*	*3*	*0*	*3*	*0.5*
Sucrets (Beecham)					
Lozenges, 1	*10*	*2*	*0.*	*2*	*0*
ANTACIDS					
Average, 1 tablet	*4*	*1*	*0*	*1*	*0*
Liquid, 1 Tbsp	*6*	*1*	*0*	*1*	*0*
Sudafed Syrup, 1 tsp	*14*	*3*	*0*	*3*	*0*
Tylenol Liquid:					
Child, 1 tsp	*17*	*4*	*0*	*4*	*0*
Extra Strength, 1 tsp	*11*	*3*	*0*	*3*	*0*
FRESH FRUIT					
ACEROLA					
1 cup, 20 Pieces, 3½ oz.	30	7.5	1.1	6.4	0.4
APPLES					
Average all Varieties					
1 small 2½"	63	16.2	2.9	13.3	0.2
Medium w/o skin	73	19.0	2.6	16.4	0.2
Caramel Apple, 1 medium	170	42	6.6	35.4	3.4

	Calories	Total Carb	Fiber	Usable Carb	Protein
APRICOTS					
1 small	*17*	*4*	*0.8*	*3.2*	*0.5*
1 medium, 2 oz.	*25*	*6*	*1.4*	*4.6*	*0.8*
1 large	35	8	2	6	1.2
AVOCADO					
w/o seed/skin: ½ oz.	*160*	*6*	*4.9*	*1.1*	*1.9*
1 salad slice, ½ oz.	*2.5*	*1*	*0.7*	*0.3*	*0.3*
Mashed Puree, ¼ C, 2 oz.	*90*	*4*	*2.7*	*1.3*	*1.1*
Californian, ½ med, 3 oz.	*160*	*8*	*4.3*	*3.7*	*1.8*
Mashed Puree, ½ c, 4 oz.	210	12	5.6	6.4	2.4
Florida, ½ med, 5½ oz.	170	14	8.2	5.8	2.5
Mashed/Puree ½ C, 4 oz.	*125*	*9*	*6.1*	*2.9*	*1.8*
Cubed, 3 oz.	*105*	*8*	*4.5*	*3.5*	*1.3*
BANANAS					
1 small, 4 oz.	55	13	1.7	11.3	0.9
1 med, 5 oz.	80	20	2.1	17.9	1.1
1 large, 7 oz.	105	25	.3	24.7	1
w/o skin, 1 med	80	20	2.4	17.6	1.0
½ C mashed	105	25	5.4	19.6	2.3
BLUEBERRIES/BLACKERRIES/BOYSENBERRIES					
½ C, 2.5 oz.	40	10	1.9	8.1	0.5
1 Pint, 14 oz.	220	56	10.9	45.1	2.7
BREADFRUIT					
½ cup, 4 oz.	115	28	5.4	22.6	1.2
CANTALOUPE					
Flesh/no skin: 1 oz.	*8*	*2*	*.2*	*1.8*	*.2*
1 slice, 2.5 oz.	*20*	*5*	*.4*	*4.6*	*.4*
CARAMBOLA (STAR FRUIT)					
1 medium	*50*	*4*	*2.5*	*1.5*	*0.5*
CASSAVA					
1 cup	330	78.3	3.7	74.6	2.7
CHERIMOYA (CUSTARD APPLE)					
4 oz.	110	27	2.7	24.3	1.5
CHERRIES					
Sweet, 8 fruit, 2 oz.	40	10	1.3	8.7	0.7
½ lb, 30 fruit	164	37.5	5.2	32.3	2.7
Sour, 8 fruit, 2 oz.	25	6	0.9	5.1	0.6
½ lb, 30 fruit	114	27.7	3.6	24.1	2.3

	Calories	Total Carb	Fiber	Usable Carb	Protein
COCONUT					
Fresh, 1 pc, 1 oz.	100	3	2.6	.4	0.9
Shredded, ½ cup	150	6	3.6	2.4	1.3
Dried, sweetened, ½ cup	235	22	2.1	19.9	1.3
CRABAPPLES,					
½ cup slices	43	11.3	.3	11	0.2
CRANBERRIES					
½ cup	*20*	*5*	*2.4*	*2.6*	*0.2*
CURRANTS					
European Black Raw, ½ cup	35	8.6	3.0	5.6	0.8
Red and White, 1 cup raw	63	15.5	4.8	10.7	1.6
CUSTARD APPLE					
Raw	110	27	2.7	24.3	1.5
DURIAN					
Flesh, 1 cup	357	65.5	9.2	56.3	3.6
ELDERBERRIES					
1 cup	106	26.7	10.2	16.5	0.9
FIGS					
Green/black: 1 med, 2.3 oz.	47	12.2	2.1	10.1	0.4
FRUIT SALAD					
Average, fresh, 1 cup	110	25	2	23	1
GOOSEBERRIES					
Raw, 1 cup	66	15	6.4	8.6	1.2
GRAPEFRUIT					
Average all types, 1 C w/ juice	74	18.4	2.3	16.1	1.4
GRAPES					
Red or green, raw, 1 C seedless	114	28.3	1.6	26.7	1.0
GRANADILLA					
1 cup	229	54.3	24.5	29.8	5.2
GROUNDCHERRIES					
Raw, ½ cup	37	7.7	2.0	5.7	1.4
GUAVA					
Fresh, 1 cup	84	19.5	8.9	10.6	1.3
HONEYDEW					
1 small wedge	44	11.5	0.8	10.7	0.5
1 cup balls	62	16.3	1.1	15.2	0.7

	Calories	Total Carb	Fiber	Usable Carb	Protein
JACKFRUIT					
1 cup sliced	155	39.6	2.6	37	2.3
JAVA-PLUM					
4 oz.	68	17.6	.1	17.5	0.8
JUJUBE					
1 oz.	22	5.7	.4	5.3	1.4
KIWIFRUIT					
1 cup	108	26.2	6	20.2	1.8
1 lg, no skin	56	13.5	3.1	10.4	0.9
KUMQUATS					
1 fruit, no refuse	*12*	*3.1*	*1.3*	*1.8*	*0.2*
LEMON					
1 slice	*2*	*0.7*	*0.2*	*0.5*	*0.1*
2⅛" diameter	*17*	*5.4*	*1.6*	*3.8*	*0.6*
Peel, 1 Tbsp	*3*	*1.0*	*0.6*	*0.4*	*0.1*
LIMES					
2" diameter	20	7.0	1.9	5.1	0.5
LOGANBERRIES					
1 cup	81	19.1	7.3	11.8	2.2
LONGANS					
1 fruit	*2*	*0.5*	*0*	*0.5*	*0*
LOQUATS					
1 cup	70	18.0	2.5	15.5	0.6
MAMEY APPLE					
1 fruit, no refuse	431	105.8	25.4	80.4	4.2
MANGOS					
1 cup sliced	107	28.0	3	25	0.8
MELON					
1 cup	57	13.7	1.2	12.5	1.4
MULBERRIES					
1 cup	60	14	2.4	11.6	2
NASHI FRUIT					
2½" diameter	51	12.9	4.4	8.5	0.6

	Calories	Total Carb	Fiber	Usable Carb	Protein
NECTARINES					
1 cup slices	68	16.1	2.2	13.9	1.2
2½ " diameter	67	15.9	2.2	13.7	1.2
OHELOBERRIES					
½ cup	*20*	*4.8*	*.9*	*3.9*	*0.3*
OLIVES					
Pickled, green, 10 large	*47*	*0.5*	*1*	*0*	*0.3*
Ripe, Greek Style,					
10 medium	*71*	*2*	*1.2*	*0.8*	*0.3*
Ripe, Black, Californian					
1 small/medium	*4*	*.3*	*.1*	*.2*	*0*
1 large	*6*	*.4*	*.1*	*.3*	*0*
1 jumbo	*7*	*.5*	*.1*	*.4*	*0*
1 colossal	*13*	*1*	*.1*	*0.9*	*0*
ORANGES					
1 small, 2⅜" diameter	45	11.2	2.3	8.9	0.9
1 large, 3 ⅙" diameter	86	21.5	4.4	17.1	1.7
1 cup Sections	85	21.1	4.3	16.8	1.6
California Valencia, 1 cup	88	21.6	4.5	17.1	1.8
California Navels,					
1 medium, 2⅞" diameter	64	16.2	3.4	12.8	1.4
Florida Orange,					
1 medium, 2¹¹⁄₁₆" diameter	69	17.4	3.6	13.8	1.1
Peel, 1 Tbsp	*6*	*1.5*	*0.6*	*0.9*	*0.1*
PAPAYA					
1 cup cubed	55	13.7	2.5	11.5	0.8
1 medium, 3" diameter	119	29.8	5.5	24.3	1.8
PASSIONFRUIT					
1 cup juice	148	35.7	0.5	35.2	1.2
PEACHES					
1 large, 5.5 oz.	68	17.3	3.1	14.2	1.1
1 cup slices, 6 oz.	73	18.7	3.4	15.3	1.2
PEARS					
Asian, 3" diameter	116	29.1	9.9	19.2	1.4
Bosc, 1 medium 6 oz.	90	22	0	22	0.5
PERSIMMONS					
Native, 1 oz.	36	9.5	.4	9.1	0.2
Japanese, 2½" diameter	118	31.2	6	25.2	1

	Calories	Total Carb	Fiber	Usable Carb	Protein
PINEAPPLE					
2 oz. slice, no skin	27	6.9	0.7	6.2	0.2
3 oz. slice, no skin	41	10.4	1.0	9.4	0.3
PITANGA					
1 fruit	*2*	*0.5*	*0*	*.5*	*.1*
PLUMS					
2⅛" diameter	36	8.6	1.0	7.6	0.5
1 cup sliced	91	21.4	2.5	18.9	1.3
1 oz.	*16*	*3.7*	*0.4*	*3.3*	*0.2*
POMEGRANATES					
3⅜" diameter	106	26.2	0.9	25.3	1.5
PUMMELLO					
1 fruit	231	58.5	6.1	52.4	4.3
1 cup sections	72	18.2	1.9	16.3	1.3
PRICKLY PEARS					
1 fruit, no refuse	42	9.9	3.7	6.2	0.9
QUINCE					
1 fruit, no refuse	52	13.8	1.8	12	0.4
RHUBARB					
Raw, 1 cup diced	*26*	*5.5*	*2.4*	*3.1*	*1.2*
SAPODILLA					
1 Fruit	141	34	9.0	25	0.7
SAPOTES					
1 Fruit	302	75.8	5.9	69.9	4.7
SOURSOP					
1 cup pulp	148	37.8	7.4	30.4	2.2
STRAWBERRIES					
1 cup halves	46	10.6	3.5	7.1	0.9
1 large, 3⅛" diameter	*5*	*1.3*	*0.4*	*0.9*	*0.1*
SOUR APPLES					
1 cup	235	59	11	48	5
TAMARIND					
1 Fruit	*5*	*1.2*	*0.1*	*1.1*	*0.1*
TANGELO					
4 oz.	31	7	1	6	1

	Calories	Total Carb	Fiber	Usable Carb	Protein
TANGERINE					
1 med, 2⅜" diameter	37	9.2	1.9	7.3	0.5
TOMATILLOS					
½ cup chopped	*27*	*3.8*	*0*	*3.8*	*1.0*
TOMATO					
1 small whole	*19*	*4.2*	*1.2*	*3.0*	*0.9*
1 med whole	*26*	*5.7*	*1.6*	*4.1*	*1.2*
WATERMELON					
Flesh only, no skin					
1 oz.	*9*	*2*	*0.1*	*1.9*	*0.2*
1 cup balls	49	11.1	0.8	10.3	0.9
1 wedge, ⅙ fruit	92	20.6	1.4	19.2	1.7
WAX JAMBU (ROSE APPLE)					
1 Fruit, 2 oz.	*14*	*3.2*	*.6*	*2.6*	*0.3*

DRIED FRUIT

	Calories	Total Carb	Fiber	Usable Carb	Protein
APPLES					
5 rings	73	19.8	2.6	17.2	0.3
APRICOTS					
8 halves	68	17.5	2.6	14.9	1.0
BANANA CHIPS					
1.5 oz.	218	24.5	3.2	21.3	1.1
CRANBERRIES					
⅓ cup	130	33	2	31	0
CURRANTS					
1 Tbsp	40	10.4	1	9.4	0.6
DATES					
1 cup pitted	490	130.8	13.3	117.5	3.6
1 large California	31	8.4	0.9	7.5	0.2
FIGS					
1 fig	48	12.4	2.3	10.1	0.6
LONGANS					
1 oz.	81	21	.6	20.4	1.4
MIXED FRUIT					
1 oz.	69	18.2	2.2	16	0.7

	Calories	Total Carb	Fiber	Usable Carb	Protein
PEACHES					
½ fruit	31	8.0	1.1	6.9	0.5
PEARS					
½ fruit	47	12.5	1.3	11.2	0.3
PRUNES					
1 cup pitted	406	106.6	12.1	94.5	4.4
3 fruit	60	15.7	1.8	13.9	0.7
RAISINS					
Seeded: 1 oz.	84	22.3	1.3	21	0.7
1 cup packed	488	129.5	7.4	122.1	4.1
Seedless: 1 oz.	85	22.5	1.3	21.2	0.9
50 fruit	78	20.6	1.2	19.4	0.8
1 cup packed	495	130.6	7.4	123.2	4.9

CANNED FRUIT & SNACKS

CANNED/BOTTLED FRUIT

Solids and Liquids, Per ½ Cup:					
Apples: sweetened	68	17	1.7	15.3	0.2
Apricots,					
In water, w/o pits	*25*	*6.2*	*1.2*	*.5*	*0.8*
In light syrup	61	15.4	2.0	13.4	0.7
In heavy syrup	107	27.7	2.1	25.6	0.7
Black/Blueberries,					
In heavy syrup	113	28.2	1.9	26.3	0.8
Cherries, pitted,					
In water	57	14.6	1.9	12.7	1.0
In light syrup	84	21.8	1.9	19.9	0.8
In heavy syrup	105	26.9	1.9	25	0.8
Pie Filling, 2.5 oz.	85	20.7	0.4	20.3	0.4
Fruit Salad: In water	37	9.6	1.2	8.4	0.4
In juice	62	16.2	1.2	15	0.6
In heavy syrup	93	24.4	1.3	23.1	0.4
Gooseberries,					
In heavy syrup	92	23.6	3.0	20.6	0.8
Grapefruit, In juice	46	11.5	0.5	11	0.9
In light syrup	76	19.6	0.5	19.1	0.6
Mixed fruit: In heavy syrup	92	23.9	1.3	22.6	0.5
Pears, In water/diet	35	10	2.0	8	0.2
In juice	62	16	2.0	4	0.4
In heavy syrup	98	25.5	2.1	23.4	0.3

	Calories	Total Carb	Fiber	Usable Carb	Protein
Pineapples: All Types					
In water	39	10.2	1.0	9.2	0.5
In juice	75	19.5	1.0	18.5	0.5
In heavy syrup	99	25.7	1.0	24.7	0.4
Plums: In water	51	13.7	1.2	12.5	0.5
In juice	73	19.1	1.3	17.8	0.6
In light syrup	79	20.5	1.3	19.2	0.5
In heavy syrup	115	30	1.3	28.7	0.5
Prunes: In heavy syrup	123	32.5	4.4	28.1	1.0
Raspberries: In heavy syrup	116	29.9	4.2	25.7	1.1
Strawberries: In heavy syrup	117	29.9	2.2	27.7	0.7
Tropical Fruit Salad					
In heavy syrup	111	28.7	1.7	27	0.5

FRUIT SNACK CUPS

	Calories	Total Carb	Fiber	Usable Carb	Protein
Mott's, per 4 oz					
Healthy Harvest	50	13	1	12	0
Blue's Clues	90	23	1	22	0
Fruitsation	90	23	1	22	0
Del Monte Fruit Cups, per 4 oz					
Fruit Cocktail:					
In light syrup	55	13.7	0.9	12.8	0
In fruit juices	55	13.7	0.9	12.8	0
Manderin Oranges:					
In light syrup	72	17.1	0	17.1	0
Pears: In pear juice	55	13.7	0.9	12.8	0
Extra light syrup	55	13.7	0.9	12.8	0
Dole Fruit Bowls:					
Per 4 oz. bowl					
Sliced Peaches	69	16.6	1.1	15.5	0.3
Mixed Fruit	80	19	1	18	0.5
Pineapples	60	18	1	17	0.5
Per 7 oz. bowl:					
Pineapple chunks	90	24	2	22	0.5
Sliced peaches	120	29	2	27	0.5
Tropical fruit	104	25	1	24	1
Tree Top					
Fruit Rocketz, 1 tube	45	11	0	11	0
Natural Apple, 1 pkg, 4 oz.	50	12	2	10	0.5
Vons: Mixed Fruit:					
In light syrup	60	13	1	12	1

	Calories	Total Carb	Fiber	Usable Carb	Protein
APPLE & FRUIT SAUCES					
Apple Sauce:					
Regular/sweetened, 4 oz.	80	19.5	1.4	18.1	0.9
Cranberry Sauce:					
Sweetened, ½ cup	209	53.9	1.4	52.5	0.3

FRESH VEGETABLES

	Calories	Total Carb	Fiber	Usable Carb	Protein
ALFALFA SPROUTS					
½ cup	*5*	*0.6*	*0.4*	*0.2*	*0.7*
ARTICHOKES					
Globe/French: 1 medium	60	13.3	6.5	6.8	4.1
1 large	100	22.2	10.8	11.4	6.8
ASPARAGUS					
1 medium spear	*4*	*0.7*	*0.3*	*0.4*	*0.4*
BAMBOO SHOOTS					
½ cup	*41*	*7.9*	*3.3*	*4.6*	*3.9*
BEANS					
Green/Snap, ½ cup	*17*	*3.9*	*1.9*	*2*	*1.1*
Kidney, 1 oz.	95	17	7.1	9.9	6.7
Lima, 1 oz.	96	18	5.4	12.6	6.1
Pinto, 1 oz.	97	18	6.9	11.1	6.0
White, 1 oz.	95	17.1	4.3	12.8	6.7
BEET					
Cooked, 1 cup slices	75	17	3.4	13.6	2.7
BEET GREENS					
½ cup	*4*	*0.7*	*0.7*	*0*	*0.3*
BOK CHOY (CHINESE CHARD)					
3 oz.	*11*	*1.8*	*0.9*	*0.9*	*1.3*
BREADFRUIT					
¼ small	99	26.0	4.7	21.3	1.0
BROADBEANS (FAVA BEANS)					
½ cup	256	43.7	10.9	32.8	19.6
BROCCOLI					
Raw, ½ cup	*12*	*2.3*	*1.3*	*1*	*1.3*
Boiled, ½ cup	*22*	*3.9*	*2.3*	*1.6*	*2.3*
Brocco Sprouts, ½ cup	*16*	*1.9*	*1.1*	*.8*	*1.4*

	Calories	Total Carb	Fiber	Usable Carb	Protein
CABBAGE					
1 cup	*18*	*3.8*	*1.6*	*2.2*	*1.0*
CARROTS					
1 medium	31	7.3	2.2	5.1	0.7
CAULIFLOWER					
Raw, 15 oz	107	22.2	10.6	11.6	8.5
Cooked, 3 oz	*20*	*3.5*	*2.3*	*1.2*	*1.5*
CELERIAC					
½ cup	33	7.2	1.4	5.8	1.2
CELERY					
½ cup diced	*10*	*2.2*	*1.2*	*1.2*	*0.4*
CHARD (SWISS)					
½ cup	*3*	*0.7*	*0.3*	*0.4*	*0.3*
CHAYOTE SQUASH					
4 oz.	*22*	*5.1*	*1.9*	*3.2*	*0.9*
CHICK PEAS (GARBANZO BEANS)					
1 cup Raw	728	121.2	34.8	86.4	39
1 cup Boiled	269	44.9	12.5	32.4	14.8
CHICORY GREENS					
½ cup	*21*	*4.2*	*3.6*	*0.6*	*1.5*
CHIVES					
1 Tbsp	*1*	*01*	*0.1*	*0*	*0.1*
COLLARDS					
3 oz.	*26*	*4.9*	*3.1*	*1.8*	*2.0*
CORN					
Raw, sweet ½ cup	66	14.6	2.1	12.5	2.5
Sweet, boiled ¼ cup	44	10.3	1.1	9.2	1.4
CRESS					
Garden ½ cup	*8*	*1.4*	*.3*	*1.1*	*0.7*
CUCUMBER					
1 lg, 9.8 oz.	*34*	*7*	*3*	*4*	*1.6*
DAIKON RADISH					
2 Tbsp	40	9	3	6	1
DANDELION GREEN					
½ cup	*12*	*2.5*	*.5*	*2*	*0.8*

	Calories	Total Carb	Fiber	Usable Carb	Protein
EGGPLANT					
¼ med, 4 oz.	30	6.9	1.5	5.4	1.1
ENDIVE					
½ cup	4	.8	.2	.6	.3
FENNEL					
2 oz.	18	4.1	0	4.1	0.6
GARLIC					
1 clove	4	1	.1	0.9	.2
GINGER					
¼ cup	20	4.3	.3	4	.5
HORSERADISH					
1 pod 15⅓"	4	0.9	.1	.8	.2
JERUSALEM ARTICHOKE					
½ cup	57	13.1	.6	12.5	1.5
JICAMA					
½ cup	25	5.7	.4	5.3	.8
KALE					
½ cup	17	3.4	.5	2.9	1.1
KOHLRABI					
boiled, ½ cup	24	5.5	.9	4.6	1.5
LEEK					
boiled/drained, 4 oz.	35	8.6	.9	7.7	1.1
LENTILS					
raw 1 oz.	96	16.2	8.7	7.5	8.0
Boiled, 1 oz.	33	5.7	2.3	3.4	2.6
LETTUCE					
Butterhead, 1 oz.	4	.7	.3	.4	0.7
Romaine, ½ cup	4	0.7	.5	.2	0.5
Iceberg, 1 oz.	3	0.6	.3	.3	0.3
LOTUS ROOT					
10 slices	60	14.0	.8	13.2	2.0
MUNG BEAN SPROUTS					
½ cup	16	3.1	.6	2.5	1.6
MUSHROOM					
Raw, ½ cup	9	1.4	.5	0.9	1.0
Cooked/Boiled	21	4.0	1.7	2.3	1.6

	Calories	Total Carb	Fiber	Usable Carb	Protein
MUSTARD GREENS					
½ cup	7	1.4	.2	1.2	0.7
OKRA					
½ cup sliced	19	3.8	.5	3.3	1.0
ONIONS					
½ cup raw	30	6.9	1.3	5.6	.9
dehydrated flakes, 1 oz.	99	23.7	1.3	22.4	2.6
Rings, breaded/fried, 4 oz.	462	43.3	.5	42.8	6.1
Scallions, ½ cup	*16*	*3.7*	*1.2*	*2.5*	*1.0*
PARSLEY					
½ cup	11	1.9	1.3	1.6	0.9
PARSNIPS					
1 oz.	*21*	*5.1*	*.6*	*4.5*	*.3*
Boiled, 4 oz.	92	22.1	3.1	19	1.5
PEAS					
Raw, edible-podded, ½ cup	*21*	*3.7*	*1.9*	*1.8*	*1.5*
Boiled/drained, 4 oz.	95	17.7	4.2	13.5	6.1
Split, raw, 1 oz.	97	17.1	1.6	15.5	7.0
Split, boiled, 4 oz.	134	23.9	2.6	21.3	9.5
Snow Peas, 3 oz. (Birds Eye)	*35*	*6.0*	*3.0*	*3.0*	*2.0*
PEPPERS					
Bell/sweet, 1 med	32	7.7	2.4	5.3	1.2
chopped, 1¾ oz.	*13*	*3.2*	*1.0*	*2.2*	*0.5*
Chile: Green/Red					
1 pepper, 1.5 oz.	*18*	*4.3*	*.8*	*3.5*	*0.9*
PIGEON PEAS					
Boiled, ½ cup	102	19.5	5.6	13.9	5.9
Poi, ½ cup	134	32.7	.7	32	0.6
PUMPKIN					
Mashed, ½ cup	25	6.0	1.0	5.0	0.9
PURSLANE					
Cooked, ½ cup	*10*	*2.0*	*.5*	*1.5*	*0.9*
POTATOES					
Raw w/ skin, 1 lb	269	61.2	5.4	55.8	7.1
Baked w/ skin	220	51	1.3	49.7	5.0
Mashed w/ milk and margarine, ½ cup	110	17.5	.3	17.2	2.1

	Calories	Total Carb	Fiber	Usable Carb	Protein
Hash Browns:					
w/ butter, ½ cup	163	16.6	.3	16.3	2.1
French Fried, frozen, heated in oven, 10 strips	111	17.0	2.1	18	1.7
Pancake, 4 oz.	738	39.3	.7	38.6	6.9
Scalloped, dry, 5.5 oz.	558	115.3	2.2	113.1	12.1
Salad, (home prepared), ½ cup	179	14.0	.5	13.5	3.4
RADISH					
½ cup slices	*10*	*2.1*	*.3*	*1.8*	*.4*
RUTABAGAS					
½ cup	25	5.7	0	5.7	.7
SALSIFY					
raw, trimmed, ½ cup	55	12.5	1.2	11.3	2.2
SAUERKRAUT					
Undrained, ½ cup	*22*	*5.1*	*1.3*	*3.8*	*1.0*
SEAWEED					
dried, Agar, 1 oz.	87	23	.2	22.8	1.6
SHALLOTS					
1 Tbsp	*7*	*1.7*	*.1*	*1.6*	*0.3*
SOYBEANS					
raw 1 oz.	118	8.6	2.6	6.0	10.4
boiled, 1 C	*149*	*8.5*	*5.2*	*3.3*	*14.2*
SPINACH					
Boiled/drained, ½ cup	*21*	*3.4*	*2.0*	*1.4*	*2.7*
Raw, 1 lb	*73*	*11.4*	*8.5*	*2.9*	*9.3*
SQUASH, WINTER					
cubes, ½ cup	*21*	*5.1*	*1.0*	*4.1*	*.8*
SUCCOTASH					
1 oz.	*28*	*5.6*	*.7*	*4.9*	*1.4*
SWEET POTATOES					
Baked in skin, no salt: 2.1 oz.	62	14.5	1.8	12.7	1.0
Boiled/mashed: ½ cup	172	39.9	3.0	36.9	2.6
Taro, cooked, ½ C	94	22	.6	21.4	0.3
TOMATO:					
1 small whole	*19*	*4.2*	*1.2*	*3*	*.8*
1 medium	*26*	*5.7*	*1.6*	*4.1*	*1.0*

	Calories	Total Carb	Fiber	Usable Carb	Protein
Boiled, ripe/red, ½ cup	32	7.0	1.0	6.0	1.3
TURNIPS					
raw ½ Cup	*18*	*4.1*	*1.2*	*2.9*	*.6*
WATERCRESS					
½ cup	*2*	*.2*	*.4*	*0*	*.4*
YAMS					
Mountain, raw, cubed, ½ cup	46	11.1	.3	10.8	.9
YUCCA ROOT					
½ cup	60	13.5	1.2	12.3	14.6
ZUCCHINI					
Baby raw, 10 oz.	58	9.0	3.2	5.8	7.7
Boiled/drained, 3 oz.	*13*	*3.3*	*1.2*	*2.1*	*0.6*

FROZEN VEGETABLES

BIRDS EYE					
Baby:					
Bean & Carrot Blend, 1 oz	*10*	*1.7*	*0.7*	*1*	*0.3*
Broccoli Florets, 1 cup	*24*	*6*	*2*	*4*	*0*
Corn & Bean, 3 oz.	65	12	2	10	3
Tiny Tender Peas, ¾ cup	40	10	2	8	0
White Corn, ⅔ cup	109	22	3	19	3
Hearty Spoonfull Soup Bowls: (per 1 bowl)					
Cheesy Cream of Broccoli	230	25	6	19	9
Chick of Noodle	140	19	2	17	11
Italian Minestrone	240	37	7	30	11

GREEN GIANT					
Vegetables:					
Asparagus Cuts, 1 cup	*38*	*4.5*	*3*	*1.5*	*3*
Corn:					
Nibblers, 1 Ear	70	14	1	13	2
Extra Sweet Niblets, 1 cup	150	30	6	24	6
Honey Glazed Carrots, 4 oz	89	12.8	2.0	10.8	0
Spinach, ½ C	*30*	*3*	*2*	*1*	*3*
Veges in Cheese & Cream Sauce: per cup					
Alfredo Vegetable	107	12.0	4.0	8.0	5.3

	Calories	Total Carb	Fiber	Usable Carb	Protein
Broccoli/Cheese	105	13.5	3	10.5	4.5
Broc/Cauliflower, Carrots,	105	15	3	12	4.5
Cauliflower/Cheese	120	16	2	14	4
Creamed Spinach	160	18	2	16	6
Green Bean Casserole	135	13.5	.3	13.2	3
Cream Corn	220	46	4	42	4
Rice & Vegetables:					
per 10 oz					
Cheesey Rice & Broccoli	301	56.2	2.0	54.2	8.0
Oriental Rice	341	52.2	4.0	48.2	7.0
Rice Medley	280	52	4.0	48	8.0
Rice Pilaf	230	44	3	41	6
White & Wild Rice	280	51	3	49	6

WILD OATS

	Calories	Total Carb	Fiber	Usable Carb	Protein
Oven Fries, 3 oz.	142	24.3	2.0	22.3	2.0
Potato Poppers 3 oz.	138	14.2	0	14.2	2.0

CANNED/BOTTLED VEGETABLES
(SOLIDS & LIQUIDS)

ARTICHOKE HEARTS

	Calories	Total Carb	Fiber	Usable Carb	Protein
Marinated, 1 oz.	53	1.8	0	1.8	0

ASPARAGUS

	Calories	Total Carb	Fiber	Usable Carb	Protein
½ cup	24	3.0	2.0	1.0	2.6

BAMBOO SHOOTS

	Calories	Total Carb	Fiber	Usable Carb	Protein
4½ oz.	24	4.1	1.8	2.3	2.2

BEANS

Per ½ cup unless indicated	Calories	Total Carb	Fiber	Usable Carb	Protein
Green	15	3.3	2.5	0.8	0.7
Baked Beans	118	26	6.3	19.7	6.3
Butter, 4½ oz.	91	16.1	4.0	12.1	6.0
Italian Cut	30	6	3	3	1
Kidney	104	18.9	4.5	14.4	6.4
Lima	95	18.1	5.8	12.3	6.0
Pinto	103	18.3	5.5	12.8	6.0

BEETS

	Calories	Total Carb	Fiber	Usable Carb	Protein
Whole ½ cup	25	5.9	1.4	4.5	0.7

CARROTS

	Calories	Total Carb	Fiber	Usable Carb	Protein
Sliced, ½ cup	37	8.0	2.2	5.8	0.9

	Calories	Total Carb	Fiber	Usable Carb	Protein
CORN					
Kernels, ½ cup	82	19.7	0.9	18.8	2.6
Creamed Style, ½ cup	92	23.2	1.5	21.7	2.2
CHICK PEAS (GARBANZO BEANS)					
3 oz.	143	27.1	5.3	21.8	6
MUSHROOMS					
½ cup	*19*	*3.9*	*1.9*	*2*	*1.6*
ONIONS					
½ cup	*21*	*4.5*	*1.2*	*3.3*	*1.0*
PEAS					
½ cup	61	11.1	2.5	8.6	3.7
PEPPERS					
Hot Chili, 4 oz.	28	6.9	1.4	5.5	1.0
Bell, sweet, 1 oz.	*5*	*1.1*	*0.3*	*0.8*	*0.3*
Jalapeno, ½ cup chop	*17*	*3.3*	*1.6*	*1.7*	*.5*
SAUERKRAUT					
undrained, ½ cup	*22*	*5.1*	*1.3*	*3.8*	*1.0*
SPINACH					
½ cup	*22*	*3.4*	*1.1*	*2.3*	*2.5*
SUCCOTASH					
Boiled/Drained, ½ cup	111	23.4	1.3	22.1	4.9
SWEET POTATO					
1 cup	258	59.2	4.3	53.9	5.1
Candied, 4 oz.	156	31.6	2.7	28.9	0.9
VEGETABLES					
Mixed/Drained, ½ cup	44	8.7	1.5	7.2	1.7

SALADS

	Calories	Total Carb	Fiber	Usable Carb	Protein
FRESH SALAD PACKS					
Pre-Packaged (Supermarkets)					
Dole: Greener Selection,					
1 bag, 12 oz.	60	12.0	4.0	8.0	4.0
Fresh Express: Salad Kits					
(per 1 cup Prepared)					
Caesar	116	6	0.7	5.3	2.0
Caesar w/ light Dressing	43	9.3	0.7	8.6	1.3
Caesar Supreme	*107*	*5.3*	*0.7*	*4.6*	*2.0*

	Calories	Total Carb	Fiber	Usable Carb	Protein
Oriental	141	13	2	11	2
Greener European	*11*	*2*	*0.7*	*1.3*	*0.7*

SALAD TOPPINGS

	Calories	Total Carb	Fiber	Usable Carb	Protein
Bacon Bits, Average, 1 Tbsp	30	0	0	0	3.0
Chow Mein Noodles, 1 cup	237	25.9	1.8	24.1	3.8
Croutons, 2 Tbsp	*20*	*3.7*	*0.3*	*3.4*	*0.6*
Potato Chips, 1 oz.	152	15.1	1.4	13.7	2.0
Sunflower Seeds, 8 oz.	*46*	*1.5*	*0.8*	*0.7*	*1.8*
Tortilla Chips, 1 oz.	141	17	1.5	15.5	2.2

FRUIT & VEGETABLE DRINKS & JUICES
(PER 8 FL. OZ. UNLESS INDICATED)

JUICES, AVERAGE ALL BRANDS

	Calories	Total Carb	Fiber	Usable Carb	Protein
Apple, unsweet	117	29	0	29	0
Carrot, canned	91	21.1	1.8	19.3	2.3
Cranberry cocktail	137	34.8	0.2	34.6	0

FRUIT, PREMIUM BLENDS

	Calories	Total Carb	Fiber	Usable Carb	Protein
All Flavors	120	29	0	29	1
Grape Juice	120	31.2	0.2	31	0.2
Grapefruit, unsweetened	94	22.1	0	22.1	1.2
Lemon/Lime, 1 Tbsp	*3*	*1*	*01*	*0.9*	*0.1*
Orange Juice	95	22.4	0.5	21.9	1.1
Peach Nectar	123	32	0	32	1.1
Pear Nectar	150	39.3	1.5	37.8	0.3
Prune Juice	170	41.9	2.4	39.5	1.2
Tangerine Juice	98	22.9	0.5	22.4	-1.1
Tomato Juice	39	9.6	1.8	7.8	2.3

JUICE BRANDS
(PER 8 FL. OZ. UNLESS INDICATED)

ARIZONA

	Calories	Total Carb	Fiber	Usable Carb	Protein
Honey Lemon	90	22	0	22	0
Pina Colada	140	34	0	34	0

CAMPBELL'S

	Calories	Total Carb	Fiber	Usable Carb	Protein
Tomato Juice	35	7	1	6	1
V-8 Splash Fruit	110	28	0	28	0

CAPRI SUN

	Calories	Total Carb	Fiber	Usable Carb	Protein
All Natural Fruit	90	24	0	24	0
Sport Drink, Berry Ice/ *Thunder, 1 pouch*	*124*	*31*	*31*	*0*	*0*

	Calories	Total Carb	Fiber	Usable Carb	Protein
DEL MONTE					
Pineapple Juice,					
Not from Concentrate	110	29	2	27	1
From Concentrate	108	13.6	0	13.6	0
Tomato Juice,					
Not from Concentrate	40	7	0	7	3
From Concentrate	50	10	1	9	2
Snap E-Tom Cocktail	54	10.8	1.4	9.4	2.7
Fruit Smoothie Blenders:					
Pineapple, Banana, Orange	281	68.9	1.3	67.6	1.3
Peach-Raspberry	225	66.4	5.1	61.3	2.6
EDEN ORGANIC APPLE					
2 Tbsp	112	28	0	28	0
FIVE ALIVE					
Citrus Beverage	115	29	0	29	0
FRESH SAMANTHA					
Big Bang	*110*	*8*	*8*	*0*	*2*
Carrot/Orange	*110*	*8*	*4*	*4*	*4*
Grapefruit	90	7	0	7	1
Mango Mama	*120*	*10*	*8*	*2*	*2*
Rasp/Dream	*120*	*10*	*8*	*2*	*2*
Protein Blast	*100*	*10*	*8*	*2*	*2*
Desperately Seeking C	*110*	*9*	*7*	*2*	*4*
FRUITOPIA					
Fruit Integration	111	25	0	25	0
Tremendously Tangerine	109	29	0	29	0
HANSEN'S					
Natural Juice Cocktail Apple	110	28	0	28	0
Lite: Cran/Rasp	37	9.6	0	9.6	0
Energy Island Blast	117	28.8	0	28.8	0
HI-C FRUIT DRINKS					
Pink Lemonade	105	26	0	26	0
JERA'S JUICE					
Per 24 oz.					
Blueberry Blitz	452	104.5	4.8	99.7	4.0
Cape Codder	388	79.9	3.0	76.9	3.0
Citrus Burst	363	84.4	4.2	80.2	3.3
Flu Fighter	292	66.9	3.8	63.1	3.6
Mango Passion	286	67.9	2.3	65.6	2.9

	Calories	Total Carb	Fiber	Usable Carb	Protein
Orange Bite	282	62	5.4	56.6	4.8
Razzle Dazzle	396	94.2	3.7	90.5	2.8
Strawberry Smile	354	83.7	3.9	79.8	3.5
Triathlete	357	71.4	5.5	65.9	15
Whey-Out Protein	343	55.5	5.4	50.1	26.9
KOOL AID					
Fruit Punch powder,					
Per serving, Unsweetened	*1*	*0.1*	*0*	*0.1*	*0*
Sweetened	64	16.3	0	16.3	0
Jammers Fruit Drink					
All Flavors 6.7 oz.	*96*	*24*	*24*	*0*	*0*
Sugar Free Fruit Drinks,					
24 oz.	*15*	*3*	*0*	*3*	*0*
KNUDSEN					
Apricot Nectar	120	30	0	30	0.5
Cream Papaya	140	10	0	10	0.5
Guava Strawberry	110	27	0	27	0.5
Just Blueberry	100	24	0	24	0
Just Boysenberry	90	23	0	23	1
Nat. Breakfast	110	27	0	27	0.5
Rasp. Peach	150	31	0	31	0.5
Razzleberry	130	33	0	33	0.5
Simply Nutritous:					
Blackberry Hibiscus Mist	100	24	0	24	1
Ginseng Boost	110	27	0	27	0.5
Inner Strength	108	26	0	26	1
MAUNA LA'I HAWAIIAN					
Guava Juice	*130*	*32*	*0*	*0*	*0*
MINUTE MAID					
Orange Juice	114	28	0	28	0
Premium Blends	120	29	0	29	0
Juices to Go	180	45	0	45	0
MOUNTAIN SUN ORGANIC					
Black Cherry	120	30	0	30	0
Lemonade: Wild Cranberry	110	27	0	27	0.5
Plain Apple Spice	120	30	0	30	0
NAKED JUICE					
Carrot-O-Copia	80	13	0	13	2
Orange, Carrot/Banana	120	27	0	27	1

	Calories	Total Carb	Fiber	Usable Carb	Protein
Power C	120	29	0	29	1
Tangerine	110	25	0	25	1
Soy Shakes: Choc	210	38	0	38	9
Vanilla	170	33	0	33	8
NANTUCKET NECTAR					
100% Juices, per serving					
Apple Raspberry	140	34	0	34	0
Grape Juice	160	39	0	39	0
Orange Passion	120	29	0	29	0
Pineapple, Orange & Banana	140	35	0	35	0
Premium Orange	170	28	0	28	0
Ruby Red Grapefruit	100	25	0	25	0
Original Peach	120	30	0	30	0
Juice Cocktails					
Cranberry	140	34	0	34	0
Cranberry Melon	110	28	0	28	0
Guava	130	33	0	33	0
Diet Green Tea	*5*	*1*	*0*	*1*	*0*
Diet Iced Tea	*5*	*1*	*0*	*1*	*0*
Fruit Punch	130	32	0	32	0
Grapeade	130	33	0	33	0
Kiwi Berry	120	30	0	30	0
Orange Mango	130	32	0	32	0
Papaya	120	30	0	30	0
Pineapple, Orange & Guava	120	31	0	31	0
Watermelon/Strawberry	120	31	0	31	0
Authentic Pink Lemonade	120	30	0	30	0
Super Nectars:					
Chili Green Tea	90	23	0	23	0
Gingko Mango	150	36	0	36	0
Green Angel	140	15	0	15	0
Protein Smoothie	170	38	0	38	2
Red Guarana Tea	110	26	0	26	0
Strawberry Smoothie	120	30	0	30	1
Vital C	130	32	0	32	0.5
Vitamin Smoothie	110	27	0	27	0
NEWMAN'S OWN					
Lemonade, 10 oz	140	34	0	34	0
OCEAN SPRAY					
Apple Juice	110	28	0	28	0

	Calories	Total Carb	Fiber	Usable Carb	Protein
Black Cherry Blast	140	33	0	33	0
Cranberry Grape	170	41	0	41	0
Cranberry Juice Cocktail	140	34	0	34	0
Fruit Punch	130	32	0	32	0
Grapefruit, Ruby Red	130	33	0	33	0
Lemonade, Pink	130	32	0	32	0
Orange Juice from concentrate	120	31	0	31	0
Kiwi Strawberry	120	31	0	31	0
Ruby Red & Strawberry	140	34	0	34	0
ODWALLA					
Carrot, Orange, Apple	100	23	0	23	2
C Monster	300	72	0	72	3
Femme Vitale	130	29	0	29	3.5
Fruitshake Blackberry	160	49	0	49	0
Grapefruit Juice	90	34	0	34	0
Lemonade	90	24	0	24	0
Orange Juice	120	34	0	34	0
Soy Milkshake	160	27	0	27	6.5
ORANGE JULIUS					
Per 16 oz.					
Original Orange	230	54	1	53	1
Pina Colada	350	70	3	67	2
Strawberry	235	57	1	56	1
Raspberry Cream	428	84.8	1.6	83.2	8.0
Tropi-Coloda	440	88	2.4	85.6	8.0
PS—PRIVATE SELECTION (RALPHS)					
Vegetable Juice Blend Cocktail	50	12	1	11	2
SNAPPLE					
Diet Ice Tea	*4*	*1*	*0*	*1*	*0*
Kiwi Strawberry Cocktail	114	28.3	0	28.3	0.2
Elements Volcano	135	34	0	34	0
TANG					
Orange Flavored Mix Prepared, 8 oz.	92	24.6	0.1	24.5	0
Fruit Frenzy Pouch	100	26	0	26	0
Sugar-Free Orange Mix, 8 oz.	*5*	*2.1*	*0.1*	*2*	*0.1*

	Calories	Total Carb	Fiber	Usable Carb	Protein
TREE OF LIFE					
Black Cherry	180	43	0	43	2
Cranberry Nectar	150	38	0	38	1
TROPICANA					
Orange Juice	100	24	0	24	1
Twister: Orange, Strawberry/Banana	458	111.6	0	111.6	1.0
V-8 SPLASH					
Diet Berry Blend	*10*	*3*	*0*	*3*	*0*
Splash Smoothie Peach Mango	120	27	0	27	3
VERYFINE					
Apple Raspberry Cherry Cocktail	126	31.2	0	31.2	0.2
WELSH'S					
Healthy Tropical Sensation	120	30	0	30	0
Mixed Berry Smoothie	175	43.0	1.5	41.5	0
Straw/ Banana Smoothie	175	43.0	1.5	41.5	0
WILD OATS					
Beautiful Juices	108	27	0	27	0
Down to Earth	136	34	0	34	0

NUTRITIONAL SHAKES/DRINKS
(PER 8 FL. OZ. UNLESS INDICATED)

BRANDS	Calories	Total Carb	Fiber	Usable Carb	Protein
ABB, Nutritional Shake, Pure Pro Chocolate, 12 oz	*175*	*6*	*2*	*4*	*35*
All Sport, All Flavors	70	18	0	18	0
AMP Energy Drink	120	32	0	32	0
Arbonne Meal Shakes (prepared w/ 7 oz water) Vanilla, 1 serving	193	24	1	23	14
Atkins: Shake Mix, per 2 scoops,					
Cappuccino	*170*	*2*	*0*	*2*	*24*
Chocolate	*180*	*3*	*2*	*1*	*24*
Strawberry/Vanilla	*170*	*1*	*0*	*1*	*24*
Biochem Shakes, Per 2 scoops	*100*	*5*	*1*	*4*	*20*

	Calories	Total Carb	Fiber	Usable Carb	Protein
Blue Thunder, 2 fl. oz.	400	68	0	68	32
Boost, High Protein, 1 cup	240	33	0	33	13.5
Carb Mate, 16 oz	28	7	0	7	0
Carnation Instant Breakfast, 1 envelope	130	28	0	28	2.5
CeraSport, 11 oz	68	17	0	17	0
Champion Nutrition Lemon Drink, 4 oz	409	56.8	0	56.8	30.7
Choice Choc Drink	220	24	3	21	9
Cytomax	80	20	0	20	0
Designer Whey	*88*	*0.5*	*0*	*0.5*	*20.3*
Endura, 8.3 oz	112	28	0	28	0
Ensure, Enlive	300	65	0	65	10
Exceed, 12 oz	105	26	0	26	0
4Kick Energy 8.5 oz	133	29.3	0	29.3	0
G-Up	211	51.8	0	51.8	0
Gatorade Frost	50	14	0	14	0
Nutritional Shake	273	45.8	0.7	45.1	13.3
Genisoy Shake, 1 scoop	128	18	0	18	14
Hansen's Energy Drink, 1 Can	144	30	0	30	0
Health Source Soy, 2 scoops	125	8	0	8	20
Herbalife (Thermogetics), 1 oz	100	14	0	14	8.8
Hydra Fuel	65	16	0	16	0
Isopure, 3.1 oz pkt	300	25	0	25	50
Jevity w/ fiber	253	37.0	3.4	33.6	10.5
Kashi GoLean Shakes, Choc., 2 Scoops	220	31	7	24	22
Powdered, 1 pkt	250	32	7	25	30
Kombucha, Wonder Drink 1 Bottle, 8.5 oz	60	15	0	15	0
Lipovitan, 8.5 oz	116	29	0	29	0
Mass Recovery	152	24	0	24	14
Metabolol, 2 scoops	230	11	0	11	42
Myoplex, Carb Sense Shake	*109*	*3.6*	*1.5*	*2.1*	*18.2*
Original	120	9.4	2.8	6.6	19.8
Low Carb Sense	*87*	*1.5*	*1.5*	*0*	*14.5*
Nitro Speed Drink	*49*	*3.1*	*0*	*3.1*	*9.1*
Nutrament	248	35.7	0	35.7	11
Optifast Powder, 1 serving	160	20	0	20	14
Power Dream, X-Treme Choc	204	34.9	1.5	33.4	7.3
Vanilla Blast	175	28.4	1.5	26.9	7.3

	Calories	Total Carb	Fiber	Usable Carb	Protein
Powerade, Rev-up	28	7.2	0	7.2	0
PowerBar Gel, 1 Serving	110	28	0	28	0
ProBalance	300	39	2.5	36.5	13.5
Pro-Cal 100, 1 Pkt	103	7	0.4	6.6	14
Pure Pro, 1 Bottle	*170*	*1*	*0*	*1*	*40*
Recharge Drink	70	18	0	18	0.5
Red Bull Energy	110	26.9	0	26.9	0
Resource Plus 1 Pkt	360	52	0	52	13
Standard	250	40	0	40	9
Fruit Beverage	180	36	0	36	9
Revenge Pro, 2 scoops	*160*	*1.5*	*0*	*1.5*	*34*
Revival Soy, Per Pkg					
Plain	*100*	*2*	*0*	*2*	*20*
Choc Daydream	240	36	2	34	20
Choc unsweetened	130	7	2	5	20
Slim-Fast Shakes, per Can					
Juice Based	220	46	5	41	7
Milk Based	220	40	5	35	10
Soy Protein Mix,					
1.7 oz serving	180	26	5	21	15
Powder Mix, 1 scoop	100	20	2	18	5
Ultra Slim-Fast, with					
Cup Fat Free Milk	220	44	5	39	11.5
SoBe Energy Power	130	32	0	32	0
Juice Elixer	96	24	0	24	0
Solaray Soytein (Protein					
Energy Meal), Per Scoop					
All Flavors	117	13	2	11	14
Natural	*81*	*5*	*1*	*4*	*14*
Spiru-Tein, Vanilla, 1 Serving	225	23	1	22	22
Synergy, Per Bottle,					
Mystic Mango	100	24	0	24	1
Tahitian Noni Shakes,					
Per 2 scoops	*140*	*7*	*4*	*3*	*21*
Total Balance, 9.5 oz					
Vanilla Drink	230	25	1	24	15
Usana, Per 2 Scoops					
Fibergy Drink	150	31	12	19	3
SoyaMax	*110*	*1*	*1*	*0*	*24*
Venom Energy	125	27.8	0	27.8	3.4
Vitamin Water	480	108	0	108	0

	Calories	Total Carb	Fiber	Usable Carb	Protein
Vita-Trim Shake, 2 oz. pkt	210	26	0	26	22
Walgreens Nutritional					
Slim Drink 1 Can	227	40	5	35	10
Weider (Powders)					
Creatine, 1 cup	208	37	0	37	15
Lean Pro, 1 cup	160	20	0	20	20
Body Shaper Pkt	140	8	2	6	25
Cell Recovery, 2 Scoops	200	25	0	25	25
Mass 1000, 1 cup	566	109.5	2.3	107.2	25.5
Worldwide, Per 20 oz.					
Carbo Rush	280	60	0	60	10
Fat Shredder	*0*	*0*	*0*	*0*	*0*
Fiber Filler	*20*	*0*	*15*	*0*	*5*
Pure Protein	*170*	*0*	*0*	*0*	*42.5*
XS Energy	*8*	*0*	*0*	*0*	*1.9*

SOFT DRINKS/SODA
(PER 12 FL. OZ. UNLESS INDICATED)

A&W					
Orange	153	38.2	0	38.2	0
BARQ'S					
Root Beer	167	42	0	42	0
COCA-COLA					
Classic	146	36	0	36	0
Cherry Coke	156	39	0	39	0
Diet, no caffeine	*1*	*0*	*0*	*0*	*0*
CRYSTAL LIGHT					
12 fl. oz.	*8*	*0*	*0*	*0*	*0*
DR. PEPPER					
Regular	145	36.3	0	36.0	0
FANTA					
Orange	177	45	0	45	0
Grape	176	43.5	0	43.5	0
FRESCA					
12 fl. oz.	*3*	*0.8*	*0*	*0.8*	*0*
HANSEN'S SODA					
Average all flavors	165	45	0	45	0
Natural Lemonade	150	39	0	39	0

	Calories	Total Carb	Fiber	Usable Carb	Protein
HEALTH VALLEY					
Ginger Ale	160	40	0	40	0
Root Beer	160	40	0	40	0
IBC ROOT BEER					
12 fl. oz.	237	62.6	0	62.6	0
MELLO YELLO					
Regular	177	43.5	0	43.5	0
Diet	*5*	*1.1*	*0*	*1.1*	*0*
MINUTE MAID					
Diet Orange	*3*	*0.8*	*0*	*0.8*	*0*
Black Cherry	174	43.5	0	43.5	0
Fruit Punch	170	42	0	42	0
Strawberry	170	42	0	42	0
Peach	165	41.3	0	41.3	0
Grape	170	42	0	42	0
Pink Grapefruit	186	46.5	0	46.5	0
MOUNTAIN DEW					
12 fl. oz.	170	45.8	0	45.8	0
MR. PIBB					
12 fl. oz	150	37	0	37	0
PEPSI					
Regular	148	31.8	0	38.1	0
Diet	*0*	*0*	*0*	*0*	*0*
Sierra Mist	150	39	0	39	0
Wild Pepsi	161	40.4	0	40.4	0
PERRIER					
6.5 oz.	*0*	*0*	*0*	*0*	*0*
SEVEN-UP					
12 fl. oz.	114	28.5	0	28.5	0
SPRITE					
Regular	114	29.7	0	29.7	0
Diet	*3*	*0.8*	*0*	*0.8*	*0*
SURGE					
12 fl. 0z.	174	43.5	0	43.5	0
TAB					
12 fl. oz.	*2*	*0.4*	*0*	*0.4*	*0*

	Calories	Total Carb	Fiber	Usable Carb	Protein
THINK					
Root Beer	170	41.8	0	41.8	0
Cola	161	41.8	0	41.8	0
Sparkling Citrus	187	44.6	0	44.6	0
WILD OATS					
Down to Earth	148	37	0	37	0
COFFEE					
INSTANT COFFEE					
Powder/Granules:					
Regular or Decaffeinated					
1 tsp	*2*	*0.5*	*0*	*0.5*	*0*
Ground, 1 cup	*5*	*1*	*0*	*1*	*0*
Brewed/Percolated, 1 cup	*5*	*1*	*0*	*1*	*0*
FLAVORED COFFEE MIXES					
Caffe' D'Vita: 1 tsp					
Coffee Essence	*16*	*4*	*0*	*4*	*0*
General Foods Int'l Regular	63	9	0	9	0
Sugar-free	*30*	*3*	*0*	*3*	*0*
Maxwell House, per envelope					
Mocha	100	17	0	17	2
Mocha sugar free	60	7	0	7	1
Vanilla	90	19	0	19	1
Nescafé Frothe, per 8 fl. oz					
Choc Mocha	80	16	1	15	1
COFFEE SUBSTITUTE MIXES					
Roasted Cereal Beverages					
(No Caffeine), per tsp:					
Cafix Instant	*6*	*1*	*0*	*1*	*0*
Kaffree Roma	*6*	*1*	*0*	*1*	*0.5*
Teeccino Caffe	*10*	*2*	*0*	*2*	*0*
COFFEE SHOPS/RESTAURANTS					
Per 8 oz. cup unless indicated					
Americano Drip Coffee	*5*	*1*	*0*	*1*	*0.5*
Café Au Lait, w/ whole milk	75	6	0	6	4
Caffe Latte: w/ whole milk	135	11	0	11	7.5
w/ 2 % milk	110	11	0	11	7.5
w/ nonfat milk	80	11.5	0	11.5	7.5
Café Mocha	200	27.2	0	27.2	2.4

	Calories	Total Carb	Fiber	Usable Carb	Protein
Cappuccino: w/ whole milk	70	6	0	6	3.5
w/ 2% milk	60	6	0	6	4.5
w/ skim milk	40	6	0	6	4
Iced Mocha	105	16.5	0	16.5	3.5
Low Fat	90	16	0	16	3.5
Espresso Regular	*3*	*0.5*	*0*	*0.5*	*0*
Espresso Double	*5*	*1*	*0*	*1*	*0.5*
Espresso w/ whipped cream	*45*	*1.5*	*0*	*1.5*	*0*
Espresso Macchiato	*8*	*1*	*0*	*1*	*0.5*
Frappuccino Mocha	145	30.5	0	30.5	2.5
Iced Latte w/ milk	80	6.5	0	6.5	4.5
IRISH & LIQUEUR COFFEES					
Irish Coffee					
1 standard cocktail	210	8	0	8	0
Coffee Liqueur, Per 1.5 oz.					
Jigger, 53 Proof	185	25.9	0	25.9	0.1
COCOA & HOT CHOCOLATE					
Cocoa: per 8 oz. cup					
w/ whole milk &					
whipped cream	210	19	0	19	2
w/ nonfat milk &					
whipped cream	*80*	*2*	*0*	*2*	*0*
Hot Chocolate: per 8 oz. cup					
w/ whole milk	200	25	0	25	2.5
w/ skim milk	140	25	0	25	5.5
COFFEE EXTRAS,					
Powdered Cocoa ½ tsp	*6*	*1.5*	*0.9*	*0.6*	*0.5*
Flavored Syrup, 2 Tbsp	70	17	0	17	0.5
Sugar Free	*0*	*0*	*0*	*0*	*0*
Hershey's Choc Syrup, 1 Tbsp	50	12	0	12	0.5
Half & Half, 1 Tbsp	*20*	*0.5*	*0*	*0.5*	*0.5*
Whipped Cream, 1 Tbsp	*8*	*0.4*	*0*	*0.4*	*0.1*
Marshmallows, 10 miniature	22	5.7	0	5.7	0.1
BOTTLED COFFEE					
Nescafe: Per 8 oz. cup					
Mocha Cooler	150	23	0	23	7
Frothes: Butterfinger:					
Per 0.7 oz.	83	13	0	13	1
Starbucks: Per 9.5 oz. Bottle:					
All Types	190	40	0	40	45

	Calories	Total Carb	Fiber	Usable Carb	Protein
TEA & ICED TEA					
TEAS					
Regular: Bag, Loose or instant					
Per 1 cup					
Brewed	*1*	*0*	*0*	*0*	*0*
Herbal, All Types	*4*	*1*	*0*	*1*	*0*
Bigelow: Apple Orchard	*5*	*1*	*0*	*1*	*0.5*
ICED TEA MIXES					
Per 1 cup serving, prepared					
4C Instant	90	22	0	22	0
Bigelow, Nice Over Ice	*1*	*0.5*	*0*	*0.5*	*0*
Crystal Light, Sugar Free	*3*	*0.4*	*0*	*0.4*	*0.1*
Kool-Aid, Per envelope					
Fruit T's	70	17	0	17	0
Lipton: Instant					
Lemon/Raspberry	*3*	*1*	*0*	*1*	*0*
Peach/Raspberry					
sugar-free	*5*	*1*	*0*	*1*	*0.5*
Nestea:					
100% instant	*2*	*0*	*0*	*0*	*0*
Decaffeinated	*6*	*1*	*0*	*1*	*0*
Ice Teasers	*6*	*1*	*0*	*1*	*0*
Peach/Raspberry	90	22	0	22	0
BOTTLED & CANNED TEAS					
Per 8 fl. oz unless indicated					
Arizona:					
Honey Lemon	90	22	0	22	0
Green Tea	70	18	0	18	0
Diet Green	*0*	*0.5*	*0*	*0.5*	*0*
Brisk: Regular	70	20	0	20	0
Unsweetened	*0*	*0*	*0*	*0*	*0*
Hansen's Original	71	21	0	21	0
Low Calorie	*10*	*3*	*0*	*3*	*0*
Lipton					
Regular mix	*0*	*0*	*0*	*0*	*0*
w/ Lemon	55	14	0	14	0
Peach/Raspberry,					
Sugar-free	*5*	*1*	*0*	*1*	*0.5*
Nantucket					
Blueberry Tea	80	19	0	19	0.5

	Calories	Total Carb	Fiber	Usable Carb	Protein
Original Lemon	90	23	0	23	0.5
Half & Half	100	25	0	25	0
Diet Lemon	*10*	*2.5*	*0*	*2.5*	*0*
Nestea Iced Tea					
Diet Lemon	*2*	*0.1*	*0*	*0.1*	*0*
Cool	82	20	0	20	0
Diet Cool	*2*	*0.2*	*0*	*0.2*	*0*
Peach	78	21	0	21	0
Snapple, Diet	*4*	*1*	*0*	*1*	*0*
SoBe: Green Tea	90	24	0	24	0
Black Tea	100	28	0	28	0

BEERS, ALES, MALT LIQUORS

BEER BRANDS

Per 12 fl. oz. Serving
Percentage alcohol listed below
is by volume, not by weight.

	Calories	Total Carb	Fiber	Usable Carb	Protein
Amber Ice (5.3%)	129	6	0	6	0
Anchor Stream (4.6%)	155	16	0	16	0
Anheuser Light (3.2%)	91	7	0	7	0
Arctic Ice (5.3%)	149	10	0	10	1
Arctic Ice Light 3.2 (3.9% alcohol)	101	6	0	6	0
Augsburger Bock (4.9%)	170	17	0	17	1
Ballard Bitter (4.7%)	178	19	0	19	1
Becks (5%)	145	10	0	10	1.7
Big Sky (4.8%)	150	12	0	12	1
Light (4.5%)	*107*	*4*	*0*	*4*	*0*
Black Label (5.6%)	152	8.7	0	8.7	1.2
Blackhook Porter (4.9%)	154	14	0	14	0
Blatz (4.6%)	139	12.5	0	12.5	1.3
Light (3.9%)	113	8.3	0	8.3	0.7
Bud Dry (4.9%)	134	7.8	0	7.8	1.1
Bud Light (3.9%)	113	6.6	0	6.6	0.9
Bud Ice (5.5%)	149	8.9	0	8.9	1.3
Bud Ice Light (4.1%)	114	6.5	0	6.5	1
Budweiser (4.9%)	144	10.8	0	10.8	1.2
Natural Light (4.2%)	112	6.6	0	6.6	0.8
Natural Ice (5.9%)	158	9.9	0	9.9	1.1
Bush (4.6%)	135	10.2	0	10.2	0.9
Light (4.2%)	113	6.7	0	6.7	0.8

	Calories	Total Carb	Fiber	Usable Carb	Protein
Ice (5.9%)	172	13	0	13	1.2
Colt 45 Malt (5.6%)	159	11	0	11	1.1
Coors Original (5%)	146	11.3	0	11.3	1.2
Light (4.2%)	93	5	0	5	0.7
Dry (4.9%)	122	6	0	6	0
Corona Extra (4.8%)	147	13	0	13	1.1
Light (4.1%)	105	5	0	5	1.1
Extra Gold Lager (5%)	148	10.7	0	10.7	1.4
Killian's (4.9%)	162	13.8	0	13.8	1.7
Goebel (4.6%)	144	12.1	0	12.1	1.2
Hamm's (4.7%)	151	12.1	0	12.1	1.1
Light (4.1%)	117	7.3	0	7.3	0.9
Heileman's (4.7%)	146	11.9	0	11.9	1.2
Heineken (5%)	150	10.8	0	10.8	1.8
Hurricane (5.8%)	161	10.3	0	10.3	1.3
Ice (7.4%)	198	11.4	0	11.4	1.8
Icehouse (5%)	138	8.7	0	8.7	1.2
Icehouse (5.5%)	156	9.8	0	9.8	1.3
Jacob Best Ice (5.9%)	163	10.6	0	10.6	1.1
Light (3.9%)	106	6.9	0	6.9	0.8
Keystone, Premium (4.4%)	115	5.6	0	5.6	1
Ice (5.9%)	145	5.1	0	5.1	1.1
Light (4.2%)	107	5	0	5	0.7
Killarney's (5.4%)	196	22.8	0	22.8	1.3
King Cobra (5.9%)`	169	12.2	0	12.2	1.1
Kirin Lager (4.9%)	144	10.7	0	10.7	1.3
Light (3.2%)	95	7.1	0	7.1	0.8
Lone Star (4.7%)	145	11.4	0	11.4	1.1
Light (3.9%)	113	8.3	0	8.3	0.7
Magnum (5.9%)	163	9.9	0	9.9	1.1
Meister Brau (4.5%)	113	4.8	0	4.8	0.8
Michelob Reg. (5%)	156	13.3	0	13.3	1.3
Light (4.5%)	136	11.7	0	11.7	1.1
Amber (5%)	164	15	0	15	1.4
Dry (4.9%)	130	8	0	8	0
Golden Draft (4.8%)	148	12.6	0	12.6	1.2
Golden Draft Light (4.2%)	113	7	0	7	1
Hefeweizen (5%)	154	11.8	0	11.8	2.3
Honey Lager (4.9%)	176	17.9	0	17.9	2
Ultra (4.2%)	*96*	*2.5*	*0*	*2.5*	*0.6*

	Calories	Total Carb	Fiber	Usable Carb	Protein
Miller					
Genuine Draft (5%)	154	13.1	0	13.1	1
Draft Light (4.5%)	122	7	0	7	0.8
High Life (5%)	154	13.1	0	13.1	1
High Life Ice (5.5%)	160	11	0	11	1.1
High Life Light (4.5%)	123	7	0	7	0.8
Milwaukee's Best (4.5%)	140	11.4	0	11.4	0.9
Ice (5.9%)	144	7.3	0	7.3	0.9
Light (4.5%)	*108*	*3.5*	*0*	*3.5*	*0.7*
Old Milwaukee (4.5%)	151	15	0	15	0
Ice (5.5%)	152	10	0	10	0
Light (4.3%)	124	10	0	10	0
Old Style (4.7%)	143	11.4	0	11.4	1.1
Light (4.2%)	116	7	0	7	0.9
LA (2.2%)	82	6.6	0	6.6	3.7
Pabst Blue Ribbon (4.7%)	145	12	0	12	0
Light (3.9%)	111	8	0	8	0.5
Piels (4.3%)	124	8.7	0	8.7	1.2
Ranier (4.7%)	143	11.3	0	11.3	1.1
Light (3.8%)	113	8.7	0	8.7	0.7
Red Dog (5%)	157	14.1	0	14.1	0.7
Red Wolf (5.4%)	152	10.3	0	10.3	1.3
Sam Adams (4.6%)	159	17	0	17	0
Lager (4.7%)	159	17	0	17	0
Sapporo (3.9%)	135	14	0	14	20
Schaefer (4.6%)	144	12.1	0	12.1	1.2
Light (3.6%)	111	7.8	0	7.8	0.7
Schlitz (4.6%)	144	12.1	0	12.1	1.2
Light (3.8%)	113	8.3	0	8.3	0.7
Malt (5.8%)	189	16.5	0	16.5	1.8
Schmidt (4.6%)	146	12.5	0	12.5	1.3
Light (3.8%)	113	8.3	0	8.3	0.7
Sierra Nevada					
Pale Ale (4.8%)	198	12.3	0	12.3	0.5
Big Foot (10.1%)	295	24.6	0	24.6	1
Porter (5.3%)	198	15.7	–	15.7	0.5
Wheat Beer (4.4%)	147	11.8	0	11.8	0.4
Silver Thunder (5.8%)	163	10.6	0	10.6	1.1
Southpaw (5%)	130	6.6	0	6.6	0.8
Stroh's (4.7%)	143	13	0	13	0
Light (4.5%)	119	7	0	7	0

	Calories	Total Carb	Fiber	Usable Carb	Protein
Wheat Hook (4.8%)	146	12	0	12	0
Zima Clear (4.8%)	150	21.4	0	21.4	0

NON-ALCOHOLIC BREWS

	Calories	Total Carb	Fiber	Usable Carb	Protein
Less than 0.5% Alcohol					
Average All Brands	65	13.3	0	13.3	1.2

CIDER, WINE, LIQUOR

HARD LEMONADE

Per 12 oz. unless indicated	Calories	Total Carb	Fiber	Usable Carb	Protein
Doc Otis (4.8%)	251	38.5	0	38.5	0.6
Mikes (5.2%)	351	15.3	0	15.3	0
Hooch (5%)	146	12	0	12	0

CIDER

Alcoholic Cider, Per 12 oz	Calories	Total Carb	Fiber	Usable Carb	Protein
Dry (5.5%)	130	12	0	12	0
Sweet (5.5%)	160	12	0	12	0
Hardcore Crisp:					
Hard Cider (6%)	195	19	0	19	0
Hornsby's (6%)	179	15	0	15	0
Woodchuck (5%)					
Per 8 oz. cup	154	14	0	14	0
Dark/Dry (5%)	142	11	0	11	0
Granny Smith (5%)	126	7	0	7	0

TABLE WINES

	Calories	Total Carb	Fiber	Usable Carb	Protein
Champagne, 4 oz	*85*	*2*	*0*	*2*	*0*
Table Wine, 4 oz	*88*	*1.8*	*0*	*1.8*	*0.3*
Sake, 3 oz.	115	7	0	7	0

DESSERT WINES

Per 4 oz.	Calories	Total Carb	Fiber	Usable Carb	Protein
Madeira (18%)	170	10	0	10	0
Marsala (18%)	140	6	0	6	0
Port (18%)	170	10	0	10	0.4
Sherry, dry (18%)	*130*	*1*	*0*	*1*	*0*
Sweet (18%)	170	10	0	10	0
Vermouth, Dry (18%)	*130*	*1*	*0*	*1*	*0*
Sweet (18%)	162	16	0	16	0

	Calories	Total Carb	Fiber	Usable Carb	Protein

COCKTAILS, LIQUEURS

COOLERS & PREMIX COCKTAILS

	Calories	Total Carb	Fiber	Usable Carb	Protein
Per 12 oz. unless indicated					
Bacardi Silver (5%)	235	35	0	35	0
Bacardi Fruit Mixers					
(with 2 oz. mix + 1 oz. Rum + ice)					
Pina Colada	249	33	0	33	0
Margarita	160	22	0	22	0
Other Varieties	200	32	0	32	0
Bartles & Jaymes					
Malt Based Coolers (3.9%)					
Berry/Black Cherry/					
Peach	210	33	0	33	0
Fuzzy Navel/Tropical	230	38	0	38	0
Margarita/Pina Colada	270	48	0	48	0
Strawberry Daiquiri	220	36	0	36	0
Captain Morgan					
Gold (5%)	240	36	0	36	0
Cruzan Island Cocktails (5%)					
Jumbie Brew	230	32	0	32	1
Mojito	300	50	0	50	0.5
Wazi Koki	285	46	0	46	1
Heublein Premium Classics					
Per 2 oz. serving					
Long Island Ice Tea (15%)	130	20	0	20	0.5
Manhattan w/ ice (22.5%)	160	20	0	20	1
Mai Tai w/ ice (22.%)	160	20	0	20	1
Pina Colada w/ ice	140	20	0	20	0.3
Jack Daniels Country					
Cocktails (5.9%)					
Average all flavors, per 6 oz.	167	25	0	25	0
Jack Daniels Hard					
Cola (5%) 12 oz.	235	34	0	34	0.5
Jose Cuervo Cocktails (5.9%)					
Margarita/Lime/					
Strawberry, 6 oz.	157	24.3	0	24.3	0
Sauza Diablo (5%)					
Cooler, 6 oz.	130	20.1	0	20.1	0
Seagram's Coolers (3.2%)					
Wild Berries	221	34.6	0	34.6	0
Skyy Blue (5%) Pre-mix, 12 oz.	280	45.3	0	45.3	0

	Calories	Total Carb	Fiber	Usable Carb	Protein
Sparks (6%) Pre-mix, 16 oz.	350	47	0	47	0
Smirnoff Ice (5%) Pre-mix, 11 oz.	225	33	0	33	0.5
TGI Friday's Frozen Cocktails (12.5%) Pre-mix & ice, 3 oz					
Margarita/Strawberry Daiquiri	145	20	0	20	0
Mudslide/Orange	240	31	0	31	0
The Club Premix Cocktails, Per 4 oz					
Long Island Ice Tea/ Manhattan	230	30	0	30	0
Margarita/Screwdriver/ Vodka/Martini	210	40	0	40	0
Mudslide	270	26	0	26	0
P. Colada/Or. Craze/ Whisky Sour	258	40	0	40	7
SHOOTERS					
Per 1.5 oz. shots					
Kamikazi	*150*	*2*	*0*	*2*	*0*
Mud Slide	154	16.3	0	16.3	0
Fuzzy Navel	120	7	0	7	0
Pineapple Bomber	130	13	0	13	0
Turbo	*110*	*3*	*0*	*3*	*0*
FLAVORINGS/SYRUPS					
Angostura Bitters, Per ¼ tsp	*3*	*0.8*	*0*	*0.8*	*0*
Grenadine, 1 Tbsp	35	8.5	0	8.5	0.3
Lime Juice, 1 oz.	*6*	*1.9*	*0.1*	*1.8*	*0.1*
Sugar Syrups, 1 oz.	91	23.8	0	23.8	0
Sour Mix, 2 Tbsp	*10*	*2*	*0*	*2*	*0.5*
Tonic Water, 8 oz.	90	22.7	0	22.7	0
COCKTAIL MIX 'N DRINKS					
No Alcohol Added					
Bloody Mary Mix	120	5	0	5	0
Pina Colada Mix , Heublein, W/Ice, 4 oz.	280	40	0	40	0.5
COCKTAILS					
(Made to Standard Recipes)					
Blushin Russian	365	47	0	47	0

	Calories	Total Carb	Fiber	Usable Carb	Protein
Bourbon & Soda	*110*	*1*	*0*	*1*	*0*
Brandy Alexander	300	11	0	11	0
Cerebral Hemorrhage	290	32	0	32	0
Chupa Naranjas	150	8	0	8	0
Collins	180	11	0	11	0
Daiquiri	*110*	*3*	*0*	*3*	*0*
Gin & Tonic	170	14	0	14	0
Harvey Wallbanger	252	11	0	11	0
Highball	*110*	*3*	*0*	*3*	*0*
Irish Coffee	210	8	0	8	0
L.A. Sunrise	280	21	0	21	0
Leprechaun's Libation	285	17	0	17	0
Long Island Ice Tea (w/ 8 oz. cola)	230	25	0	25	0
(w/ 8 oz. diet cola)	*130*	*0*	*0*	*0*	*0*
Mai Tai (2 oz. rum)	260	17	0	17	0
Manhattan	*130*	*3*	*0*	*3*	*0*
Margarita	*170*	*4*	*0*	*4*	*0*
Martini	*160*	*1*	*0*	*1*	*0*
Mind Eraser	160	10	0	10	0
Mint Julep	165	8	0	8	0
Mojito (2 oz. rum)	170	10	0	10	0
Pina Colada	260	12	0.8	11.2	0
Screwdriver	180	20	0	20	0
Spritzer (3 oz. wine)	*70*	*3*	*0*	*3*	*0*
Tequila Sunrise	190	14	0	14	0
Tom Collins	*120*	*2*	*0*	*2*	*0*
Whiskey Sour	125	5	0	5	0
LIQUEURS/CORDIALS					
Per 1 fl. oz					
Baileys Irish Cream (34 proof)	95	5	0	5	0.5
Cherry Brandy (48 proof)	78	9	0	9	0
Coffee Liqueur (53 proof)	101	14.1	0	14.1	0
Amaretto (56 proof)	110	17	0	17	0
Benedictine (80 proof)	90	5	0	5	0
Cointreau (80 proof)	98	7	0	7	0
Crème de Cacao (54 proof)	100	15	0	15	10
Crème de Menthe (60 proof)	120	14	0	14	3.8
Drambuie (80 proof)	106	9	0	9	0
Grand Marnier (80 proof)	98	7	0	7	0

	Calories	Total Carb	Fiber	Usable Carb	Protein
Kahlua (53 proof)	90	11	0	11	0
Kirsch (68 proof)	80	6	0	6	0
Midori (42 proof)	79	11	0	11	0

RESTAURANTS & FAST FOODS

A & W

Burgers					
Baby Burger	264	28	0	28	15
Mama Burger	480	36	0	36	26
Papa Burger	700	36	.1	35.9	47
Grandpa Burger	910	36	.1	35.9	68
Add Cheese to the above	*53*	*0*	*0*	*0*	*3*
Teen Burger	565	36	1	35	31
Double Teen Burger	790	36	1	35	52
Mozza Burger	630	38	1	37	33
Double Mozza Burger	830	38	2	36	54
Chicken					
Chicken Grill	344	40	2	38	22
Chubby Chicken Burger	486	48	3	45	21
Chubby Chicken Pieces					
Thigh	411	9	2	7	24
Breast	328	10	3	7	28
Wing	204	6	1	5	13
Drumstick	*139*	*5*	*1*	*4*	*12*
Chubby Chicken Strips, 1	121	10	2	8	7
Chicken Strip Dipping Sauces					
Dijon Honey Mustard, 1 oz.	104	11	0	11	1.5
Barbeque, 1oz.	32	7	1	6	1
Sweet and Sour, 1 oz.	47	11	0	11	0
Hot Dogs					
Hot Dog	375	31	1	30	12
Whistle	490	39	2	37	17
Fries					
Small, 2.9 oz.	225	33	2	31	2.5
Regular, 4.75 oz.	375	54	3	51	4
Large, 6 oz.	470	68	4	64	5
Salads					
Coleslaw, individual	88	7	2	5	1
Potato Salad, individual	158	22	2	20	2
Macaroni Salad, individual	173	22	5	21.5	3

	Calories	Total Carb	Fiber	Usable Carb	Protein
Breakfast					
Bacon 'n Egger	509	32	1	31	17
Sausages & Egger	595	34	0	34	20
Bacon & Eggs	573	28	1	27	23
Hash Brown	175	18	2	16	1
Toast, wholewheat					
2 pieces, 3½ oz.	182	7.5	1	6.5	5.5
French Toast,					
2 pieces, 10 oz.	400	49	1	48	11.5
Cinnamon Bun	388	65	2	63	7
Apple Turnover	193	29	3	26	3
Desserts					
Soft ice cream Cone:					
Regular	219	30	0	30	4
Large	298	40	0	40	5
Fountain Beverages					
A & W Root Beer	216	56	0	56	0
Diet A&W Root Beer	*3*	*0*	*0*	*0*	*1*
Coco-Cola	190	47	0	47	0
Diet Coke	*3*	*0*	*0*	*0*	*0*
Sprite	195	50	0	50	0
Nestea Ice Tea	186	50	0	50	0
Beverages					
Orange Juice, 10 fl. oz.	136	33	1	32	2
Apple Juice, 10 fl. oz.	141	35	0	35	0
2% Milk, 250 ml	124	12	0	12	8
2% Chocolate Milk, 250 ml	188	28	0	28	9
Hot Chocolate, 8 fl. oz.	104	18	0	18	1
Coffee, 8 fl. oz.	*4*	*1*	*0*	*1*	*0*
Milkshakes & Floats					
Chocolate Milkshake	459	76	0	76	13
Strawberry Milkshake	454	76	0	76	13
Vanilla Milkshake	450	74	0	74	13
A & W Root Beer Milkshake	458	78	0	78	13
A & W Root Beer Float	300	60	0	60	4
APPLEBEE'S					
Low Fat Menu					
Asian Chicken Salad	714	121	9.6	111.4	37.5
Half Portion	426	69	5.4	63.6	20.5
Blackened Chicken Salad	424	39	4.7	34.3	48
Half Portion	226	21	2.6	18.4	26

	Calories	Total Carb	Fiber	Usable Carb	Protein
Chicken Quesadilla	742	89	10.7	78.3	65
Chicken Roma Rollup	642	83	5.6	77.4	54
Garlic Chicken Pasta	532	76	7	69	34
Veggie Quesadilla	595	86	10.7	75.3	36.5
Whitefish w/ Mango Salsa	437	53.5	6.4	47.1	34.5
Desserts, Sundaes					
Low Fat Brownies Sundae	326	72	4.6	67.4	3
Bikini Banana Strawberry					
Shortcake	229	49	2.5	46.5	1.5
ARBY'S					
Breakfast Items					
Biscuit: w/ Butter	280	27	.5	26.5	5
w/ Bacon	325	27	1	26	7
w/ Sausage	445	27	1	26	10
Croissant: Plain	225	25	0	25	4
w/ Bacon	325	28	0	28	8
w/ Ham	340	29	0	29	13
w/ Sausage	445	28	0	28	11
Sourdough					
w/ Bacon	235	29	2	27	14
w/ Ham	230	30	1	29	12
w/ Sausage	325	29	1	28	10
French-Toastix, no syrup	375	48	4	44	7
Swiss Cheese, 1 slice	*40*	*0*	*0*	*0*	*3*
Roast Beef Sandwiches					
Arby-Q	350	40	2	38	16
Arby's Melt w/ Cheddar	345	36	2	34	16
Beef 'N Cheddar	480	43	2	41	23
Big Montana	630	41	3	38	47
Giant Roast Beef	500	41	3	38	32
Junior Roast Beef	315	34	2	32	16
Regular Roast Beef	365	34	2	32	21
Super Roast Beef	485	47	3	44	22
Sub Sandwiches					
French Dip	440	42	2	40	28
Hot Ham 'N Cheese	540	45	3	42	29
Italian	790	49	3	46	29
Other Sandwiches					
Chicken Bacon 'n Swiss	615	49	2	47	31
Chicken Breast Fillet	555	47	2	45	24
Chicken Cordon Bleu	640	47	2	45	34

	Calories	Total Carb	Fiber	Usable Carb	Protein
Grilled Chicken Deluxe	460	37	2	35	29
Hot Ham 'N Swiss	350	35	1	34	23
Roast Chicken Club	520	38	2	36	29
Market Fresh Sandwiches					
Roast Beef & Swiss	820	73	5	68	37
Roast Chicken Caesar	815	75	5	70	43
Roast Ham & Swiss	745	74	5	69	36
Roast Turkey & Swiss	770	75	5	70	43
Market Fresh Salads					
(no dressing)					
Caesar Salad	95	8	3	5	7
Caesar Side Salad	*50*	*4*	*2*	*2*	*4*
Chicken Finger Salad	580	39	3	36	30
Grilled Chicken Caesar Salad	235	8	3	5	33
Turkey Club Salad	355	9	3	6	33
Light Menu					
Garden Salad	70	14	6	8	4
Grilled Chicken	280	30	6	24	29
Grilled Chicken Salad	210	14	6	8	30
Roast Chicken Deluxe	260	33	3	30	23
Roast Chicken Salad	160	15	6	9	20
Roast Turkey Deluxe	260	33	3	30	23
Side Salad	*25*	*6*	*3*	*3*	*2*
Sides					
Cheddar Curly					
Fries w/ Sauce	455	54	4	50	6
Chicken Finger 4-Pack	650	42	0	42	31
Chicken Finger	585	55	3	52	19
Snack					
Jalapeno Bites	335	30	2	28	7
Mozzarella Sticks	470	34	2	32	18
Onion Petals	405	43	2	41	4
Potato Cakes (2)	255	26	3	23	2
Baked Potato: Plain	355	82	7	75	7
w/ Butter & Sour Cream	510	65	6	59	8
w/ Broccoli 'N Cheddar	550	71	7	64	12
Deluxe Baked Potato	655	67	6	61	20
Shakes					
Chocolate, 14 oz.	520	84	0	84	10
Jamocha/Vanilla, 14 oz.	505	82	0	82	10
Strawberry, 14 oz.	510	87	0	87	11

	Calories	Total Carb	Fiber	Usable Carb	Protein
Condiments					
Arby's Sauce	*15*	*4*	*0*	*4*	*0*
Au Jus Sauce	*5*	*1*	*0*	*1*	*.3*
BBQ Vinaigrette	155	9	0	9	0
Bronco Berry Sauce™	90	23	0	23	0
Buttermilk Ranch Dressing	*285*	*3*	*0*	*3*	*1*
Reduced Calorie	105	12	1	11	1
Caesar Dressing	*315*	*1*	*0*	*1*	*1*
Croutons: Cheese & Garlic	105	10	0	10	2.5
Seasoned	35	5	1	5	1
Honey French Dressing	290	18	.5	17.5	0
Horsey Sauce, Packet	*55*	*3*	*0*	*3*	*0*
Italian Dressing,					
Reduced Calorie	*21*	*3*	*.5*	*2.5*	*0*
Marinara Sauce	*30*	*4*	*0*	*4*	*1*
Mayonnaise	*90*	*0*	*0*	*0*	*0*
Light Cholesterol Free	*20*	*1*	*0*	*1*	*0*
Tangy Southwest Sauce	*245*	*3*	*0*	*3*	*0*
ATLANTA BREAD COMPANY					
Bagel: Per Bagel					
Asiago	350	65	2	63	14
Banana	350	65	3	62	13
Blueberry; Plain	340	68	2	66	13
Chocolate Chip	330	62	2	60	11
Cinnamon Raisin	340	69	3	66	12
Everything	310	61	2	59	12
Honey Wheat	330	66	5	61	12
Jalapeno	330	66	2	64	13
Onion	300	60	2	58	12
Pumpernickel	300	60	3	57	11
Poppy Seed	310	60	2	58	12
Sesame Seed	310	60	2	58	12
Bread: Per Thick Slice, 2 oz					
Asiago	150	26	1	25	6
Cinnamon Raisin	170	31	2	29	6
Cracked Wheat	160	30	2	28	6
French	140	29	1	28	6
Honey Wheat;					
Nine Grain; Rye	150	29	2	27	6
Pesto	150	29	1	28	6
Pumpernickel	150	28	2	26	6

	Calories	Total Carb	Fiber	Usable Carb	Protein
Sourdough	140	29	1	28	5
Sundried Tomato	150	30	1	29	5
Muffins: Each					
Apple Cinnamon	400	52	1	51	6
Banana Walnut	440	53	1	52	8
Blueberry	430	55	1	54	7
Chocolate Chip	460	60	1	59	7
Chocolate Mocha	470	61	2	59	7
Cranberry Apple	390	51	2	49	6
Cranberry Orange Walnut	440	51	2	49	7
Honey Raisin Bran	460	65	6	59	8
Lemon Poppy Seed	460	57	1	56	9
Low Fat Apple Cinnamon	310	60	2	58	7
Low Fat Banana Blueberry	310	60	2	58	7
Low Fat Chocolate	340	64	2	62	8
Low Fat Pumpkin	290	58	2	56	5
Peaches/Crème	530	68	1	67	8
Pumpkin	370	58	2	56	4
Zucchini	480	60	2	58	7
Muffin Tops					
Blueberry	320	41	1	40	5
Banana Walnut	330	40	1	39	6
Chocolate Chip	340	45	1	44	5
Chocolate Mocha	350	45	1	44	5
Pumpkin	280	43	1	42	5
Rolls					
French	180	37	1	36	7
Sourdough	190	38	1	37	7
Salads					
Caesar, no dressing	35	8	2	6	2
Chicken	*303*	*.5*	*0*	*.5*	*28*
Chicken Caesar, no dressing	115	8	2	6	20
Chicken Curry	340	10	2	8	21
Chicken House, no dressing	115	8	2	6	21
Chopstix Chicken, no dressing	470	38	6	32	30
Fruit	140	32	2	30	2
Greek Chicken, no dressing	210	12	2	10	20
Greek, no dressing	120	12	2	10	20
House	35	8	2	6	2
Tuna	*240*	*0*	*0*	*0*	*22*

	Calories	Total Carb	Fiber	Usable Carb	Protein
Sandwiches (sourdough)					
ABC Special, no dressing	450	67	2	65	47
Avocado, no dressing	630	75	7	68	15
Chicken Curry, no dressing	630	70	4	66	32
Chicken Salad, no dressing	600	61	2	59	40
Honey Maple Ham, no dressing	310	66	2	64	30
Pastrami, no dressing	440	62	2	60	32
Roast Beef, no dressing	450	62	2	60	40
Tuna, no dressing	530	61	2	59	33
Turkey Breast, no dressing	420	60	2	58	36
Veggie, no dressing	290	60	2	58	11
Soup: Per Cup					
Baked Potato	210	20	1	19	2
Black Bean & Rice	110	14	9	5	6
Chicken Gumbo	110	15	9	5	1
Black Bean w/ Ham	200	32	16	16	15
Chicken 'n Dumpling	240	21	0	21	9
Chicken Chili	220	27	8	19	18
Chicken Noodle	110	12	1	11	7
Chicken Tortilla	140	15	1	14	7
Chili w/ Beans	280	24	8	16	20
Clam Chowder	270	22	1	21	8
Country Bean	140	24	3	21	6
Cream of Broccoli	150	14	1	13	5
French Onion	60	9	1	8	2
Garden Vegetable	60	15	1	14	2
Mushroom	80	15	3	12	2
Barley & Sage	75	13	1	12	3
Italian Style Wedding	120	19	1	18	6
Lentil & Roasted Garlic	200	33	14	19	11
Pasta Fagioli	160	17	2	15	8
Seven Bean w/ Ham	240	27	9	18	12
Southwest Chicken	180	20	0	20	6
Szechuan Hot & Sour	80	12	1	11	3
Tomato Florentine	120	17	2	15	5
Tomato, Fennel & Dill	100	8	1	7	2
Vegetable Chili	180	31	6	25	8
Wisconsin Cheese	210	20	0	20	8

	Calories	Total Carb	Fiber	Usable Carb	Protein
AU BON PAIN					
Bagels: Per bagel					
Plain	301	61	3	58	12
Asiago Cheese	380	59	3	56	18
Cinnamon Crisp	482	96	3	93	11
Cinnamon Raisin	341	71	3	68	12
Dutch Apple Walnut	484	99	5	94	13
Everything	331	63	3	60	13
French Toast Bagel, 4.6 oz.	411	76	3	73	11
Honey 9 Grain	374	75	6	69	14
Jalapeno Cheddar	350	56	2	54	18
Sesame Seed	336	62	3	59	13
Spreads, 2 oz					
Smoked Salmon	*113*	*3*	*0*	*3*	*5*
Plain Cream	*131*	*4*	*0*	*4*	*4*
Cheese Honey Walnut	141	12	0	12	3
Sundried Tomato	*174*	*4*	*0*	*4*	*1*
Veggie	*144*	*3*	*0*	*3*	*6*
Breakfast Sandwiches: Per Sandwich					
Bagel & Egg	388	63	3	60	25
Bagel & Egg w/ Bacon or cheese	480	63	3	60	30
Bagel & Egg w/ Bacon & cheese	554	63	3	60	35
Wraps					
Chicken Caesar	609	63	5	58	33
Fields & Feta	597	91	13	78	20
Southwestern Tuna	724	69	7	62	49
Soups: Per 8 oz. Serving					
Black Bean	172	32	17	15	11
Broccoli Cheddar	220	13	2	11	6
Chicken Noodle	90	11	0	11	7
Clam Chowder	231	16	1	15	8
Corn Chowder	271	28	2	26	6
Curried Rice & Lentil	133	24	6	18	7
Garden Vegetable	45	7	2	5	2
Old Fashioned Tomato	129	17	2	15	4
Potato Leek	192	17	2	15	4
Split Pea	141	23	8	15	10
Tomato Florentine	70	10	1	9	3

	Calories	Total Carb	Fiber	Usable Carb	Protein
Vegetarian Chili	165	30	15	15	9
Breads					
Country White					
Sandwich Loaf	112	23	1	22	5
Bread Bowl	647	127	6	121	28
Focaccia (1)	733	137	7	130	26
Four Grain Bread, 1 Slice	315	58	2	56	14
Rosemary Garlic Breadstick	201	33	2	31	6
Bread Rolls:					
Hearth (1)	238	44	2	42	11
Petit Pain (1)	192	40	2	38	8
Yogurt & Fruit Cups:					
Per Serving					
Plain Yogurt	186	36	0	36	6
Fruit cup: Small	68	16	1	15	1
Large	145	32	2	30	2
Salads (Container Per Serving)					
Caesar Salad	236	19	4	15	13
Charbroiled Salmon					
Filet, Yellow Peppers	195	9	2	7	24
Chef's Salad	287	11	3	8	27
Chicken Caesar	310	20	4	16	26
Garden Salad, large	164	26	5	21	6
Mediterranean Chicken	228	12	3	9	18
Tomato, Mozzarella					
w/ Basil Pesto	279	11	3	8	16
Tuna Garden	445	28	6	22	27
Cookies: Per Cookie					
Chocolate Chip	266	41	1	40	3
Chocolate Macadamia	244	38	0	38	4
Oatmeal Raisin	242	43	2	41	4
Shortbread	275	48	1	47	5
Cakes & Bars					
Chocolate Chip Brownie	489	61	2	59	5
Apple Strudel	410	56	1	55	6
Cherry Strudel	391	49	1	48	6
Pecan Roll	765	112	4	108	14
Croissants					
Ham & Cheese	346	46	2	44	18
Spinach & Cheese	249	32	2	30	10
Filled: Plain	262	44	2	42	8

	Calories	Total Carb	Fiber	Usable Carb	Protein
Almond	529	63	3	60	13
Apple	239	47	2	45	6
Chocolate	411	61	3	58	8
Cinnamon Raisin	332	66	2	64	8
Raspberry	290	55	2	53	9
Sweet Cheese	370	52	1	51	9
Muffins					
Blueberry	492	71	3	68	7
Carrot Walnut Spice	563	71	4	67	9
Double Chocolate	563	80	3	77	9
Old Fashioned Corn	450	64	2	62	8
Raisin Bran	571	97	10	87	12
Lowfat					
Chocolate Cake	330	74	4	70	4
Triple Berry	282	61	2	59	5
Drinks					
Mocha Blast, 16 oz.	339	56	0	56	13
Iced Cappuccino, 16 oz.	216	22	0	22	14
Frozen Mocha Blast, 12 oz.	266	43	0	43	10

AUNTIE ANNE'S

	Calories	Total Carb	Fiber	Usable Carb	Protein
Pretzels w/ Butter					
Almond Crunch	400	72	2	70	9
Cinnamon Sugar	450	83	3	80	8
Garlic	350	68	2	66	9
Sour Cream & Onion	340	66	2	64	9
Glazin' Raisin	510	107	4	103	11
Jalapeno	310	59	2	57	8
Kidstix, 4 sticks	247	48	2	46	7
Original Pretzel	370	72	3	69	10
Parmesan Herb	440	72	9	63	10
Sesame Pretzel	410	64	7	57	12
Whole Wheat	370	72	7	65	11
Pretzels: Without Butter					
Almond Pretzel	350	72	7	67	11
Cinnamon Sugar	350	74	2	72	9
Garlic Pretzel	320	66	2	64	9
Sour Cream & Onion	310	66	2	64	9
Glazin' Raisin	470	104	3	109	11
Jalapeno	270	58	2	56	8
Kidstix, 4 sticks	227	48	2	46	7
Original Pretzel	340	72	3	69	10

	Calories	Total Carb	Fiber	Usable Carb	Protein
Parmesan Herb	390	74	4	70	11
Sesame Pretzel	350	63	3	60	11
Dipping Sauces					
Caramel Dip	135	27	0	27	1
Cheese Sauce	*100*	*4*	*0*	*4*	*3*
Hot Salsa Cheese	*100*	*4*	*0*	*4*	*2*
Chocolate Flavored Dip	130	24	1	23	1
Light Cream Cheese	*70*	*1*	*0*	*1*	*3*
Marinara Sauce	*10*	*4*	*0*	*4*	*0*
Strawberry Cream Cheese	*110*	*4*	*0*	*4*	*2*
Sweet Mustard	60	8	0	8	.5
Beverages: Per Serving					
Dutch Ice, 20 oz					
Kiwi Banana	270	63	0	63	0
Blue Raspberry	250	57	2	55	0
Lemonade	450	110	0	110	0
Mocha	570	105	0	105	0
Orange Cream	400	92	0	92	0
Pina Colada	360	82	0	82	0
Strawberry	315	72	0	72	0
Wild Cherry	330	75	0	75	0
BAJA FRESH					
Burritos: Includes Cheese					
Baja Burrito					
Chicken	810	75	11	64	14
Steak	914	75	9	66	59
Burrito Mexicano					
Chicken	817	124	20	104	51
Steak	900	124	19	105	56
Bean & Cheese					
w/ Chicken/Steak	860	104	20	84	41
Burrito Ultimo					
Steak	929	90	8	82	59
Chicken	850	90	10	80	55
Grilled Vegetarian	770	100	16	84	32
Burrito "Dos Manos"					
Chicken	736	101	14	87	38
Steak	784	101	13	88	41
Tacos: Includes Cheese and					
Sour Cream					

	Calories	Total Carb	Fiber	Usable Carb	Protein
Baja Style Tacos					
Steak	223	26	3	23	14
Chicken	200	26	4	22	13
Shrimp	90	26	3	23	12
Tres Tacos Combo					
3 Steak	636	78	3	75	14
2 Steak, 1 Chicken	636	79	9	70	35
3 Chicken	606	78	10	68	33
2 Chicken, 1 Fish	665	80	8	72	30
3 Fish	775	82	8	74	24
Baja Mahi Mahi Taco	270	32	6	26	13
Baja Taco Combos					
2 Steak	362	50	9	41	27
1 Steak, 1 Chicken	349	50	9	41	26
1 Steak, 1 Fish	396	51	11	40	21
Taco Chilito					
Chicken	322	58	9	49	20
Steak	344	38	8	30	21
Taquitos: Includes Sour Cream					
Chicken/Beans	740	66	19	47	38
Steak/Beans	814	69	20	49	40
Baja Fajita Combos					
Tortillas Not Included					
Chicken	900	101	16	85	55
Steak	968	101	16	85	60
Quesadilla	1113	80	9	71	48
Steak	1355	80	9	71	81
Chicken	1263	80	10	70	76
Mini Quesadita	612	81	15	66	27
Steak	683	87	15	72	38
Chicken	661	81	16	65	37
Nachos	851	166	33	133	65
Steak	2073	166	33	133	98
Chicken	1901	166	34	132	93
Baja Ensalada, No dressing					
Steak	450	17	5	12	55
Chicken	310	17	7	10	47
Tostada					
Steak	1212	102	28	74	66
Chicken	1120	102	30	72	61

	Calories	Total Carb	Fiber	Usable Carb	Protein
Mini Tostadita					
Steak	606	67	12	55	35
Chicken	549	67	13	54	32
Torta					
Steak	916	72	5	67	49
Chicken	863	72	5	67	47
Extras					
Corn Chips (15), 1 oz.	143	18	2	16	2
BIG APPLE BAGELS					
Bagels: All Types, 5 oz.	380	77	4	73	14
My Favorite Muffin Bagels:					
Per Bagel (4 oz)					
Blueberry	320	66	2	64	11
Cinn. Raisin Sour Dough	315	66	3	63	11
Plain, Sour Dough	310	64	2	62	11
Honey Grain	315	61	4	57	11
Russian Black Bread	320	67	4	63	11
Whole Wheat	325	66	5	61	12
My Favorite Muffin					
Per Muffin (6 oz)					
Plain	600	75	3	72	6
Plain, Fat Free	390	90	3	87	6
Chocolate	510	69	3	66	6
Chocolate, Fat Free	375	87	3	84	6
Cream Cheese:					
Per 2 Tbsp (1 oz)					
Plain; Garden					
Vegetable, avg	*100*	*1*	*.5*	*.5*	*2*
Onion Chive	*105*	*2*	*0*	*2*	*2*
Honey Cinnamon	*130*	*3*	*0*	*3*	*2*
Lite, plain	*65*	*3*	*0*	*3*	*2*
BLIMPIE					
Cold Subs: Per 6"					
Blimpie Best	476	52	3.3	48.7	30
Club Sub	440	50.5	3.3	47.2	27.5
Ham & Swiss	436	51.5	3.3	48.2	28
Roast Beef	468	49	3.3	45.7	37
Turkey Sub	424	49	3.3	45.7	24.5
Grilled Chicken	373	50	3.3	46.7	29
Italian Meatball	572	55	1.7	53.3	28
Mexi Max	425	65	7.3	57.7	25

	Calories	Total Carb	Fiber	Usable Carb	Protein
Vegi Max	395	60	8.3	51.7	24
Salads					
Chef	212	9	3	6	20
Coleslaw, ½ cup	180	13	1	12	1
Potato Salad, 5 oz.	270	19	2	17	19
Wraps					
Zesty Italian	638	74	3	71	26
Chicken Caesar	646	56	3	53	25
BOJANGLES					
Cajun Spiced Chicken					
Breast	275	12	.5	11.5	18
Leg	265	11	.5	10.5	19
Thigh	310	11	.5	10.5	15
Wing	355	11	.5	10.5	21
Southern Style Chicken					
Breast	255	12	.5	11.5	16
Leg	255	11	.5	10.5	19
Thigh	310	14	.5	13.5	16
Wing	335	19	.5	18.5	17
Sandwiches					
Cajun Filet: w/o mayo	350	41	3	38	22
w/ Mayo	450	41	3	38	22
Grilled Filet, w/o mayo	235	25	2	23	23
w/ Mayo	335	25	2	23	23
Snacks: Buffalo Bites	175	5	0	5	27
Chicken Supremes	330	26	1	25	21
Biscuit Sandwiches					
Bacon	290	26	1	25	8
Bacon, Egg & Cheese	555	27	1	26	17
Biscuit (plain)	240	29	2	27	4
Cajun Filet	455	46	1	45	20
Country Ham	275	26	1	25	9
Egg	405	26	1	25	8
Sausage	345	26	1	25	9
Smoked Sausage	380	27	1	26	10
Steak	645	37	1	36	14
Fixins': Per Serving					
Botato Rounds	235	31	3	28	3
Cajun Pintos	95	18	6	12	6
Corn on the Cob	175	34	2	32	5
Dirty Rice	170	24	1	23	5

	Calories	Total Carb	Fiber	Usable Carb	Protein
Green Beans	20	5	0	5	2
Macaroni & Cheese	200	12	.5	11.5	7
Marinated Cole Slaw	135	26	3	23	1
Potatoes, no Gravy	80	16	1	15	2
Seasoned Fries	345	39	4	35	5
Sweet Biscuits					
Bo Berry	220	29	1	28	3
Cinnamon	325	37	1	36	4
BOSTON MARKET					
Entrees					
¼ Chicken:					
White meat w/ skin	*275*	*2*	*0*	*2*	*40*
No skin	*175*	*2*	*0*	*2*	*33*
Dark meat w/ skin	*315*	*2*	*0*	*2*	*30*
No skin	*180*	*1*	*0*	*1*	*22*
½ Chicken w/ Skin	1190	8	0	8	140
Chicken Pot Pie, 1 pie	745	57	2	55	26
Grilled Chicken BBQ	400	16	.5	15.5	41
Grilled Chicken Teriyaki	280	14	.5	13.5	34
Honey Glazed Ham (lean), 5 oz.	210	5	0	5	24
Marinated Grilled Chicken, 1 breast	*225*	*1*	*0*	*1*	*33*
Meatloaf, 5 oz.	325	16	1	15	22
Meatloaf & Brown Gravy	375	19	1	18	23
Meatloaf & Chunky Tomato Sauce	365	25	2	23	24
Rotisserie Turkey Breast: no skin	*165*	*3*	*0*	*3*	*36*
Turkey Pot Pie	715	58	2	56	28
Soup					
Chicken Noodle, ¾ cup	95	8	0	8	6
Chicken Tortilla w/ toppings, 6.5 oz.	175	18	.2	16	8
Turkey Tortilla w/ toppings, 6.0 oz.	170	18	2	16	9
Salads					
Caesar Side Salad, 6.4 oz.	510	21.7	.8	19.9	8.4
Caesar Salad Entrée	485	17	3	14	14
No dressing	185	17	3	14	14

	Calories	Total Carb	Fiber	Usable Carb	Protein
Chunky Chicken					
Salad, ¾ cup	**465**	**4**	**0**	**4**	**25**
Grilled Chicken Caesar	710	18	3	15	47
Old Fashioned Potato Salad	210	22	2	20	3
Oriental Grilled Chicken,					
No dressing/noodles	320	20	7	13	37
Sandwiches					
BBQ Chicken	625	102	4	98	30
No cheese/mayo					
Chicken w/ cheese & sauce	655	61	4	56	38
No cheese or sauce	420	60	4	56	32
Ham w/ cheese & sauce	685	67	4	63	32
No cheese or sauce	445	65	4	61	26
Meatloaf w/ Cheese					
Open-Faced	755	85	5	80	39
w/ Sides	735	74	5	69	29
Turkey: Bacon Club	790	64	4	59	50
Open faced	715	93	5	88	41
Turkey w/ cheese & sauce	650	64	4	60	40
No cheese or sauce	420	61	4	57	34
Side Dishes					
Rice Pilaf, 1 cup	140	24	1	23	2
Whole Corn, ¾ cup	175	30	2	28	5
Hot Cinnamon					
Apples, ¾ cup	265	56	3	53	0
Macaroni & Cheese, ¾ cup	285	33	1	32	13
Mash Potatoes (¾ cup)					
& Gravy	225	32	3	29	4
Creamed Spinach, ¾ cup	260	11	2	9	9
BRUEGGER'S BAGELS					
Bagels					
Classic Blueberry,					
Cranberry, Orange	330	68	4	64	11
Classic Cinnamon Raisin	320	68	4	64	11
Classic Egg	320	68	4	64	12
Classic Everything	320	64	4	60	12
Sandwiches					
Deli-Style Ham					
w/ Honey Mustard	440	77	4	73	24
Garden Veggie	390	70	5	65	17
Grilled Chicken Breast	590	74	4	70	46

	Calories	Total Carb	Fiber	Usable Carb	Protein
Grilled Chicken Club					
w/ Mayo	750	65	4	61	51
Herby Turkey	530	73	4	69	28
Hot Shot Turkey	430	70	4	66	28
Leonardo da Veggie	460	69	4	65	19
Medterranean	540	74	6	68	19
Olivia De Hamiland	560	71	4	67	32
Roadhouse Chicken	710	77	4	73	51
Santa Fe Turkey	480	71	4	67	29
Turkey Club with Mayo	590	65	4	61	31
Turkey with Mayo	480	65	4	61	25
BURGER KING					
Burgers					
Whopper	720	52	4	48	31
Without Mayo	555	52	4	48	31
w/ Cheese	805	53	4	49	36
w/ Cheese, w/o Mayo	650	53	4	49	35
Double Whopper	975	52	4	48	52
Without Mayo	820	52	4	48	52
w/ Cheese, w/o Mayo	910	53	4	49	57
Whopper JR	395	32	2	30	17
Without Mayo	310	31	2	29	17
w/ Cheese	440	32	2	30	19
w/ Cheese, w/o Mayo	355	32	2	30	19
Hamburger	310	31	2	29	17
Double Hamburger	450	31	2	29	28
Cheeseburger	355	31	2	29	19
Double Cheeseburger	535	32	2	30	32
w/ Bacon	575	32	2	30	35
BK Homestyle Griller	480	35	2	33	26
King Supreme Sandwich	555	32	2	30	30
BK Veggie Burger	390	46	4	42	15
w/ Reduced Fat Mayo	335	47	4	43	14
Chicken & Fish Sandwiches					
BK Fish Sandwich	520	44	2	42	18
Chicken Sandwich	560	52	3	49	25
Without Mayo	460	52	3	49	25
Chicken Whopper	580	48	3	45	39
Without Mayo	420	47	3	44	38
Chicken Whopper Jr	350	30	2	28	26
Without Mayo	275	30	2	28	25

	Calories	Total Carb	Fiber	Usable Carb	Protein
Chicken Tenders					
4 pieces	165	10	0	10	11
5 pieces	215	13	.5	12.5	14
6 pieces	250	15	.5	14.5	16
8 pieces	340	20	.5	19.5	22
Dipping Sauces (1 oz)					
Barbecue	35	9	0	9	0
Honey Flavored	90	23	0	23	0
Honey Mustard	90	9	0	9	0
Ranch	*145*	*1*	*0*	*1*	*1*
Sweet & Sour	40	10	0	10	0
Zesty Onion Ring	*145*	*3*	*0*	*3*	*0*
French Fries (Salted)					
Small, 2.6 oz	225	29	2	27	3
Medium, 4 oz	360	46	4	42	4
Large, 5.6 oz	500	63	5	58	6
King Size, 6 oz	600	76	6	70	7
Salad Dressings: Per ½ oz					
Kraft Catalina	185	10	0	10	0
Kraft Ranch	*215*	*2*	*0*	*2*	*0*
Kraft Thousand Island	113	7	0	7	1
Light Done Right					
Light Italian	*55*	*4*	*0*	*4*	*0*
Signature Creamy Caesar	*135*	*4*	*0*	*4*	*1*
Salads, no dressing					
Chicken Caesar	*175*	*5*	*3*	*2*	*25*
Garden Salad	*25*	*5*	*2*	*3*	*1*
Onion Rings					
Small, 1.8 oz	175	22	2	20	2
Medium, 3.2 oz	320	40	3	37	4
Large, 5 oz	475	60	5	55	7
King Size, 5.6 oz	555	70	5	65	8
Sides/Condiments					
Croutons, ¾ oz	90	14	0	14	2
American Cheese,					
2 Slices, 25g	*95*	*1*	*0*	*1*	*5*
Bacon, 3 pieces, 8g	*40*	*0*	*0*	*0*	*3*
Ketchup, ½ oz	*15*	*4*	*0*	*4*	*0*
Breakfast					
Biscuit, 3 oz	300	35	.5	34.5	6
Croissan'wich					

228

	Calories	Total Carb	Fiber	Usable Carb	Protein
w/ Egg & Cheese	315	24	.5	23.5	12
w/ Sausage & Cheese	425	23	.5	22.5	14
w/ Sausage, Egg & Cheese	525	24	1	23	19
French Toast Sticks (5), 4 oz	390	46	2	44	6
Hash Brown Rounds:					
Small, 2.6 oz	235	23	2	21	2
Large, 4.5 oz	390	38	4	34	3
Cini-Minis Roll w/out icing	109	12.8	3	9.8	1.5
Grape/Strawberry Jam	30	7	0	7	0
Desserts					
Hershey's Sundae Pie, 2.6 oz	300	31	1	30	3
Fresh Baked Cookies	435	57	2	55	44
Beverages					
Sprite, med., 22 fl. oz	220	55	0	55	0
Coca-Cola, med, 22 fl. oz	225	56	0	56	0
Minute Maid Orange Juice, 10 fl. oz	130	33	0	33	0
Reduced Fat Milk, 1% Fat, 8 fl. oz	105	12	0	12	8
Chocolate Shake w/ syrup:					
Small, 11 oz	625	72	2	70	12
Medium, 14 fl. oz	795	89	2	87	15
Strawberry Shake w/ syrup:					
Small, 11 oz	615	71	1	70	11
Medium, 14 fl. oz	780	88	1	87	15
Vanilla Shake:					
Small, 11 fl. oz	555	56	1	55	11
Medium, 14 oz	720	73	1	72	15

CARVEL ICE CREAM

	Calories	Total Carb	Fiber	Usable Carb	Protein
Soft Serving Ice Cream					
Chocolate: Regular	195	22	0	22	4
Vanilla: Regular	195	21	0	21	5
No Sugar Added:					
Regular, 4 oz	145	25	0	25	5
No Fat: Regular,					
Avg all flavors	120	28	0	28	2
Sherbet: Regular,					
Avg all flavors	140	31	0	31	2

	Calories	Total Carb	Fiber	Usable Carb	Protein
Cakes & Novelties					
Flying Saucers: Chocolate	235	33	2	31	5
Flying Saucers: Vanilla	240	33	1	32	5
CHICK-FIL-A					
Breakfast: Per Serving					
Plain Biscuit	265	38	1	37	4
Hot Buttered Biscuit	275	38	1	37	4
Biscuit:					
w/ Bacon	302	38	1	37	6
w/ Bacon & Egg	390	38	1	37	13
w/ Bacon, Egg & Cheese	430	38	1	37	16
w/ Egg & Cheese	390	38	1	37	13
w/ Sausage	410	42	1	41	9
w/ Sausage & Egg	500	43	1	42	15
w/ Sausage, Egg & Cheese	540	43	1	42	18
Chicken Biscuit	400	43	1	42	16
Chicken Biscuit w/ Cheese	450	43	2	41	19
Danish	430	63	2	61	6
Hashbrowns	170	20	2	18	2
Chick-Fil-A Sandwiches					
Chicken Sandwich	410	38	1	37	28
No butter	375	37	1	36	28
Chicken Deluxe	410	39	2	37	28
Chicken, 1 fillet					
(no bun/pickles)	230	10	0	10	23
Chargrilled Chicken					
Sandwich	285	30	1	29	26
No butter	245	28	1	27	26
Deluxe	295	31	2	29	27
Chargrilled Chicken,					
1 fillet (no bun/pickles)	***100***	***1***	***0***	***1***	***22***
Club Sandwich	370	31	2	29	32
Chicken Salad Sandwich	345	32	5	27	20
Cool Wraps					
Spicy Chicken	380	52	3	49	30
Chargrilled Chicken	385	54	5	49	29
Chicken Caesar	440	52	2	50	36
Salads					
Chick-n-Strips Salad	385	22	4	18	34
Chargrilled Chicken Garden	180	9	3	6	22

	Calories	Total Carb	Fiber	Usable Carb	Protein
Strips, Nuggets: Per Serving					
Chick-n-Strips (4- count)	290	14	1	13	29
Nuggets (8-pack)	260	12	.5	11.5	26
Salad Dressing: Per 1.25 oz					
Caesar	*195*	*1*	*0*	*1*	*1*
Bleu Cheese;					
Buttermilk Ranch	*190*	*2*	*0*	*2*	*1*
Fat Free Dijon					
Honey Mustard	55	14	0	14	0
Light Italian	*15*	*3*	*0*	*3*	*0*
Spicy	*165*	*2*	*0*	*2*	*1*
Thousand Island	170	6	0	6	0
Sides: Per Serving					
Carrot & Raisin Salad, small	135	22	2	22	1
Coleslaw, small	215	14	2	13	1
Garlic and Butter					
Croutons, ½ oz	50	6	0	6	1
Roasted, Unsalted					
Sunflower Kernel,					
½ oz serving	*85*	*3*	*1*	*2*	*3*
Sauces					
Polynesian, 1 oz	105	13	0	13	0
Dijon Honey					
Mustard, ½ oz	*55*	*2*	*0*	*2*	*0*
Barbecue, 1 oz	45	11	0	11	0
Honey Mustard, 1 oz	45	10	0	10	0
Desserts					
Cheesecake, 3.3 oz	335	30	2	28	6
w/ Fruit Topping	370	39	2	37	6
Icedream Cup, Small	225	38	0	38	5
Icedream Cone, Small	165	28	0	28	4
Lemon Pie, 4 oz	320	51	3	48	7
Fudge Nut Brownie, 2.6 oz	330	45	2	43	4
Drinks: 9 fl. oz					
Lemonade	170	41	0	41	0
Diet Lemonade	20	5	0	5	0
Iced Tea, Sweetened	75	19	0	19	0
Iced Tea, Unsweetened	*0*	*0*	*0*	*0*	*0*
Coca-Cola Classic	110	28	0	28	0
Diet Coke	*0*	*0*	*0*	*0*	*0*

	Calories	Total Carb	Fiber	Usable Carb	Protein
CARL'S JR.					
Burgers/Sandwiches					
Bacon Swiss Crispy Chicken	760	72	3	69	31
Carl's Catch Fish Sandwich	530	55	1	54	18
Charbroiled BBQ Chicken Sandwich	290	41	2	39	25
Charbroiled Chicken Club Sandwich	470	37	2	35	31
Charbroiled Santa Fe Chicken Sandwich	540	37	2	35	28
Charbroiled Sirloin Steak	550	52	2	50	30
Double Sourdough Bacon Cheeseburger	880	37	2	35	50
Double Western Bacon Cheeseburger	920	65	2	63	51
Famous Bacon Cheeseburger	700	51	3	48	31
Famous Star Hamburger	590	50	2	48	24
Hamburger	280	36	1	35	14
Ranch Crispy Chicken S'wich	660	71	3	68	24
Sourdough Bacon Cheeseburger	640	37	2	35	30
Sourdough Ranch Bacon Cheeseburger	720	43	3	40	33
Spicy Chicken Sandwich	480	47	2	45	14
Southwest Spicy Chicken Sandwich	620	48	2	46	16
Super Star Hamburger	790	51	2	49	41
Western Bacon Cheeseburger	660	64	2	62	31
Western Bacon Crispy Chicken Sandwich	750	91	3	88	31
Cheese:					
American Cheese, large	*60*	*1*	*0*	*1*	*3*
Swiss style Cheese	*50*	*0*	*0*	*0*	*4*
Great Stuff Potatoes:					
Plain	290	68	6	62	6
Bacon & Cheese	640	75	6	69	21
Broccoli & Cheese	530	76	7	69	11
Sour Cream & Chives	430	70	6	64	7

	Calories	Total Carb	Fiber	Usable Carb	Protein
Breakfast					
Breakfast Burrito	550	36	2	34	29
Breakfast Quesadilla	370	38	2	36	16
English Muffin w/ margarine	210	28	2	26	5
French Toast Dips, no syrup	370	42	1	41	6
Sourdough Breakfast	410	33	1	32	26
Scrambled Eggs	*180*	*1*	*0*	*1*	*13*
Sunrise Sandwich,					
No Bacon/Sausage	360	28	2	26	13
Bakery/Desserts					
Cheese Danish	400	49	1	48	5
Blueberry Muffin	340	49	1	48	5
Bran Raisin Muffin	370	61	6	55	7
Chocolate Chip Cookie	350	46	1	45	3
Strawberry Swirl Cheesecake	290	30	0	28	6
Side Orders					
Chicken Stars, 6 pces	260	14	0	14	13
Crisscut Fries, 5 oz	410	43	16	27	5
French Fries, small, 3 oz	290	37	12	25	5
Hash Brown Nuggets, 3.8 oz	330	32	13	19	3
Onion Rings, 4.5 oz	430	53	13	40	7
Salads: no dressing					
Charbroiled Chicken					
Salad-to-go	200	12	3	9	25
Garden Salad-to-go	*50*	*4*	*2*	*2*	*3*
CHUCK E. CHEESE					
Appetizers					
Blended Pizza	140	28	4	24	4
Buffalo Wings, 4 pieces	*220*	*1*	*0*	*1*	*20*
Lamb Wesson French Fries	285	43	3	40	5
Sargento Mozzarella					
Sticks, 2	380	26	2	24	13
Sandwiches: Fries not Included					
Grilled Chicken Sub	740	57	5	52	41
Ham & Cheese	770	60	6	54	39
Hot Dog	430	27	2	25	15
Italian Sub	770	52	4	48	35
Pizza (Medium): Per Slice					
BBQ Chicken	205	25.5	1.5	24	11
Beef	205	43	2	41	9
Cheese	165	21.5	1.5	20	7.5

	Calories	Total Carb	Fiber	Usable Carb	Protein
Pepperoni	185	21.5	1.5	20	8.5
Sausage	193	22	1.5	20.5	9.5
Salad Dressings: Per 2 Tbs					
Kraft Catalina	35	8	0	8	0
NF Bleu Cheese	*170*	*1*	*0*	*1*	*0*
NF Lite Ranch	*80*	*1*	*0*	*1*	*0*
NF Olive Oil & Vinegar	*90*	*2*	*0*	*2*	*0*
NF Thousand Island	*110*	*4*	*0*	*4*	*0*
Birthday Items:					
Per Slice (½ Cake)					
8" Chocolate Cake					
w/ Whip Cream	210	25	1	24	2
8" White Cake					
w/ Whip Cream	210	26	0	26	2
Breakfast: Per Serving					
Kellogg's Snack Um's:					
Cinn Blast	140	24	1	23	2
Froot Loops	120	26	0	26	2
Rice Krispy	130	26	0	26	2
PCB Banana Loaf Cake	350	50	2	48	5
PCB Cinnamon Crumb					
Pound Cake	385	55	1	54	4
Desserts: Per Serving					
PCB Brownie	380	46	1.4	44.6	4
PCB Choc Chunk Cookie	410	56	0	56	5
PCB Original Krispy Treat	340	50	1	49	3

CINNAMONSTER

Cinnamon Roll: Per Roll					
Carmel Pecan	840	120	8	112	16
Original	880	100	4	96	20

CHURCH'S FRIED CHICKEN

Fried Chicken					
Breast, 1 piece	*200*	*4*	*0*	*4*	*19*
Leg, 1 piece	*140*	*2*	*0*	*2*	*13*
Thigh, 1 piece	230	5	0	5	16
Wing, 1 piece	250	8	0	8	19
Krispy Tender Strips, 1 piece	135	11	.4	10.6	11
Tender Crunchers,					
6-8 pieces	411	32	1	31	34
Chicken Fried Steak,					
w/ White Gravy	470	36	1	35	21

	Calories	Total Carb	Fiber	Usable Carb	Protein
Side Items: Per Serving					
Apple Pie, 1 piece	280	41	1	40	2
Honey Butter Biscuits	250	26	1	25	2
Cajun Rice, Regular	130	16	.5	15.5	.1
Cole Slaw, Regular	90	8	2	6	4
Corn on the Cob, 1 ear	140	24	9	15	4
French Fries, Regular	210	29	2	27	3
Okra, regular	210	19	3	16	4
Mashed Potatoes					
& Gravy, regular	90	14	1	13	1
COUSIN'S SUBS					
Italian 7½" Subs					
Cappocolla & Cheese	635	48	1	47	28
Cappocolla & Genoa	630	48	1	47	23
Special	795	48	1	47	36
Genoa & Cheese	730	48	1	47	29
Regular	685	48	1	47	28
Mini 4" Subs					
Chicken Salad	320	37	2	35	14
Italian Special	430	31	1	30	18
Provolone (Cheese)	420	30	1	29	15
Ham & Cheese	380	30	1	29	15
Meatball & Cheese	330	32	1	31	22
Seafood w/ Crab	310	33	1	32	9
Tuna	475	30	1	29	15
Turkey Breast	345	31	1	30	15
Cold 7½" Subs					
BLT	615	45	1	44	17
Club Sub	745	48	2	46	43
Club Sub,					
No mayo/cheese	369	48	2	46	34
Cold Veggie	365	49	2	47	20
Cold Veggie,					
No mayo/cheese	245	49	2	47	11
Chicken Salad	570	61	3	62	25
Ham	309	47	2	45	22
Ham & Cheese	645	47	2	45	28
Provolone (Cheese) Sub	685	46	2	44	25
Roast Beef	620	46	1	45	33
Roast Beef,					
No mayo/cheese	363	46	1	45	33

	Calories	Total Carb	Fiber	Usable Carb	Protein
Seafood with Crab	560	53	1	52	15
Tuna	830	46	2	44	28
Turkey Breast	560	48	1	47	25
Turkey Breast, No mayo/cheese	304	48	1	47	25
Hot 7½" Subs					
Cheese Steak	540	46	1	45	36
Double Cheese Steak	850	46	1	45	61
Chicken Breast	620	46	1	45	35
Chicken Breast, No mayo/cheese	363	46	1	45	35
Gyro	680	55	2	53	31
Hot Veggie	490	49	2	47	25
Italian Sausage	480	50	3	47	22
Meatball & Cheese	585	50	2	48	36
Pepperoni Melt	785	47	2	45	33
Philly Cheese Steak	680	50	1	49	42
Steak	420	46	1	45	27
French Fries					
Medium	400	55	1	54	5
Large	525	72	1	71	7
Extras					
Hot Dog	300	29	0	29	12
Italian/Wheat Bread, Half loaf	210	42	0	42	9
Soups					
Cheese Broccoli	190	15	3	12	6
Cheese	240	18	2	16	7
Chicken w/ Wild Rice	230	21	2	19	10
Chicken Dumpling	170	19	3	16	11
Chili	250	26	14	12	18
Clam Chowder	150	19	3	16	8
Cream of Potato	190	24	3	21	5
Salads					
Chef Salad	***190***	***7***	***7***	***0***	***20***
Garden	***135***	***7***	***7***	***0***	***10***
Italian	***295***	***7***	***7***	***0***	***20***
Seafood	175	12	7	5	14
Side Salad	***70***	***4***	***2***	***2***	***5***
Tuna Salad	***310***	***7***	***7***	***0***	***19***
Cookies: Chocolate Chip	210	25	1	24	2

	Calories	Total Carb	Fiber	Usable Carb	Protein
CULVER'S					
Butterburgers					
Dbl. Bacon Deluxe	785	35	3	32	46
Cheese, Single	500	32	2	30	23
Deluxe, Single	420	29.8	2.1	27.6	24.4
Double	470	32	2	30	34
Double Cheese	575	32	2	30	40
Double Mushroom & Swiss	588	33	3	30	42
Single	350	32	2	30	20
Double Sourdough Melt	545	37	2	35	41
Dbl. Wisconsin Swiss Melt	555	36	3	33	42
Favorite Sandwiches					
Chicken Filet	515	61	4	57	24
Chicken Tenders	465	28	0	28	34.7
Grilled Chicken Breast	310	35	1.6	33.4	26.8
Grilled Ham & Swiss	405	35	2	33	21
Norwegian Cod Filet	605	52	1.7	50.3	25.8
Philly Ribeye Steak	345	43	2	41	36
Pork Tenderloin	530	72	4	68	27
Smoked Turkey	315	44	2	42	26
Turkey Sourdough BLT	525	38	2	36	30
Garden Fresh Salads					
Chef	405	17	3.6	13.4	34.5
Grilled Chicken Caesar	410	18	3	15	25
Grilled Chicken Cashew	525	21	5	16	31
Taco: w/ Shell	701	52	7	45	22
Tossed Salad, Small	105	7.5	1.8	5.7	5.7
Seafood & Chicken					
CheckerBasket Chicken	895	40	0	40	40.2
Norwegian Cod Sandwich	625	52	2	50	32
Fries, Rings & Things					
Dinner Roll	90	16	1	15	3
Cheese Curds	600	54	3	51	28
Chili Cheddar Fries	620	52	5	47	22
French Fries, Regular	355	44	3	41	5
Mashed Potatoes					
& Gravy, small	100	32	3	29	5
Onion Rings	395	73	3	70	7
Frozen Custard, Single:					
Vanilla Cake Cone	340	38	0	38	6
Vanilla Dish	310	32	0	32	6

	Calories	Total Carb	Fiber	Usable Carb	Protein
Vanilla Waffle Cone	410	53	0	53	8
Desserts					
Lemon Ice	210	46	0	46	0
Hot Fudge Sundae Jr	570	53	2	51	9
Old Fashioned Soda, Choco	445	64	1.2	62.8	6.5
Rasberry Cooler	480	116	2.5	113.5	.4
Root Beer Float	465	116	.5	115.5	6
Smoothie, Lemon	668	94	.5	93.5	10
DAIRY QUEEN					
Burgers/Sandwiches					
BBQ Beef Sandwich	293	37	2	35	16
BBQ Pork Sandwich	284	36	2	34	17
Chicken Breast					
Filet Sandwich	500	48	4	44	19
Chili 'n' Cheese Dog	330	22	2	20	14
DQ Homestyle:					
Hamburger	290	29	2	27	17
Bacon Double Cheeseburger	610	31	2	29	41
Cheeseburger	340	29	2	27	20
Double Cheeseburger	540	30	2	28	35
Ultimate Burger	670	29	2	27	40
Grilled Chicken Sandwich	310	30	3	27	24
Hot Dog, regular	240	19	1	18	9
Sides					
Chicken Strip					
Basket w/ Gravy	1000	102	5	97	35
Onion Rings	320	39	3	36	5
Ice Cream Cones/Soft Serve					
DQ Van. Soft Serve, ½ cup	140	22	0	22	3
DQ Choc. Soft Serve, ½ cup	150	22	0	22	4
Dipped Cone, Medium	490	59	1	58	8
Novelties					
Buster Bar	450	41	2	39	10
Chocolate Dilly Bar	210	21	0	21	3
DQ Fudge Bar,					
No Sugar Added	50	13	0	13	4
DQ Sandwich	200	31	1	30	4
DQ Vanilla Orange Bar,					
No Sugar Added	60	17	0	17	4
Lemon DQ Freez'r, 1 cup	160	40	0	40	0
Starkiss	80	21	0	21	0

	Calories	Total Carb	Fiber	Usable Carb	Protein
Blizzards & Sundaes					
Choc. Chip Cookie Dough, medium	950	143	2	141	17
Chocolate Sandwich Cookie, medium	640	97	1	96	12
DQ Treatzza Pizza, 1/8 cake	180	28	1	27	3
Royal Treats:					
Banana Split	510	96	3	93	8
Peanut Buster Parfait	730	99	2	97	16
Strawberry Shortcake	430	70	1	69	7
Frozen Yogurt					
Cup of Yogurt, Medium	230	48	0	48	8
DQ Nonfat Frozen Yogurt, 1/2 cup	100	21	0	21	3
Yogurt Cone, Medium	260	56	0	56	9
Yogurt Strawberry Sundae, Medium	280	61	1	60	8
Misty Slushes, Medium	290	74	0	74	0
DAYLIGHT DONUTS					
Raised Donuts:					
Glazed	140	20	1	19	2
Chocolate Iced	190	23	1	19	3
Cholesterol Free:					
Glazed	140	20	1	19	2
Iced	190	23	1	19	3
Cake Donuts:					
Plain, no topping	210	27	2	25	3
Iced Cake	340	48	3	45	4
Low Cholesterol	210	27	2	25	3
DIPPIN DOTS					
Ice Cream, Per 5 oz containers					
Average all types	190	22	0	22	4
Non-fat Yogurt	110	23	0	23	4
No Sugar, reduced fat	120	17	0	17	4
Fat-free, no sugar, Fudge	60	14	0	14	1
Flavored Ice	50	13	0	13	1
Flavored Sherbet	100	21	0	21	1
DEL TACO					
Breakfast:					
Breakfast Burrito	250	24	1	23	10

	Calories	Total Carb	Fiber	Usable Carb	Protein
Bacon & Egg Quesadilla	450	40	2	38	21
Egg & Cheese Burrito	450	39	3	36	23
Macho Bacon & Egg Burrito	1030	82	6	76	40
Steak & Egg Burrito	580	39.2	2.9	36.3	31.6
Tacos:					
Big Fat Chicken Taco	340	38	3	35	18
Big Fat Crispy Chicken Taco	620	52	3	49	21
Big Fat Steak Taco	390	38	3	35	18
Big Fat Taco	320	39	3	36	16
Chicken Soft Taco	210	16	1	15	11
Soft Taco, average	160	11	1	10	7
Ultimate Taco	260	13	2	11	14
Burritos:					
Combo Burrito	530	61	11	50	28
Bean & Cheese Red/Green Burrito	270	38	6	32	11
Chicken Works Burrito	520	57	4	53	26
Del Beef Burrito	550	42	3	39	31
Del Classic Chicken Burrito	560	41	3	38	24
Deluxe Combo Burrito	570	64	12	52	29
Deluxe Del Beef Burrito	590	45	4	41	32
Half Pound Red/Green Burrito	430	65	13	52	20
Macho Beef Burrito	1170	89	7	82	60
Macho Combo Burrito	1050	113	17	96	49
Spicy Chicken/ Veggie Works, Avg	490	69	9	60	18
Steak Works Burrito	590	58	5	53	27
Quesadillas:					
Chicken	530	41	2	39	33
Regular	500	39	2	37	23
Spicy Jack Chicken	570	40	2	38	32
Spicy Jack Regular	490	38	2	36	23
Salads:					
Deluxe Chicken Salad	740	75	14	61	33
Deluxe Taco Salad	780	76	14	62	33
Taco Salad	350	10	2	8	9
Burgers:					
Cheeseburger	330	37	3	34	16
Double Del Cheeseburger	560	35	4	31	26
Del Cheeseburger	430	35	4	31	16

	Calories	Total Carb	Fiber	Usable Carb	Protein
Nachos: Regular	380	40	2	38	5
Sides:					
Beans 'n Cheese Cup, 7.7 oz	265	44	16	28	16
Rice Cup, 4 oz	140	27	1	26	3
Fries:					
Chili Cheese, 10.5 oz	670	50	5	45	17
Deluxe Chili Cheese, 12 oz	720	53	6	47	17
Large, 7 oz	490	47	5	42	5
Regular, 5 oz	350	34	3	31	3
DENNY'S					
Breakfast					
All American Slam,					
no bread/potato	*800*	*3*	*1*	*2*	*46*
Dogwood Breakfast,					
no bread	1460	81	1	80	82
Farmer's Slam	1250	82	3	79	51
French Slam, no syrup	1160	71	3	68	46
Grand Slam Slugger,					
no bread/potato	927	74	3	71	34
Lumberjack Slam, no syrup	1020	73	3	70	51
Moons Over My Hammy,					
No potato	843	42	2	40	54
Original Grand Slam	677	33	2	31	26
Breakfast Skillets (no Bread)					
Chicken Fajita	665	30	11	19	26
Meat Lover's Skillet	930	27	10	17	39
Breakfast Sides					
Applesauce	60	15	1	14	0
Bacon, 4 strips	*210*	*0*	*0*	*0*	*12*
Bagel	230	46	0	46	9
Biscuit, Buttered w/					
Sausage Gravy	400	45	0	45	8
Country Fried Potatoes, 5 oz	284	23	10	13	3
Cream Cheese, 1 oz	*100*	*1*	*0*	*1*	*2*
Egg: 1 only	*115*	*.5*	*0*	*.5*	*6*
Egg Beaters					
(egg substitute)	*69*	*1*	*0*	*1*	*5*
English Muffin	125	24	1	23	5
Flour Tortillas and Salsa	290	50.5	4	46.5	6
Grits, 4 oz	80	18	0	18	2
Ham, grilled slice, 3 oz.	*95*	*2*	*0*	*2*	*15*

	Calories	Total Carb	Fiber	Usable Carb	Protein
Hashed Browns, 4 oz	195	20	2	18	2
Covered, 6 oz	283	21	2	19	7
Covered & Smothered, 8 oz	500	54	3	51	14
Kellogg's Dry Cereal, Average, 1oz	100	23	1	22	2
Quaker Oatmeal, 4 oz	100	16	3	13	5
Sausage, 1 link	*88*	*0*	*0*	*0*	*4*
Sausage Gravy, 4 oz	125	6	0	6	3
Syrup: 3 Tbsp					
Maple Flavored	145	36	0	36	0
Sugar-free	35	9	0	9	0
Toast, 1 slice dry	90	17	1	16	3
Toppings, avg. 3 oz	105	26	1	25	0
Whipped Cream, Dollop, 2 oz	*25*	*2*	*0*	*2*	*0*
Whipped Margarine, ½ oz	*90*	*0*	*0*	*0*	*0*
French Toast					
Cinnamon Swirl	1030	124	4	120	23
Omelette (no extras)					
Ham'n Cheddar	610	5	0	5	41
Ultimate	630	11	3	8	34
Veggie-Cheese	515	11	2	9	30
Waffles					
Plain Belgian	305	23	0	23	7
Buttermilk Hot Cakes Plain (3)	475	47	2	45	20
Steak & Eggs (no extras)					
Country Fried Steak	475	13	6	7	29
Sirloin Steak	*657*	*1*	*1*	*0*	*62*
T-Bone Steak	*989*	*1*	*1*	*0*	*73*
Soup					
Chicken Noodle	60	8	0	8	2
Clam Chowder	625	55	4	51	7
Cream of Broccoli	575	41	2	39	6
Vegetable Beef	80	11	2	9	6
Sandwiches (no fries/sides)					
Albacore Tuna Melt	640	42	3	39	30
BBQ Chicken	1095	86	5	81	48
BLT	600	50	2	48	15
Bacon Cheddar Burger	910	58	5	53	53
BBQ Burger	965	72	4	68	52

	Calories	Total Carb	Fiber	Usable Carb	Protein
Boca Burger	630	64	9	55	32
Buffalo Chicken Sandwich	720	80	5	75	37
Classic Burger	700	56	4	52	40
w/ Cheese	856	57	4	53	49
Club Sandwich	720	62	3	59	32
Garlic Mushroom					
Swiss Burger	900	63	5	58	51
Grilled Chicken	480	53	4	49	35
Ham & Swiss on Rye	430	39	5	34	32
Patty Melt	790	37	4	33	45
The Super Bird Sandwich	620	48	2	46	35
Turkey Breast w/ Multigrain	290	41	5	36	23
Appetizers					
Buffalo Chicken Strips (5)	734	43	0	43	48
Buffalo Wings (12)	*858*	*1*	*1*	*0*	*92*
Chicken Strips (5)	709	56	0	56	47
Mozzarella Sticks (8)	710	49	6	43	36
Onion Rings, 4 oz	380	38	1	37	5
Sampler, no condiments	1405	124	4	120	47
Entrees (no sides)					
Chicken Strips, 10 oz	635	55	0	55	47
Fried Shrimp Dinner	230	18	1	17	17
Country Fried Steak	645	30	11	29	28
Fried Shrimp & Scampi	350	15	1	14	27
Shrimp Scampi					
Skillet Dinner	*283*	*3*	*.3*	*2.7*	*25*
Grilled Chicken					
Breast Dinner	*130*	*0*	*0*	*0*	*24*
Pot Roast Dinner w/ Gravy	290	5	0	5	42
Roast Turkey &					
Stuffing w/ Gravy	365	38	2	36	46
Sirloin Steak Dinner	*330*	*1*	*1*	*0*	*18*
Steak & Shrimp Dinner	646	31	2	29	36
T-Bone Steak Dinner	*845*	*0*	*0*	*0*	*65*
Sides					
Bread Stuffing, Plain	100	19	1	18	3
Fries: 6 oz Unsalted	432	57	5	52	6
Fries: 6 oz Seasoned	270	35	0	35	5
Green Beans w/ Bacon	*65*	*6*	*3*	*3*	*1*
Potato: Baked, plain w/ skin	225	51	5	46	5
Mashed	170	23	2	21	3

	Calories	Total Carb	Fiber	Usable Carb	Protein
Salads (no dressing/bread unless indicated)					
Garden Deluxe Salad:					
w/ Chicken Breast	270	10	4	6	32
w/ Fried Chicken Strips	470	26	4	22	33
w/ Tuna	450	12	4	8	35
Grilled Chicken Caesar					
w/ Dressing	595	19	4	15	37
Side Caesar w/ Dressing	360	20	3	17	11
Side Garden Salad,					
No Dressing	110	16	3	13	3
Dressings					
BBQ Sauce, 1.5 oz	55	11	0	11	0
Blue Cheese, 1 oz	*170*	*1*	*0*	*1*	*1*
Caesar, 1 oz	*135*	*1*	*0*	*1*	*1*
French, regular, 1 oz	*100*	*3*	*0*	*3*	*0*
Honey Mustard, 1 oz	215	20	0	20	0
Italian Dressing,					
Low Calorie	*15*	*3*	*0*	*3*	*0*
Marinara Sauce, 1.5 oz	50	7	1	6	1
Ranch, 1 oz	*130*	*1*	*0*	*1*	*0*
Salsa, 2 oz	*10*	*2.5*	*1*	*1.5*	*0*
Sour Cream, 1.5 oz	*95*	*2*	*0*	*2*	*1*
Tarter Sauce, 1.5 oz	235	5	0	5	0
Thousand Island, 1 oz	120	5	0	5	0
Desserts					
Pies: Per ⅛ Whole					
Apple, 7 oz	484	64	1	63	3
Cheesecake,					
No topping, 7 oz	578	51	0	51	8
Chocolate Peanut Butter	667	64	3	61	15
Sundaes					
Single Scoop, no topping	195	14	0	14	3
Double Scoop, no topping	385	29	0	29	6
Banana Split	931	121	6	115	15
Dessert Toppings					
Blueberry, 3 oz	105	26	11	15	0
Chocolate, 2 oz	340	27	0	27	2
Fudge, 2 oz	214	30	1	29	1
Strawberry, 3 oz	117	26	1	25	1

	Calories	Total Carb	Fiber	Usable Carb	Protein
Drinks					
Cappuccino, 8 oz avg	105	17	0	17	2
Floats, Rootbeer/Cola	290	47	0/.5	47/46.5	3/12
Malted Milk-shake,					
Vanilla/Chocolate	610	82	0	82	6
Ruby Red GrapeFruit, 10 oz	165	41	0	41	0
Raspberry Iced Tea, 16 fl. oz	85	21	0	21	0
DOMINO'S					
Buffalo Chicken Kickers					
1 avg piece, 24g	***47***	***3.2***	***.1***	***3.1***	***3.8***
1 order, 10 pieces, 240g	470	32	1.4	30.6	37.5
Hot Sauce, 1.5 oz cup	***16***	***3.6***	***.3***	***3.3***	***.3***
Blue Cheese; Ranch, 1.5 oz	***222***	***1.8***	***0***	***1.8***	***1.1***
Classic Hand Tossed Pizza					
Medium (12") Pizza:					
Per 2 Slices (¼ Pizza)					
Cheese Pizza (base only)	380	54.7	3	51.7	15.4
America's Favorite Feast	514	57.4	3.6	53.8	21.5
Bacon Cheese Burger Feast	554	55	3	52	25.4
Barbeque Feast	511	61.7	3	58.7	21.8
Deluxe Feast	471	57.4	3.5	53.9	19.5
Hawaiian Feast	458	58.3	3.3	55	21.2
MeatZZa Feast	567	57	3.4	53.6	26.2
Pepperoni Feast	541	56	3.2	52.8	23.7
Vegi Feast	448	57.3	3.7	53.6	19.2
Crunchy Thin Crust Pizza					
Medium (12") Pizza:					
Per 2 Slices (¼ Pizza)					
Cheese Pizza (base only)	279	31	1.8	29.2	12
Large (14") Pizza:					
Per 2 Slices (¼ Pizza)					
Cheese Pizza (base only)	391	43.5	2.5	41	16.8
Deep Dish Pizza					
Medium (12") Pizza:					
Per 2 Slices (¼ Pizza)					
Cheese Pizza (base only)	495	56.2	3.3	52.9	18.7
Large (14") Pizza:					
Per 2 Slices (¼ Pizza)					
Cheese Pizza (base only)	694	80.3	4.7	75.6	26.4
Sides: 1 piece					
Breadstick	118	17.5	.8	16.7	2.9

	Calories	Total Carb	Fiber	Usable Carb	Protein
Cheesey Bread	144	17.7	.8	16.9	4.4
Barbecue Wings	*50*	*1.6*	*.2*	*1.4*	*5.5*
Hot wings	*46*	*.5*	*.2*	*.3*	*5.5*
Cinnastix	112	15.3	.7	14.6	2.1

DUNKIN DONUTS

Donuts: Each	Calories	Total Carb	Fiber	Usable Carb	Protein
Apple/Blueberry					
Crumb Donut	230	34	.5	33.5	3
Apple N' Spice Donut	200	29	.5	28.5	3
Black Rasberry/					
Strawberry Donut	210	32	0	32	3
Blueberry Cake Donut	290	35	.5	34.5	3
Boston Kreme Donut	240	36	.5	35.5	3
Butternut Cake Donut	300	36	.5	35.5	3
Chocolate Coconut					
Cake Donut	300	31	1	30	4
Chocolate Frosted					
Cake Donut	360	40	1	39	4
Chocolate Frosted Donut	200	29	.5	28.5	3
Chocolate Glazed					
Cake Donut	290	33	1	32	3
Cinnamon Cake Donut	330	34	1	33	4
Coconut Cake Donut	290	33	.5	32.5	3
Double Chocolate					
Cake Donut	310	37	2	35	3
Dunkin' Donut	240	25	.5	24.5	3
Glazed/Powdered					
Cake Donut	350	41	1	40	4
Glazed Donut	180	25	.5	24.5	3
Jelly Filled Donut	210	32	.5	31.5	3
Jelly Stick Donut	290	44	.5	43.5	3
Lemon Donut	200	28	.5	27.5	3
Marble Frosted Donut	200	29	.5	28.5	3
Old Fashioned Cake Donut	300	28	1	27	4
Strawberry/Vanilla Frosted;					
Bavarian	210	30	.5	29.5	3
Sugar Raised Donut	170	22	.5	21.5	3
Toasted Coconut					
Cake Donut	300	35	.5	34.5	3
Whole Wheat Glazed					
Cake Donut	310	32	2	30	4

	Calories	Total Carb	Fiber	Usable Carb	Protein
Muffins					
Apple Danish, 3 oz	250	36	0	36	4
Banana Nut	540	73	3	70	10
Blueberry: Regular	490	76	2	74	8
Reduced Fat	450	74	2	72	9
Blueberry Scone, 4 oz	410	55	1	54	5
Cheese Danish, 3 oz	270	32	0	32	4
Chocolate Chip	585	85	3	82	9
Coffeee Cake Muffin, 6.5 oz	710	102	2	100	11
Corn	515	81	1	80	9
Cranberry Orange	460	71	3	68	8
Honey Raisin Bran	490	81	5	76	10
Maple Walnut Scone, 4 oz	470	62	1	61	6
Raspberry White Chocolate	450	59	2	57	6
Strawberry Cheese					
Danish, 3 oz	250	33	0	33	4
Crullers					
Glazed Cruller	290	37	.5	36.5	3
Glazed Chocolate Cruller	280	35	1	34	3
Plain Cruller	240	25	.5	24.5	3
Powdered Cruller	270	30	.5	29.5	3
Sugar Cruller	270	30	.5	29.5	3
Sandwiches					
Biscuit Sandwiches:					
Egg/Cheese Sandwich	360	31	1	30	14
Sausage/Egg/Cheese					
Sandwich	560	31	1	30	23
Croissant: Plain	330	37	0	37	5
Spanish Cheese	520	33	2	31	18
English Muffin Sandwich:					
Ham/Egg/Chse	310	31	1	30	21
Bagels					
Biscuit Bagel	255	29	1	28	5
Garlic	410	79	3	76	16
Everything	430	75	3	72	17
Poppyseed	443	72	3	69	17
Onion	375	71	4	67	14
Sesame	455	71	3	68	18
Plain	360	69	2	67	14
Cream Cheese: Plain	***180***	***3***	***0***	***3***	***4***

	Calories	Total Carb	Fiber	Usable Carb	Protein
Cake Munchkins					
Plain (4)	270	27	1	26	3
Cinnamon	270	31	1	30	3
Powdered	270	31	1	30	3
Sugared	240	28	.5	27.5	2
Coconut	200	23	.5	22.5	2
Other types, avg (3)	200	26	.5	25.5	2
Fancies, Buns, Rolls, Fritters					
Apple Fritter	300	41	1	40	4
Bismark Chocolate Iced Donut	340	50	.5	49.5	3
Bow Tie Donut	300	34	.5	33.5	4
Cinnamon Bun	510	85	0	85	8
Coffee Roll: Regular	270	33	1	32	4
Frosted (Chocolate/ Maple/Vanilla)	290	36	1	35	4
Éclair Donut	270	39	.5	38.5	3
Glazed Fritter	260	31	1	30	4
Cookies					
Chocolate varieties, avg (1)	220	28	1	27	3
Oatmeal Raisin Pecan	220	29	1	28	3
Drinks					
Dunkaccino, 10 fl. oz	240	35	0	35	2
Hot Chocolate, 10 fl. oz	230	38	2	36	2
Iced Coffee, 16 fl. oz	*5*	*1*	*0*	*1*	*0*
w/ Cream	*50*	*1*	*0*	*1*	*0*
w/ Milk	115	14	0	14	1
Vanilla Chai, 10 fl. oz	235	40	0	40	1
Coolatta: Per 16 fl. oz					
Coffee Coolatta: w/ Cream	370	40	0	40	3
w/ Milk	220	42	0	42	4
w/ 2% Milk	200	42	0	42	4
Orange Mango Frt Coolatta	270	66	2	64	1
Strawberry Fruit Coolatta	290	72	1	71	0
Vanilla Bean Coolatta	440	70	1	69	1
DON PABLOS					
Appetizers: Per Serving					
Acapulco Nachos	1640	84.8	14.1	70.7	70.4
Beef Fajita Nachos	1465	99	14.8	83.2	72
Chicken Fajita Nachos	1405	86.8	14.1	72.7	83.1
Cholula Buffalo Wings	1045	24	2.9	21.1	43.1

	Calories	Total Carb	Fiber	Usable Carb	Protein
Burritos:					
Beef & Bean	1390	123	19.1	103.9	66.2
Chicken	1252	133	21.4	111.6	58.8
Chimichangas:					
Beef	1190	109	15.1	93.9	50.8
Chimi de Oro w/ Queso	1398	116	15.5	100.5	63.8
Pollo (Chicken)	1090	117	17.1	99.9	43.8
Combinations:					
Conquistador	1977	179	19.3	159.7	97
El Matador	1407	110	18.3	91.7	63.3
El Presidente	940	77.6	12.8	64.8	40.3
Mexican Dinner	1047	75.2	14.2	61	49.6
Primo Combo	1184	90.6	10.4	80.2	41.9
Primo Combo All Chicken	1134	93	11.1	81.9	44.7
Dressings: Per 4 oz					
Blue Cheese	**601**	**3.4**	**0**	**3.4**	**4.5**
Chipolte Ranch	340	5.7	0	5.7	2.3
Creamy Cilantro	**544**	**4.5**	**1.1**	**3.4**	**2.3**
Don's House Vinaigrette	476	19.3	3.4	15.9	7.9
Honey Mustard	420	22.6	0	22.6	0
Italian	397	32	0	32	5.7
Low-Fat-French	200	40	1	39	45
Enchiladas:					
Mama's Skinny	580	57	11.3	65.7	32.6
Chicken Fajita Enchiladas	1350	77.4	13.8	63.6	58.5
Real Enchiladas Beef	1135	64	6.2	57.8	35.3
Real Enchiladas Combo	995	58	6.2	51.8	38
Steak Fajita Enchiladas	1106	67	13.8	53.2	63.5
Three Amigos	991	63.6	13.1	50.5	46.4
Fajitas:					
BBQ Chicken Melt	1683	180	17.8	162.2	81.3
Classic Chicken	1350	139	16.8	122.2	60.8
Classic Steak	1771	157	16.8	140.2	52.4
Pepper Cheese Steak	1945	167	18.8	148.2	60.5
Peso Valley Vegetables	1355	155	22.9	132.1	34.7
Shrimp & Chicken	1398	142	17.4	124.6	57.2
Shrimp & Steak	1608	151	17.4	133.6	53.1
Favorites:					
Chipolte BBQ Ribs	1890	103	12.3	90.7	88.7
Flautas Y Taquitos	1145	103	18.3	84.7	48.1
Parilla Chicken	530	63	7.3	55.7	52.2

	Calories	Total Carb	Fiber	Usable Carb	Protein
Steak & Enchiladas	1375	68	8.8	59.2	79.4
Steak & Shrimp	1171	71.6	9.2	61.8	75.5
Lunch Specials:					
El Favorito	760	59.6	32.5	27.1	42.9
Cheese Quesadilla Salad	838	63.4	5.1	58.3	31.4
Dos Enchilladas	732	63.5	12.4	51.1	31.2
Vegetable Quesadilla Salad	854	76.3	8.2	68.1	29
Salads:					
Grilled Chicken	472	26.1	3.5	22.6	39.4
Grilled Chicken Caesar	1454	95.1	12.2	82.9	38.7
Grilled Steak Caesar	1735	107	12.2	94.8	38.7
Soup & Salad Infinito	1422	136	18.1	117.9	40.8
Taco	1390	103	21.6	81.4	61.3
Tortilla Tossed	1050	101	11.2	89.8	19.8
Desserts:					
Chocolate Volcano	1380	161	1.8	159.2	11.1
Iron Skillet Pie	740	86.5	3	83.5	3.6
Sopapillas	527	62.7	1	61.7	6.1

DONATO'S PIZZA

	Calories	Total Carb	Fiber	Usable Carb	Protein
Pizza: Per 7" Individual					
Chicken Vegy Medley	505	56	11	45	28
Founders Favorite	815	71	10	61	38
Hawaiian	620	58	4	54	30
Mariachi Beef/Chicken	590	56	11	45	35
Original Pepperoni	650	58	6	52	30
Serious Cheese	635	62	6	56	34
Serious Meat	875	68	10	58	45
The Works	810	75	12	63	35
Vegy	560	60	12	48	26
Salads:					
Side Salad w/ Lite Italian Dressing	*110*	*6*	*2*	*4*	*6*
Subs:					
Big Don w/ Italian Dressing	705	68	3	65	34
Big Don w/ Lite Italian Dressing	635	69	3	66	34
Grilled Chicken Club	785	68	3	65	31
Ham & Cheese/Lite Italian	535	70	3	67	32
Vegy w/ Lite Italian Dressing	670	78	6	72	26

	Calories	Total Carb	Fiber	Usable Carb	Protein
EAT 'N PARK					
Breakfast					
Cornbeef Hash, 7.5 oz.	340	16.3	1.4	14.9	16.3
Egg Beaters Breakfast	*75*	*5.6*	*1.6*	*4*	*13.2*
Eggs Benedict	600	35	1.7	33.3	42.5
Fruit Cup	60	14.5	1.2	13.3	1.1
Hash Browns, 6 oz	235	28.1	2.9	25.2	5.4
Homefries, 6 oz	210	24.2	2.3	21.9	2.2
Omelette:					
Bacon & Cheese	*500*	*2.4*	*0*	*2.4*	*32.8*
Cheese	*390*	*2.3*	*0*	*2.3*	*27*
Ham & Cheese	*465*	*3*	*0*	*3*	*37.5*
Supreme	420	8.6	1.7	6.9	28
Western	345	7	1	6	30
Pancake, Plain, 1	225	42.6	1.6	41	5.9
Waffle, Apple	960	125.6	4.3	121.3	17.5
Burgers					
American Grill	785	36.7	2.4	34.3	50.4
Amer./Swiss/Provolone					
Gourmet	770	36.7	2.4	34.3	49.8
American Bacon & Cheese		32.4	1.4	31	37.2
Cheeseburger	540	32.3	1.4	30.9	33.4
Garden	355	60	5.8	54.2	15.8
Hamburger	495	32.1	1.4	30.7	30.6
Southwest	680	56.3	4	52.3	31.4
Super	705	37.6	2.6	35	27.7
Swiss	580	34.2	1.7	32.5	36.9
Turkey	500	37.6	3.2	34.4	38.1
Sandwiches					
Bacon Turkey Swiss	525	16	1.8	14.2	12.5
Chicken Bacon Deluxe	565	50.2	2	48.2	36
Chicken Breaded	515	50	2	48	33.3
Chicken Chargrill	320	35	1.4	33.6	30.9
Spicy	320	32.2	1.7	30.5	31.3
Chicken Fiesta	325	21	2.1	18.9	33.6
Cod	670	67	3.3	63.7	41.1
Croissant					
Grilled Cheese	505	26.2	1.4	24.8	20.7
Chicken Salad	595	36	2.2	33.8	25.6
Tuna	580	35	2.1	32.9	23.6
Turkey	390	31	1.2	29.8	24.5

	Calories	Total Carb	Fiber	Usable Carb	Protein
Dutch Ham & Swiss	570	35.3	5.5	29.8	41
Hot Roast Beef	280	25	1.4	23.6	30
Pita					
Chicken Fajita	620	68.5	3.6	64.9	42.4
Tuna	640	72	3.9	68.1	29.5
Turkey	445	67.4	3	64.4	30.4
Reuben	720	31.1	3.7	27.4	37.6
Shredded Pot Roast	530	27.6	1.3	26.3	35.4
Steak'n Cheese	765	42.6	2.8	39.8	34.3
Tuna Melt	610	35.2	4.2	31	26
Turkey Club	775	50	2.5	47.5	39
Turkey Pastrami	715	40	6.2	33.8	38.5
Whitefish (Breaded)	790	69	3.4	65.6	45.3
Appetizers					
Cheese Fries	880	93.1	8.1	85	18.2
Cheese Sticks	410	17	.5	16.5	29.6
Onion Rings	210	19.5	1.3	18.2	4.2
Wings	***400***	***.5***	***.4***	***.1***	***34.4***
Dinners					
Chicken Breast, Stuffed	370	27.3	1.3	26	26.3
Chicken Fillets, 5	530	28	1	27	42.6
Chicken Milano	***215***	***3.7***	***.1***	***3.6***	***25.4***
Chicken Naturelle	***140***	***0***	***0***	***0***	***24.9***
Chicken Parmigiana:					
Marinara	840	90.4	5.8	84.6	47.5
Meat	900	86	5.4	80.6	51.7
Chicken Stir-Fry	555	47.3	7.6	39.7	38.5
Chicken'n Biscuits	495	30	1	29	46.2
Chicken, 3 piece	1195	57.6	2	55.6	78
Cod, breaded	925	56.3	2	54.3	69.1
Floridian Scrod	***120***	***4***	***.3***	***3.7***	***21.7***
Spaghetti Marinara	620	119.7	7.4	112.3	19.1
Veal Parmigiana					
w/ Meat Sauce	820	107.4	6.2	101.2	41.1
Whitefish (Breaded)	790	69	3.4	65.6	45.3
Ziti w/ Meat Balls					
& Meat Sauce	960	102	5.6	96.4	44.5
Salads & Dressings					
Chef Salad	460	10.3	3.1	7.2	47.6
Chicken Salad	440	29.6	5.2	24.4	37.1
Chicken Caesar Salad	270	15.6	4.1	11.5	32.5

	Calories	Total Carb	Fiber	Usable Carb	Protein
Chicken Portabella Salad	345	22.6	5.2	17.4	37.6
Fruit w/ Sherbert	310	73	7.5	65.5	4.6
Garden Salad	100	16.5	3.6	12.9	3.4
Steak Salad	615	29.6	5.1	24.5	37.5
Taco Salad	385	36.1	7.6	28.5	17.8
Dressings					
Bleu Cheese	90	7	0	7	1
French Fat Free	70	17	0	17	.2
Fruit Salad	145	5.4	.1	5.3	.3
Italian Fat Free	*10*	*3.1*	*1*	*2.1*	*.1*
Light Burgundy Vinaigrette	35	6	0	6	0
Thousand Island	*95*	*3.1*	*0*	*3.1*	*.2*
Desserts:					
Cheesecake	505	39.6	.2	37.4	8.1
Banana Fudge Sensation	975	47.3	5.4	41.9	13.7
Grilled Sticky Loaf	485	53.2	1.6	51.6	6.4
Ice cream Pies:					
Apple, Reduced Fat	340	61.3	3.7	57.6	2.8
Peach Lite	300	50	1.8	48.2	3
Pudding (Sugar Free)	90	12.5	.8	11.7	4.5
Strawberry Shortcake	685	13.8	2.1	11.7	6.6
EINSTEIN BROS					
Bagels:					
Average all types, 4 oz	320	71	2	69	11
Chocolate Chip Bagel, 4 oz	370	76	3	73	11
Egg Bagel, 3½ oz	340	69	2	67	11
Sesame Dip	380	75	3	72	11
Cream Cheese: 2 Tbsp					
Plain	*70*	*1*	*0*	*1*	*1*
Plain Lite	*60*	*2*	*0*	*2*	*1*
Smoked Salmon	*60*	*1*	*0*	*1*	*1*
Flavors, average	70	.5	0	5	1
Spreads: 2 Tbsp Fruit	75	19	0	19	0
Honey Butter, 1 Tbsp	*90*	*4*	*0*	*4*	*0*
Peanut Butter	190	8	2	6	7
Sandwiches					
Chicago Bagel Dog Asiago	740	78	2	76	29
Classic NY Lox & Bagel	660	79	3	76	26
Egg Santa Fe	650	78	2	76	30
Ham Deli	450	74	3	71	25
Holey Cow	900	77	3	74	36

	Calories	Total Carb	Fiber	Usable Carb	Protein
Mediterranean Hummus	540	89	5	84	18
Roast Beef Deli	480	76	3	73	31
Smoked Turkey Deli	420	75	3	72	25
The Veg-Out	490	77	3	74	17
Tuna Salad Deli	500	77	3	74	32
Turkey Pastrami Deli	440	76	3	73	31
Turkey Pastrami Reuben Deli	660	83	4	79	39
Bagel Shtick:					
Asiago	450	72	2	70	20
Cinnamon Sugar	570	79	2	77	11
Everything	380	73	3	70	12
Potato	350	69	2	67	10
Sesame Bagel Shtick	420	75	5	70	13
Bagel Chips					
Plain, 1 oz Serving	90	15	0	15	2
Roll-Ups:					
Albuquerque Turkey	790	81	5	76	31
Cookies					
Big Brownie	500	76	2	74	4
Chocloate Chunk, 4 oz	600	78	3	75	8
Oatmeal Raisin, 4 oz	550	82	4	78	8
Muffins					
Banana Nut	520	59	3	56	9
Blueberry	460	57	2	55	6
Chocolate Chip	240	28	0	28	3
Lowfat Lemon Poppyseed	370	69	1	68	8
Coffee					
Café Latte, Regular	140	13	0	13	9
Cappuccino	90	9	0	9	6
EL POLLO LOCO					
Flame Broiled Chicken					
Breast	*160*	*0*	*0*	*0*	*26*
Leg	*90*	*0*	*0*	*0*	*11*
Thigh	*170*	*0*	*0*	*0*	*16*
Wing	*100*	*0*	*0*	*0*	*12*
Tortillas					
6" Corn	70	14	1	13	1
6.5" Flour	100	13	0	13	3
Burritos					
Bean, Rice & Cheese	505	73	10	63	17
Chicken Lover's	475	47	8	39	29

	Calories	Total Carb	Fiber	Usable Carb	Protein
Classic	585	66	9	55	31
Mexican Chicken Caesar	720	65	2	63	36
Ranch	610	45	7	38	40
Spicy	635	80	10	70	31
Ultimate	625	66	5	61	39
Tacos					
Chicken Soft Taco	235	15	0	15	17
Taco Al Carbon	180	20	2	18	7
Bowls					
Flame Broiled Chicken Salad	375	39	4	35	25
Mexican Chicken					
Caesar Salad	500	32	3	29	26
Nacho Pollo Bowl	700	64	11	53	37
Smokey Black Bean					
Pollo Bowl	625	75	6	69	29
Specialties					
Chicken Nachos	1425	105	15	90	47
Chicken Quesadilla	595	48	0	48	36
Chicken Sticks (kids), 4 oz	185	11	2	9	12
Chicken Tamale	185	21	2	19	7
Chicken Taquito	385	43	3	40	15
Chicken Tostada Salad	990	91.5	9.5	82	39
Tortilla Chips, Unsalted	400	44.6	3.7	40.9	4.6
Tostada Salad, w/out shell					
& sour cream	305	28	4	24	29
Tostada, shell only	440	42	0	42	7
Side Dishes					
Cole Slaw	200	12	2	10	2
Corn Cobbette (3")	95	18	1	18	3
French Fries	440	61	0	61	6
Garden Salad	110	7	1	6	5
Macaroni & Cheese	245	24	3	21	10
Pinto Beans	195	29	8	21	11
Potato Salad	260	30	3	27	3
Smokey Black Beans	310	35	5	30	7
Spanish Rice	130	24	1	23	2
Dressings					
Bleu Cheese	*230*	*2*	*0*	*2*	*2*
Creamy Cilantro	*270*	*1*	*0*	*1*	*1*
Hidden Valley Ranch	*105*	*1*	*0*	*1*	*1*
Light Italian	*15*	*2*	*0*	*2*	*0*

	Calories	Total Carb	Fiber	Usable Carb	Protein
Thousand Island	215	7	0	7	0
Condiments					
Guacamole	*30*	*3*	*0*	*3*	*0*
House	*5*	*1*	*0*	*1*	*0*
Spicy Chipotle Salsa	*5*	*1*	*0*	*1*	*0*
Jalapeno Hot Sauce, 1 pkt	*5*	*1*	*0*	*1*	*0*
Sour Cream	*53*	*1*	*0*	*1*	*1*
Pico de Gallo Salsa	*10*	*1.5*	*0*	*1.5*	*0*
Desserts					
Banana Split	730	107	3	104	12
Churros	185	18	1	17	3
Foster's Freeze without cone	180	30	0	30	4
Smoothies, all types	345	67	2	65	4

FAZOLI'S ITALIAN FOOD

	Calories	Total Carb	Fiber	Usable Carb	Protein
Soup; Bread					
Minestrone Soup	105	23	8	15	1
Breadstick, dry	95	17	1	16	4
Breadstick	140	18	1	17	4
Salads: No Dressing					
Unless indicated					
Chicken & Pasta					
Caesar Salad	345	33	3	30	24
Chicken Finger Salad	195	8	2	6	20
w/ Bacon Honey					
Mustard Dressing	400	17	2	15	20
Chicken Caesar Salad	415	17	4	13	22
Garden Salad	*30*	*6*	*2*	*4*	*2*
Italian Chef Salad	300	13	3	10	15
Pasta Salad	575	70	5	65	18
Side Pasta Salad	235	29	2	27	7
Dressing: Per 1 oz					
Honey French	145	9	0	9	0
House Italian	100	5	0	5	0
Reduced Calorie Italian	*55*	*3*	*0*	*3*	*0*
Ranch	*155*	*1*	*0*	*1*	*0*
Thousand Island	*135*	*4*	*0*	*4*	*0*
Submarinos: Per ½ Sandwich					
Original	1170	124	8	116	45
Meatball	1265	128	8	120	55
Turkey	960	121	7	114	43
Club	1085	121	7	114	51

	Calories	Total Carb	Fiber	Usable Carb	Protein
Ham & Swiss	990	120	7	113	44
Pepperoni Pizza	1110	133	6	127	55
Pizza: Per Double Slice					
Cheese	465	58	2	56	24
Combination	595	63	3	60	29
Pepperoni	550	61	2	59	27
Pasta: Per Serving					
Fettucine Alfredo:					
Small	525	80	3	77	17
Regular	775	19	5	14	25
Peppery Chicken Alfredo	590	80	3	77	31
Small Spaghetti:					
w/ Marinara	410	74	5	69	15
w/ Meat Sauce	425	74	5	69	14
w/ Meatballs	710	80	6	74	28
Regular Spaghetti:					
w/ Marinara	600	111	7	104	21
w/ Meat Sauce	625	111	8	103	21
w/ Meatballs	1010	119	8	111	39
Italian Specialities: Per Serving					
Baked Chicken Alfredo	775	82	3	79	46
Baked Chicken Parmesan	745	99	6	93	42
Baked Spaghetti Parmesan	680	76	5	71	38
Baked Ziti:					
Small	370	32	4	28	0
Regular	575	49	6	43	0
Broccoli Fettucine Alfredo:					
Regular	815	125	8	117	27
Cheese Ravioli:					
w/ Marinara	480	65	4	61	21
w/ Meat Sauce	495	65	4	61	20
Classic Sampler	675	90	7	83	29
Lasagna:					
Homestyle	430	27	6	21	29
Broccoli	515	34	8	26	34
Pizza Baked Spaghetti	750	78	5	73	40
Shrimp & Scallop Fettucine	595	81	3	78	32
Paninis: Per Serving					
Chicken Caesar Club	675	51	3	48	39
Chicken Pesto	515	51	3	48	33
Four Cheese & Tomato	720	55	3	52	28

	Calories	Total Carb	Fiber	Usable Carb	Protein
Ham & Swiss	605	53	2	51	31
Italian Deli	695	61	4	57	34
Italian Club	670	54	3	51	30
Smoked Turkey	700	57	3	54	32
Desserts: Per Serving					
Cheesecake:					
Plain	290	17	0	17	6
Turtle	435	24	2	22	8
Chocolate Chip	315	22	1	21	7
Lemon Ice	180	45	0	45	0
Milk Chocolate					
Chunk Cookie	375	54	0	54	6
Strawberry Topping, 1 oz	30	8	0	8	0

FRESHENS

	Calories	Total Carb	Fiber	Usable Carb	Protein
Yogurt Smoothies: Per 21 oz					
Blueberry Sunset	385	84	4.2	79.8	10.6
Jamaican Jammer	475	110	4.1	105.9	11.5
Peachy Pineapple	405	91	1.7	89.3	10.7
Pina Collider	560	126	3.7	122.3	11.4
Raspberry Rapture	575	121	4.5	116.5	12.2
Raspberry Rocker	490	113	4.5	108.5	12.3
Strawberry Squeeze	390	88	2.1	85.9	10.7
Tropical Fruit Juice					
Smoothies: Per 21 oz					
Blueberry Wave	330	82	3	79	.6
Caribbean Craze	330	84	3.9	80.1	1.6
Peach Sunset	365	93	2.5	90.5	1.2
Pineapple Passion	440	100	3.5	96.5	1.4
Raspberry Rhapsody	345	88	4.3	83.7	2.4
Raspberry Rumba	375	95	4.3	90.7	2.3
Strawberry Shooter	245	63	1.9	61.1	.8
Orange Smoothies: Per 21 oz					
Aruba Orange	420	97	3.2	93.8	2.6
Orange Shooter	370	81	3.4	77.6	2.7
Orange Sunrise	415	90	2.8	87.2	3
Orange Wave	420	98	1	97	2.8
Coffee Smoothies: Per 21 oz					
Original Coffee	340	70	0	70	6.6
Caramel Coffee	425	89	0	89	7.9
Mocha Coffee	375	79	.9	78.1	7.2
Oreo Coffee	520	96	.9	95.1	8.3

	Calories	Total Carb	Fiber	Usable Carb	Protein
Decadent Smoothies: Per 21 oz					
Fudge Oreo Supreme	640	126	2	124	14.7
Peanut Butter Cup	980	141	2.6	138.4	27.5
Pretzel Logic Pretzels,					
½ Pretzel, 3 oz	255	49	2	47	7

GODFATHER'S PIZZA

	Calories	Total Carb	Fiber	Usable Carb	Protein
Original Crust, Per Slice:					
Combo	350	38	1	37	18
Cheese	260	35	0	35	13

GRETEL'S PRETZELS

	Calories	Total Carb	Fiber	Usable Carb	Protein
Cinnamon/Sugar	195	38	.6	37.4	3
Original	170	31	.5	30.5	3
Poppy Seed	175	31	.6	30.4	3
Raisin Danish/Icing	350	79	3.3	75.7	6.5
Sesame Seed	175	31	.6	30.4	3
Sweet Dough	115	23	1.6	21.4	4

HÄAGEN-DAZS

	Calories	Total Carb	Fiber	Usable Carb	Protein
Per ½ cup					
Baileys Irish Cream	270	23	0	23	5
Banana Foster	260	28	0	28	4
Belgian Choc	330	29	3	26	5
Butter Pecan	310	21	1	20	5
Cherry Vanilla	240	23	0	23	4
Chocolate	270	22	1	21	5
Chocolate Brownie/					
w/ walnuts	290	25	1	24	5
Chocolate Cheescake	300	29	1	28	5
Chocolate, Chocolate Chip	300	26	2	24	5
Chocolate Cookies					
and Cream	270	24	1	23	5
Chocolate Peanut Butter	360	27	2	25	8
Chocolate Raspberry	270	29	1	28	4
Coffee	270	21	0	21	5
Coffee Almond	320	27	1	26	5
Cookie Dough Chip	310	29	0	29	4
Cookies n' Cream	270	23	0	23	5
Cream Carmel Pecan	320	29	0	29	5
Dulce De Leche	290	28	0	28	5
German Chocolate Cake	290	28	1	27	5
Macadamia Brittle	300	25	0	25	4

	Calories	Total Carb	Fiber	Usable Carb	Protein
Mint Chip	300	26	0	26	5
Peanut Butter Fudge Chunk	340	25	1	24	7
Pineapple Coconut	230	25	0	25	4
Pistachio	290	22	0	22	5
Rocky Road	300	29	1	28	5
Rum Raisin	270	22	0	22	4
Strawberry Cheesecake	270	28	0	28	4
Vanilla Carmel Brownie	300	30	0	30	5
Vanilla Chocolate Chip	310	26	0	26	5
HOT DOG ON A STICK					
Fries, 1 order	550	113	6	107	9
American Cheese on a Stick	240	22	1	21	9
Hot Dog on a Stick	250	23	1	22	9
Lemonade, regular, 16 fl. oz	180	45.3	0	45.3	0
Pepper Jack on a Stick	235	21	1	20	9
IN-N-OUT BURGER					
Burgers					
Hamburger	390	39	3	36	16
w/ Mustard/Ketchup,					
no Spread	310	41	3	38	16
Protein Style, no Bun	240	10	2	8	12
Cheeseburger	480	39	3	36	22
w/ Mustard/Ketchup,					
no Spread	400	41	3	38	22
Protein Style, no Bun	330	11	2	9	18
Double Double (2 patty/					
2 slices cheese)	670	40	3	37	37
w/ Mustard/Ketchup,					
no Spread	590	42	3	39	7
Protein Style, no Bun	520	11	2	9	33
French Fries, 125g	400	54	2	52	7
Drinks:					
Milk, 10 fl. oz	180	18	0	18	12
Coca-Cola; Dr. Pepper,					
16 fl. oz	200	54	0	54	0
Diet Coca-Cola, 16 fl. oz	*0*	*0*	*0*	*0*	*0*
Lemonade, 16 fl. oz	180	40	0	40	0
Root Beer, 16 fl. oz	220	60	0	60	0
Seven-Up, 16 fl. oz	215	54	0	54	0
Shakes: 15 fl. oz					
Chocolate	690	83	0	83	9

	Calories	Total Carb	Fiber	Usable Carb	Protein
Strawberry	690	91	2	89	8
Vanilla	680	78	2	76	8
INTERNATIONAL HOUSE OF PANCAKES					
Pancakes: (Syrup/Butter extra)					
Buttermilk, Full Stack, 5	550	85	5	80	15
Buckwheat, 1 (1.7 oz)	110	15	1	14	3
Country Griddle, 1 (2 oz)	120	19	1	18	3
Harvest Grain 'N Nut, 1 (2¼ oz)	180	20	2	18	5
Crepes (Egg Pancakes), 1 (2 oz)	120	14	0	14	3
Syrup: 1 Tbsp	230	58	0	58	0
Whipped Butter, 1 Tbsp	*80*	*0*	*0*	*0*	*0*
Waffles (Plain),					
Regular, 1 (3 oz)	310	37	1	36	6
Belgian: Regular, 1 (4 oz)	390	48	1	47	8
JACK IN THE BOX					
Breakfast					
Biscuit	190	24	1	23	3
Breakfast Jack	310	34	1	33	14
Extreme Sausage Sandwich	720	35	2	33	26
French Toast Sticks, 4 pces	430	57	2	55	8
Hash Brown	150	13	2	11	1
Sausage Biscuit	380	25	2	23	11
Sausage Croissant	680	41	2	39	18
Sausage, Egg & Cheese Biscuit	760	33	2	31	25
Sourdough Breakfast Sandwich	450	36	2	34	18
Supreme Croissant	570	41	1	40	19
Ultimate Breakfast Sandwich	730	66	2	64	30
Country Crock Spread	*25*	*0*	*0*	*0*	*0*
Grape Jelly, 1 packet	35	9	0	9	0
Syrup	130	32	0	32	0
Burgers					
Hamburger	315	30	1	29	17
Hamburger w/ cheese	360	31	1	30	19
Bacon Bacon Cheeseburger	910	58	3	55	38
Bacon Ultimate Cheeseburger	1120	59	2	57	52

	Calories	Total Carb	Fiber	Usable Carb	Protein
Big Cheeseburger	700	59	2	57	26
Big Texas Cheeseburger	610	55	2	53	26
Ultimate Cheeseburger	990	59	2	57	41
Jumbo Jack: Regular	600	58	3	55	22
w/ cheese	690	60	3	57	26
Sourdough Jack	700	36	3	33	30
Mexican Food:					
Monster Taco	255	21	3	18	9
Taco	165	15	2	13	6
Snacks					
Onion Rings	500	51	3	48	6
Bacon Cheddar					
Potato Wedges	770	52	3	49	21
Cheese Sticks:					
3 piece	240	21	1	20	11
5 piece	400	35	1.7	33.3	18.3
Chicken Breast Pieces,					
5 piece	360	24	1	23	27
Curly Fries:					
Chili Cheese, 8.3 oz	630	54	6	49	13
Seasoned, 4.4 oz	400	45	5	40	6
French Fries: Small	330	44	3	41	3
Medium	410	55	4	51	4
Large	580	77	6	71	6
Egg Rolls: 1 piece	130	15	2	13	5
3 piece	388	44.7	6	38.7	14.9
Stuffed Jalapenos: 3 piece	230	22	2	20	7
7 piece	537	51.3	4.7	46.6	16.3
Taquitos: 3 piece	320	28	1	27	14
5 piece	491	43	1.5	41.5	21.5
Sandwiches					
Chicken Fajita Pita	330	35	3	32	24
Chicken Sandwich	410	39	2	37	15
Jack's Spicy Chicken	730	69	4	65	30
Sourdough Grilled					
Chicken Club	520	33	3	31	33
Salads: No Dressing					
Side Salad	*55*	*4*	*2*	*2*	*3*
Condiments					
Cheese: 1 slice American	*45*	*1*	*0*	*1*	*2*
Swiss-style	*40*	*1*	*0*	*1*	*2*

	Calories	Total Carb	Fiber	Usable Carb	Protein
Dipping Sauce:					
Buttermilk, 1 oz	*130*	*3*	*.5*	*2.5*	*0*
Frank's Red Hot					
Buffalo, 1 oz	*10*	*2*	*0*	*2*	*0*
Marinara, 1 oz	*15*	*3*	*0*	*3*	*0*
Barbeque; Sweet					
& Sour, 1 oz	45	11	0	11	1
Tartar	*210*	*2*	*0*	*2*	*1*
Packet Sauce					
Soy Sauce	*5*	*1*	*0*	*1*	*1*
Taco	*0*	*0*	*0*	*0*	*0*
Desserts					
Cheesecake	310	34	0	34	7
Double Fudge Cake	310	49	4	45	3
Ice Cream Shakes					
Chocolate, 11 oz	660	89	1	88	1
Strawberry, 11 oz	630	84	0	84	10
Vanilla, 10 fl. oz	570	65	0	65	12
Drinks					
Barq's Root Beer, 20 fl. oz	180	50	0	50	0
Coca-Cola Classic, 20 fl. oz	170	46	0	46	0
Dr Pepper, 20 fl. oz	190	49	0	49	0
Lowfat Milk (2 %), 8 fl. oz	140	14	0	14	10
Orange Juice, 10 fl. oz	140	32	2	30	2
JAMBA LA JUICE					
Smoothies: Per 24 fl. oz					
Aloha Pineapple	470	89	5	84	7
Banana Berry	470	112	5	107	5
Berry Lime Sublime	450	104	6	98	3
Caribbean Passion	440	102	4	98	4
Orange-A-Peel	440	102	5	97	9
Chocolate Moo'd	690	141	2	139	16
Citrus Squeeze	450	93	5	88	4
Coldbuster	440	100	5	95	5
Cranberry Craze	420	97	4	93	6
Jamba Powerboost	440	103	7	96	9
Kiwi-Berry Burner	470	112	5	107	4
Mango-A-Go-Go	500	117	4	113	4
Orange Blitz	410	94	5	89	5
Orange Dream Machine	545	112	1	111	18
Peach Pleasure	460	108	5	103	4

	Calories	Total Carb	Fiber	Usable Carb	Protein
Peanut Butter Moo'd	860	145	5	140	23
Peenya Kowlada	650	118	3	115	8
Protein Berry Pizazz	460	92	6	86	20
Razzmatazz	480	112	4	108	3
Strawberries Wild	450	105	4	101	6

JIMMY JOHN'S

Gourmet Subs
Made on 8" French Bread

	Calories	Total Carb	Fiber	Usable Carb	Protein
Sorry Charlie w/ Mayo/Sauce	501	58.4	2.7	55.7	22.5
The Pepe w/ Mayo/Cheese	663	53.7	.9	52.8	27.2
Turkey Tom w/ Mayo	538	52.6	1.2	51.4	23.6
Vegetarian w/ Mayo/Cheese	720	58.1	2.4	55.7	26.3
Vito w/ Italian Dressing/ Cheese	556	55.6	1.2	54.4	29.4

Gourmet Club Sandwiches
Made on 8" French Bread

	Calories	Total Carb	Fiber	Usable Carb	Protein
Beach Club w/ Mayo/Cheese	900	78.4	3.1	75.3	42.1
Billy Club w/ Mayo/Cheese	844	75	1.4	73.6	43
Bootlegger's w/ Mayo, No Cheese	693	71.1	.9	70.2	37.9
Country Club w/ Mayo/Cheese	813	73.8	1.2	72.6	43.3
Hunter's Club w/ Mayo/Cheese	818	73.3	1.2	72.1	44.2
Italian Night w/Dressing/ Mayo/Cheese	951	75.1	1.2	73.9	42.3
Smoked Ham Club w/ Mayo/Cheese	832	73.2	.9	72.3	40
Tuna Club w/ Mayo/ Sauce/Cheese	792	79.4	2.7	76.7	40.6
Veggie Club w/ Mayo/Cheese	1020	79.1	2.4	76.7	44.3

Gourmet Club Sandwiches
Made on 7-Grain Wheat Bread

	Calories	Total Carb	Fiber	Usable Carb	Protein
Beach Club w/ Mayo/Cheese	917	73.4	7.6	65.8	41
Billy Club w/ Mayo/Cheese	854	68.9	5.6	63.3	41.6
Bootlegger's w/ Mayo, No Cheese	710	66.1	5.5	60.6	36.9

	Calories	Total Carb	Fiber	Usable Carb	Protein
Country Club					
w/ Mayo/Cheese	831	68.8	7.2	61.6	39.5
Hunter's Club					
w/ Mayo/Cheese	835	68.3	5.8	62.5	43.1
Italian Night w/ Dressing/					
Mayo/Cheese	969	70.2	5.8	64.4	41.2
Smoked Ham Club					
w/ Mayo/Cheese	849	68.2	5.5	62.7	39
Tuna Club w/ Mayo/					
Sauce/Cheese	818	74.4	7.2	67.2	39.5
Veggie Club					
w/ Mayo/Cheese	1038	74.1	7	67.1	43.3
KFC					
Crispy Strips					
Blazin Strips, 3 pce, 4.5 oz	315	21	1	20	26
Colonel's Crispy Strips,					
3 pce, 4 oz	340	20	0	20	28
Honey BBQ Strips,					
3 pce, 6.3 oz	377	33	0	33	28
Spicy Crispy Strips,					
3 pce, 4 oz	335	23	.5	22.5	25
Extra Crispy Breast, 6 oz	470	19	0	19	34
Drumstick, 2.4 oz	160	5	0	5	12
Thigh, 4.2 oz	370	12	0	12	21
Whole Wing, 1.9 oz	190	10	0	10	10
Hot & Spicy Breast, 6.5 oz	450	20	0	20	33
Drumstick, 2.3 oz	***140***	***4***	***0***	***4***	***13***
Thigh, 3.8 oz	390	14	0	14	22
Whole Wing, 1.9 oz	180	9	0	10	11
Original Recipe Breast	370	11	0	11	40
Drumstick, 2.1 oz	***140***	***4***	***0***	***4***	***14***
Thigh, 3.2 oz	360	12	0	10	22
Whole Wing, 1.6 oz	145	5	0	5	11
Entrées					
Chunky Chicken					
Pot Pie, 13 oz	770	69	5	64	29
Honey BBQ Wings, 6 pieces	607	33	1	32	33
Hot Wings, 6 pieces, 4.8 oz	470	18	2	16	27
Popcorn Chicken, large, 6 oz	620	36	0	36	30
Popcorn Chicken,					
small, 3.5 oz	362	21	.2	20.8	17

	Calories	Total Carb	Fiber	Usable Carb	Protein
Sandwiches					
Blazin Twister, 8.7 oz	719	56	4	52	30
Chicken Twister, wrap, 8.5 oz	600	52	4	48	22
Crispy Caesar Twister, 9.5 oz	744	66	5	61	27
Honey BBQ Crunch Melt, 8.1 oz	556	48	2	46	33
Chicken w/ sauce, 6.3 oz	310	37	2	35	28
Original Recipe:					
w/ sauce, 7 oz	450	33	2	31	29
without sauce, 6.6 oz	360	21	.5	20.5	29
Triple Crunch Chicken:					
w/ sauce 6.6 oz	490	39	2	37	28
without sauce, 6.2 oz	390	29	2	27	25
Triple Crunch Zinger:					
w/ sauce, 7.4 oz	550	39	2	37	28
without sauce, 6.2 oz	390	36	2	34	25
Side Dishes: Per Serving					
BBQ Baked Beans, 5.5 oz	190	33	6	27	6
Biscuit, 2 oz	180	20	.5	19.5	4
Coleslaw, 5 oz	232	26	3	23	2
Green Beans, 4.6 oz	*45*	*7*	*3*	*4*	*1*
Macaroni & Cheese, 5.4 oz	180	21	2	19	7
Mashed Potatoes w/ Gravy, 4.8 oz	120	17	2	15	1
Mean Greens, 5.4 oz	70	11	5	6	4
Potato Salad, 5.6 oz	230	23	3	20	4
Potato Wedges, 4.8 oz	376	53	4.5	48.5	6.2
Dessert					
Colonel's Pies: Per Slice					
Apple Pie, 4 oz	310	44	0	44	2
Pecan Pie, 4 oz	490	66	2	64	5
Strawberry Crème Pie, 2.7 oz	280	32	2	30	4
Double Chocolate Chip Cake, 2.7 oz	320	41	1	40	4
Little Bucket Parfaits					
Chocolate Cream, 4 oz	290	37	2	35	3
Fudge Brownie, 3.5 oz	280	44	1	43	3

	Calories	Total Carb	Fiber	Usable Carb	Protein
Lemon Crème, 4.5 oz	410	62	4	58	7
Strawberry Shortcake, 3.5 oz	200	33	1	32	1

KILWIN'S

	Calories	Total Carb	Fiber	Usable Carb	Protein
Ice cream: Per 1 cup					
Black Cherry; Caramel Revel	180	44	0	44	6
Butter Pecan	380	32	0	32	6
Butter Pecan Yogurt	260	34	0	34	6
Chocolate	340	34	0	34	6
Chocolate Chip					
Cookie Dough	380	44	0	44	6
Chocolate Ripple	200	46	0	46	6
French Silk; Mud	380	40	0	40	6
Lemon/Raspberry Sorbetto	100	25	0	25	0
Old Fashioned Vanilla	360	40	0	40	6
Toppings:					
Caramel, 40g	160	31	0	31	1
Fudge, 40g	110	28	1	27	2
Fudge: Per Piece (40g)					
Butter/Vanilla Pecan	160	29	0	29	0
Chocolate	150	30	0	30	1
Chocolate Peanut Butter	160	27	1	26	0
Chocolate Pecan/					
Walnut; Peanut Butter	160	28	1	27	1
German Chocolate	160	27	1	26	1
Heavenly Hash	200	24	2	22	1
Walnut Maple	160	29	1	28	0
Chocloate Bars: Per 1 oz Bar					
Chocolate Sea Foam,					
Dark/Milk	190	28	1	27	2
Happy Birthday;					
Teacher; Thank You	160	17	1	16	2
Kilwin's Molded	270	24	1	23	2
Cluster: Per Serving					
Almond Cluster: Dark (4)	250	20	4	16	5
Milk (3)	211	17	4	13	2
Cashew Cluster: Dark (4)	254	21.4	5.3	16.1	5.3
Milk (3)	188	15	3	12	3.8
Coconut Cluster: Dark (4)	230	24	3	21	2
Milk (4)	211	21	1	20	2
Peanut Cluster (3)	132	9.6	1.2	8.4	3.6
Dark/Milk (4)	220	19	2	17	5

	Calories	Total Carb	Fiber	Usable Carb	Protein
Pecan Cluster: Dark (4)	241	20.1	3	17.1	3
Milk (4)	251	21	1	20	3
Raisin Cluster: Dark (3)	190	28	2	26	2
Milk (4)	170	25	1	24	2
Choclate-Coated Candy:					
Per Serving					
Coated almonds:					
Dark (5); Milk (6)	221	20	2	18	4
Coated Brazils: Dark (6)	229	14	2	12	4
Milk (7)	249	15	2	13	4
Coated Cashews: Dark (6)	221	16.1	5	11.1	5
Milk (7)	240	17	5	12	5
Coated Pecans: Dark (7)	229	14	3	11	3
Milk (8)	273	17.2	3	14.2	2
KOO KOO ROO					
Original Skinless					
Flame Broiled Chicken					
3 Piece Original Dark	**320**	**4.8**	**0**	**4.8**	**38.9**
Breast & Wing					
(skin on wing)	**345**	**1**	**.1**	**.9**	**49**
Original Breast, 3.4 oz	**185**	**.3**	**0**	**.3**	**34.1**
Half Original Chkn					
(skin on wing)	**635**	**2**	**.3**	**1.7**	**80**
Fresh Roasted Carved Turkey					
¼ lb Sliced White Meat	**175**	**0**	**0**	**0**	**25.3**
Hand-Carved Turkey Dinner					
w/ potatoes, vegetables,					
stuffing, gravy, sauce	695	66.9	7.6	59.3	41.5
Turkey Pot Pie, 5.5 oz	870	83	6.3	76.7	36.7
Salads: Per Regular					
(no dressing)					
BBQ Chicken Salad, 15½ oz	365	21.8	6.1	15.7	37.5
Chicken Caesar Salad, 12 oz	285	15	3.5	11.5	33.9
Chinese Chicken Salad, 17 oz	570	38.8	9.7	29.1	39.7
Koo Koo Roo House					
Salad, 16 oz	125	16.4	5.1	11.3	5.5
Chicken Chop Bowls:					
Chargrilled: w/out Sauce	560	57.2	3.5	53.7	41.4
Southwestern, w/out Sauce	580	66.7	8.1	58.6	36.9
Soup:					
Ten Vegetable	100	16.3	4.1	12.2	3.2

	Calories	Total Carb	Fiber	Usable Carb	Protein
Sandwiches:					
BBQ Chicken w/ Sauce	565	71	2.7	68.3	44.6
Original Chicken Breast w/ Dressing	670	62.6	2.5	60.1	41
Wraps:					
Caesar Chicken	755	59.4	3.7	55.7	41.7
Cold Sides:					
Cucumber Salad 5 oz	40	8.7	1.9	6.8	1.3
Creamy Cole Slaw, 5 oz	240	14	2.3	11.7	1.4
Tangy Tomato Salad, 4.5 oz	*65*	*6*	*1.4*	*4.6*	*1.1*
Hot Sides:					
Baked Yams, 6 oz	200	47	6.6	40.4	2.5
Black Beans, 6 oz	145	22.5	6.3	16.2	8
Creamed Spinach, 5 oz	115	10	2.9	7.1	4.3
Hand-Mashed Potaotes, 6.5 oz	190	32.3	2.8	29.5	3.5
Macaroni & Cheese, 6 oz	335	31.9	1.2	30.7	14.5
Roasted Garlic Potatoes, 5 oz	135	21.3	2	19.3	2.2
Dressings: Per Serving					
BBQ, 2 oz	90	14.1	0	14.1	0
Caesar, 1.5 oz	*240*	*1.4*	*0*	*1.4*	*0*
Chinese Chicken Salad, 3 oz	340	26	0	26	0
Cranberry Sauce, 1 oz	45	11	0	11	0
Gravy, 2 oz	*50*	*2.8*	*0*	*2.8*	*.9*
KOHR BROS					
Frozen Custard: Per ½ cup					
Chocolate	140	18	0	18	4
Orange Sherbert	105	21	.5	20.5	1
Vanilla	135	16	0	16	4
KRISPY KREME					
Yeast Doughnuts					
Glazed Rings:					
Doughnut	205	22	.5	21.5	2
Chocolate Iced w/ Sprinkles	270	38	.5	37.5	3
Chocolate Iced	250	33	.5	32.5	3
Maple Iced	245	32	.5	31.5	2
Cinnamon Bun	270	28	.5	27.5	3
Sugar Doughnut (3)	200	21	0	20	2

	Calories	Total Carb	Fiber	Usable Carb	Protein
Cinnamon Twist	225	33	.5	32.5	3
Glazed Twist, 1 piece	205	28	.5	27.5	3
Cake Doughnuts:					
Traditional Cake Doughnut	230	25	.5	24.5	3
Chocolate Iced	280	36	.5	35.5	3
Powdered Sugar	285	37	.5	36.5	3
Glazed Cruller	240	26	.5	25.5	2
Chocolate Iced	210	24	.5	23.5	2
Old Fashioned:					
Glazed Blueberry	340	42	.5	41.5	3
Glazed Devil's Food	340	42	.5	41.5	3
Honey & Oat	340	42	.5	41.5	3
Vanilla Iced Cake					
w/ Sprinkles	269	35	.5	34.5	3
Filled Doughnuts:					
Apple-Filled Cinnamon					
Sugar Coated	285	32	.5	31.5	3
Blueberry-Filled					
Sugar Coated Yeast	295	35	.5	34.5	3
Chocolate Iced:					
Crème-Filled	355	39	.5	38.5	3
Custard-Filled	315	35	.5	34.5	3
Glazed:					
Crème-Filled	350	39	1	38	3
Raspberry-Filled	310	39	.5	38.5	3
Yeast:					
Powdered Raspberry-Filled	300	36	.5	35.5	3
Vanilla Iced Crème-Filled	345	38	.5	37.5	3
Vanilla Iced Custard-Filled	290	33	.5	32.5	3
Glazed Lemon-Filled	292	34	.5	33.5	3
Glazed Custard-Filled	290	34	.5	33.5	3
Powdered Strawberry-Filled	260	26	.5	25.5	3
KRYSTAL					
Breakfast					
Biscuit: Plain	260	27	2	25	4
Bacon, Egg & Cheese	385	28	2	26	12
Chik	335	34	1	33	11
Sausage	445	27	3	24	12
Country Breakfast	660	46	8	38	24
Hash Browns	190	17	2	15	1
Sunriser	230	14	2	12	12

	Calories	Total Carb	Fiber	Usable Carb	Protein
Sandwiches					
Regular	160	17	1	16	7
Double	265	24	2	22	13
Bacon Cheese	195	16	2	14	10
Cheese	180	16	2	14	9
Double Cheese	312	26	1	25	16
Chik	240	24	2	22	11
Chili Cheese Pup	210	17	2	15	9
Corn Pup	265	19	1	18	5
Plain Pup	165	15	1	14	6
Fries					
Regular	375	49	6	43	4
Chili Cheese	540	59	6	53	13
LITTLE CAESAR'S					
Pizza: Per Slice					
12" Round:					
Cheese, 1/8 Pizza	170	23	1	22	10
Pepperoni, 1/8 Pizza	190	23	1	22	11
12" Deep Dish:					
Cheese, 1/8 Pizza	140	27	1	26	11
Pepperoni, 1/8 Pizza	160	27	1	26	12
12" Thin:					
Cheese, 1/8 Pizza	120	13	0	13	8
Pepperoni, 1/8 Pizza	150	13	0	13	9
14" Round:					
Cheese, 1/10 Pizza	200	25	1	24	10
Meatsa, 1/10 Pizza	250	26	2	24	15
Pepperoni, 1/10 Pizza	220	25	1	24	12
Supreme, 1/10 Pizza	230	31	3	28	13
Veggie, 1/10 Pizza	190	32	3	29	12
14" Deep Dish:					
Cheese, 1/10	290	37	2	35	15
Pepperoni, 1/10 Pizza	340	38	2	36	17
14" Thin:					
Cheese, 1/10 Pizza	130	14	0	14	8
Pepperoni, 1/10 Pizza	160	14	0	14	9
16" Round:					
Cheese, 1/12 Pizza	210	27	1	26	11
Pepperoni, 1/12 Pizza	230	27	1	26	12
18" Round:					
Cheese, 1/12 Pizza	220	30	1	29	12

	Calories	Total Carb	Fiber	Usable Carb	Protein
Pepperoni, ½ Pizza	250	30	1	29	13
Baby Pan! Pan!	348	34	2	32	17
Pizza By the Slice:					
Cheese, ⅙	290	42	2	40	17
Pepperoni, ⅙ medium pizza	340	42	2	40	20
Sandwiches (Cold)					
Italia	690	66	3	63	35
Ham & Cheese: Turkey	600	66	3	63	32
Veggie	720	67	3	64	24
Salads					
Antipasto	*130*	*6*	*2*	*4*	*9*
Caesar; Greek	80	12	3	9	5
Tossed Salad	50	15	3	9	2
Dressings					
Caesar, 1.5 oz	*230*	*1*	*0*	*1*	*1*
Buttermilk Ranch, 1 oz	*270*	*2*	*0*	*2*	*1*
Creamy Caesar;					
Golden Ital.; Blue Cheese	*210*	*2*	*0*	*2*	*0*
Fat Free Italian, 1 oz	25	5	0	5	0
Sides					
Chicken Wings, 1 piece	*50*	*0*	*0*	*0*	*5*
Crazy Bread, 1 stick, 1.2 oz	100	15	0	15	3
Crazy Sauce, 4 oz	60	9	3	6	0
Italian Cheese Bread,					
1 piece	110	13	0	13	7
Cinnamon Stick	340	19	0	19	3
LONG JOHN SILVER'S					
Sandwiches					
Ultimate Fish	480	51	3	48	20
Chicken Sandwich	340	41	3	38	12
Flatbread Fish	560	48	6	42	29
Side Items					
Fries: Regular	240	34	3	31	3
Cheese Sticks (3)	135	12	1	11	4
Coleslaw, 4 oz	200	15	3	12	1
Corn Cobbette; no butter	95	14	3	11	3
Hushpuppy, 1 piece	65	9	1	8	1
Rice, 4 oz	180	34	3	31	3
Soup, Clam Chowder: 1 cup	220	23	.5	22.5	9
Chicken Battered Plank,					
1 piece	140	9	0	9	8

	Calories	Total Carb	Fiber	Usable Carb	Protein
Seafood					
Battered Fish	225	16	0	16	11
Battered Shrimp, 1 piece	*45*	*3*	*0*	*3*	*2*
Breaded Clams, 1 order	235	22	1	21	8
Desserts: Per Piece					
Chocolate Crème Pie	315	24	1	23	5
Pecan Pie	370	55	2	53	4
Pineapple Crème Pie	290	39	1	38	4
Beverages: Per Medium					
Diet Coke	*0*	*0*	*0*	*0*	*0*
Sprite	195	49	0	49	0

MAGGIE MOO'S ICE CREAM & TREATERY

	Calories	Total Carb	Fiber	Usable Carb	Protein
Ice cream: Per ½ cup					
No Sugar Added 10%	90	13	0	13	3
Non Fat	85	18	0	18	3
Sorbet: Per ½ cup					
Non Fat, Non Dairy	90	22	0	22	0
Yogurt: Per ½ cup					
Non Fat	100	20	0	20	3
Non Fat, No Sugar Added	60	11	0	11	4

MCDONALD'S

	Calories	Total Carb	Fiber	Usable Carb	Protein
Burgers/Sandwiches					
Big Mac	580	47	3	44	24
Big N' Tasty	530	37	2	35	24
with cheese	585	37	2	35	26
BBQ Chicken Sandwich	340	48	4	44	18
Cheeseburger	330	36	2	34	15
Chicken Fajita: w/ Cheese	190	21	1	20	11
w/out Cheese	170	19	1	18	12
Chicken McGrill	400	37	2	35	25
plain (no mayo)	300	34.2	1.9	32.3	22.2
Crispy Chicken	505	46	2	44	22
Double Cheeseburger	490	37	2	35	25
Filet-O-Fish	475	45	1	44	15
Hamburger	280	35	2	33	12
Quarter Pounder w/ Cheese	535	38	2	36	28
Sourdough Crispy Chicken	580	54	3	51	26
Sourdough Supreme Burger	660	44	4	40	31
French Fries					
Small, 2.4 oz	205	26	2	24	3
Medium, 5 oz	443	56.2	4.3	51.9	6.5

	Calories	Total Carb	Fiber	Usable Carb	Protein
Large, 6 oz	531	68	5.2	62.8	7.8
Super Size, 7 oz	597	75.7	5.8	69.9	8.7
Chicken McNuggets:					
4 pieces	205	12	1	11	10
6 pieces	308	18	1.5	16.5	15
10 pieces	515	30	3	27	25
Sauces: BBQ, 1 oz pkg	40	10	0	10	0
Honey (1 pkg), ½ oz	50	12	0	12	0
Honey Mustard					
(1 pkg), ½ oz	*55*	*3*	*0*	*3*	*0*
Hot Mustard (1 pkg), 1 oz	65	7	0	7	1
Light Mayonnaise (1 pkg)	*45*	*1*	*0*	*1*	*0*
Sweet 'N' Sour	45	11	0	11	0
Breakfast Menu: Per Serving					
Bacon, Egg & Cheese Biscuit	485	31	1	30	20
Biscuit, 2.7 oz	235	30	1	29	4
Breakfast Sourdough	560	41	2	39	22
Chorizo & Egg Breakfast					
Burrito	290	24	1	23	13
Egg McMuffin	295	29	2	27	18
English McMuffin, 2 oz	145	27	2	25	5
Ham, Egg & Cheese Bagel	545	58	2	56	26
Hash Browns, 2 oz	130	14	1	13	1
Hotcakes: Plain, (3)	340	58	3	55	9
w/ margarine,					
2 pats & syrup	605	104	3	101	9
Sausage Biscuit With Egg	410	30	1	29	10
Sausage Breakfast					
Burrito, 4 oz	290	24	2	22	13
Sausage McMuffin	380	29	2	27	14
Sausage Patty, 1.5 oz	*170*	*0*	*0*	*0*	*6*
Scrambled Eggs (2), 3½ oz	*155*	*1*	*0*	*1*	*13*
Spanish Omelette Bagel	705	59	3	56	27
Steak, Egg & Cheese Bagel	630	57	2	55	31
McSalad Shaker					
Salads/Dressings					
Caesar Salad	*90*	*7*	*3*	*4*	*7*
Grilled Chicken Caesar Salad	210	11	3	8	26
Croutons (1 pkg)	50	8	0	8	1
Desserts/Cookies					
Baked Apple Pie, 2¾ oz	265	34	.5	33.5	3

	Calories	Total Carb	Fiber	Usable Carb	Protein
Chocolate Chip Cookies (1)	180	23	.5	22.5	2
Fruit 'n Yogurt Parfait:					
w/ Granola	390	76	2	74	10
w/out Granola	280	53	1	52	8
McDonaldland Cookies,					
2 oz bag	235	38	1	37	3
McFlurry: Butterfinger	620	90	0	90	16
M&M	912	130.3	1.4	128.9	23.2
Nestlé Crunch	920	128.9	0	128.9	23.2
Oreo	824	118.5	0	118.5	21.7
Sundaes/Cone Sundae:					
Hot Caramel Sundae	360	61	0	61	7
Hot Fudge Sundae, 6.3 oz	350	52	1	51	8
Strawberry Sundae	290	50	0	50	2
Nuts (Sundae/					
Topping), ¼ oz	**50**	**2**	**0**	**2**	**2**
Cone: Vanilla Reduced Fat	150	23	0	23	4
Drinks					
1% Lowfat Milk, 8 fl. oz ctn	105	13	0	13	8
Orange Juice, 17.9 oz	243	57.3	0	57.3	3.5
Root Beer Float, 16 oz	310	57	0	57	6
Thick Creamy Shakes,					
16 fl. oz cup:					
Chocolate	573	93.3	1.3	92	14.7
Strawberry	560	89.3	.7	88.6	14.7
Vanilla	560	89.3	0	89.3	14.7
Coca-Cola Classic (25% Ice):					
Childs, 12 fl. oz	115	29	0	29	0
Small, 16 fl. oz	153	38.7	0	38.7	0
Medium, 21 fl. oz	201	50.8	0	50.8	0
Large, 32 fl. oz	307	77.3	0	77.3	0
Super Size, 42 fl. oz	403	101.5	0	101.5	0
Diet Coke (25% Ice):					
Childs, 12 fl. oz	**0**	**0**	**0**	**0**	**0**
Small, 16 fl. oz	**0**	**0**	**0**	**0**	**0**
Medium, 21 fl. oz	**0**	**0**	**0**	**0**	**0**
Large, 32 fl. oz	**0**	**0**	**0**	**0**	**0**
MAZZIO'S PIZZA					
Pizza: Per Slice (⅛ Med. Pizza)					
Pepperoni:					
Thin Crust	160	18	2	16	10

	Calories	Total Carb	Fiber	Usable Carb	Protein
Large Pizzeria Crust	330	42	3	39	17
Sausage:					
Thin Crust	190	19	2	17	11
Original Crust	250	30	3	27	13
Large Pizzeria Crust	380	43	3	40	19
Combo:					
Thin Crust	200	20	2	18	11
Original Crust	250	31	3	28	12
Large Pizzeria Crust	370	44	3	41	18
Supremebuster:					
Thin Crust	190	19	2	17	10
Original Crust	240	30	3	27	12
Deep Pan Crust	340	38	3	25	13
Large Pizzeria Crust	360	43	3	40	18
Meatbuster:					
Thin Crust	220	19	2	17	12
Original Crust	270	30	3	27	13
Deep Pan Crust	370	38	3	35	15
Large Pizzeria Crust	410	43	3	40	21
Chicken Club:					
Thin Crust	180	19	2	17	13
Original Crust	250	30	3	27	15
Deep Pan Crust	350	38	3	35	16
Large Pizzeria Crust	360	40	3	37	21
California Alfredo:					
Thin Crust	210	17	1	16	12
Original Crust	260	28	1	27	14
Deep Pan Crust	370	36	2	34	15
Large Pizzeria Crust	320	42	3	39	18
Mexican:					
Thin Crust	280	25	4	21	14
Original Crust	330	36	4	32	16
Deep Pan Crust	440	44	5	39	18
"Mazzio's Works":					
Thin Crust	220	20	3	17	11
Deep Pan Crust	380	39	4	36	14
Large Pizzeria Crust	410	44	3	41	20
Appetizers: Per Serving					
Cheese Nachos, ½ container	440	19	1	18	18
Cheese Dippers,					
¼ container	330	38	3	35	11

	Calories	Total Carb	Fiber	Usable Carb	Protein
Wings of Fire: Large	*370*	*2*	*0*	*2*	*24*
Small	*260*	*3*	*0*	*3*	*24*
Cinnamon Sticks, 3.2 oz	350	45	2	43	5
Breadsticks, 2.8 oz	120	25	2	23	5
Pasta: Per Serving					
Calzone:					
Pepperoni, ⅒ whole	240	33	2	31	9
Ham-Bacon-Cheddar, ⅒	280	32	2	30	9
Italian Sampler, 24 oz	1640	218	11	207	63
Spaghetti:					
w/ Meatballs, 21 oz	1560	206	11	195	64
w/ Meat Sauce, 17 oz	1210	200	10	190	43
w/ Marinara, 16 oz	940	208	16	192	36

MIMI'S CAFÉ

	Calories	Total Carb	Fiber	Usable Carb	Protein
Per Serving					
Broiled 10 oz Halibut Steak	625	51	9	42	69
Capellini w/ Tomatoes					
& Basil	680	130	11	119	21
EggBeater Fitness Omelette	655	110	14	96	36
Half-A-Turkey Sandwich	410	55	2	53	33
Maggie's Chicken					
and Fruit	545	59	6	53	57
Roasted Turkey Breast	540	52	8	44	65
Two "AA" Large Eggs	395	62	3	59	19

MRS FIELDS COOKIES

	Calories	Total Carb	Fiber	Usable Carb	Protein
Per 1 Cookie, 1.7 oz					
Butter; Butter Toffee	290	40	.5	39.5	3
Cinnamon Sugar	285	41	.5	40.5	3
Coconut Macadamia	285	39	.5	38.5	3
Debra's Special	280	39	2	37	4
Milk Chocolate	280	38	.5	37.5	3
Milk Choc w/ Walnuts/					
Macadamia	320	36	1	35	4
Oatmeal Chocolate Chip	290	40	1	39	3
Oatmeal Raisin w/ Walnuts	280	39	2	37	4
Peanut Butter	300	34	1	33	5
Peanut Butter Milk Chocolate	315	35	1	34	5
Semi-Sweet Chocolate	295	40	.5	39.5	2
w/ Pecans/Walnuts	310	38	2	36	3
White Chunk Macadamia	315	37	.5	36.5	4

	Calories	Total Carb	Fiber	Usable Carb	Protein
Bite Size Nibbler:					
Per 2 Cookies, 1 oz					
Butter	105	15	0	15	1
Chewy Chocolate Fudge	110	15	1	14	1
Cinnamon Sugar	115	17	0	17	1
Debra's Special	95	13	0	13	1
Milk Choc w/ Walnuts	102	12.5	0	12.5	.9
Peanut Butter	115	13	0	13	2
Triple Chocolate	120	15	1	14	1
Milk/Semi-Sweet Chocolate	110	15	1	14	.1
White Chunk Macadamia	120	13	0	13	1
Brownies: Each (76g)					
Double Fudge	385	49	2	47	4
Frosted Fudge	455	62	2	60	4
Pecan Fudge	365	40	2	38	4
Walnut Fudge	405	45	1	44	5
Pecan Pie Brownie	360	40	2	38	5
Bundt Cakes: Per Piece (83g)					
Banana Walnut	355	35	3	32	6
Banana Walnut					
w/ Chocolate Chip	380	39	3	36	6
Blueberry	270	36	1	35	4
Raspberry	270	36	1	35	4
MR SUB					
Breads and Wraps					
Cheese Tortilla, 2.6 oz	235	34	1.1	32.9	6.5
Harvest Wheat, reg 4.5 oz	380	70	12	58	15
Hearty Multi-Grain, reg 5 oz	370	69	5	64	12
Mozza Cheddar, reg 5.6 oz	430	70	9	61	20
Spinach Tortilla, 2.6 oz	220	37	1.7	35.3	6.4
Sundried Tomato					
Tortilla, 2.6 oz	220	37	1.8	35.2	6.9
Traditional, regular, 4.9 oz	365	70	8.7	61.3	15
Whole Wheat Tortilla, 2.6 oz	220	37	3.6	33.4	6.3
Cheese (Processed), 1 slice	*85*	*3.4*	*0*	*3.4*	*5*
Classic Subs: Per Regular Sub					
Assorted	650	82	10	72	36
Ham	500	87	10	77	28
Meatball	735	78	8.7	69.3	39
Pizza	590	72	8.7	63.3	28
Vegetarian	395	73	10	63	16

	Calories	Total Carb	Fiber	Usable Carb	Protein
Premium Subs: Per Regular Sub					
Breaded Chicken	755	100	10	90	41
Canadian Club	555	78	10	68	41
Grilled Chicken	570	80	10	70	42
Louisiana Chicken	585	71	9.3	61.7	38
Seafood with Crab	515	89	9.3	79.7	26
Specialty Subs: Per Regular Sub					
BBQ Rib	695	73	8.7	64.3	40
BLT	540	75	10	65	26
Roast Beef	500	70	8.7	61.3	34
Tuna	565	81	20	79	36
Turkey	462	75	5	70	30
Wraps:					
Louisiana Chicken	350	39	4.4	34.6	22
Roast Beef	305	38	3.8	34.2	20
Seafood with Crab	320	52	4.4	47.6	15
Tuna	350	46	5.1	40.9	22
Turkey	280	41	5	36	17
Sauces: Per ½ oz					
BBQ Sauce	15	3.9	.2	3.7	.1
Louisiana	10	2.3	.1	2.2	.2
Mr SUB Secret Sauce	**80**	**0**	**0**	**0**	**0**
Mayo Lite	**55**	**2**	**0**	**2**	**0**
Meatball	10	2.8	.1	2.7	.1
Pizza	10	2.3	.1	2.2	.2
Soups and Chili:					
Bean and Spring Vegetable	124	23	.5	22.5	5.9
Caribbean and Black Bean	110	22.2	.4	21.8	4.5
Chicken Noodle	95	14.7	.1	14.6	4
Chili with Beef	185	31.5	.3	31.2	11.7
Clam Chowder	175	21	.1	20.9	5
Cream of Mushroom	65	10.7	.2	10.5	2.3
Cream of Potato and Leek	170	20.7	.1	20.6	3.5
French Canadian Pea	145	23	.3	22.7	7.4
Garden Vegetable	50	11	.5	10.5	1.4
Italian Wedding Style	125	21.4	.1	21.3	3.8
Minestrone	80	15.4	.4	15	3.4
Pasta Fagioli	140	25.6	.3	25.3	6.3
Vegetable Beef and Barley	85	16.3	.3	16	2.9
Cookies					
Gourmet Choc Chunk	175	24	.7	23.3	2

	Calories	Total Carb	Fiber	Usable Carb	Protein
Gourmet Double Choc Chip	180	23	.9	22.1	2
Gourmet Oatmeal Raisin	155	23	.9	22.1	2

PANDA EXPRESS

	Calories	Total Carb	Fiber	Usable Carb	Protein
Chicken, 5 oz:					
Black Pepper	180	10	2	8	13
Orange Chicken	473	50	2	48	21
Chicken w/ Mushrooms	135	7	2	5	11
Chicken w/ String Beans	175	11	2	9	12
Spicy Chicken w/ Peanuts	205	19	4	15	18
Beef:					
Beef & Broccoli, 5 oz	150	9	1	8	11
Pork:					
Sweet & Sour Pork, 4 oz	415	17	3	14	19
Sweet & Sour Sauce, 2 oz	62	15	0	15	.5
Vegetables:					
Mixed Vegetables, 5 oz	70	8	1	7	3
Chow Mein & Rice:					
Per 8 oz Serve					
Vegetable Fried Rice	390	61	2	59	9
Steamed Rice	330	74	2	72	7
Vegetable Chow Mein	330	48	4	44	10
Egg Rolls: 2 pieces, 3 oz	188	21	3	18	8

PANERA BREAD

	Calories	Total Carb	Fiber	Usable Carb	Protein
Bagels					
Asiago	330	57	2	55	15
Blueberry	330	69	3	66	12
Choc. Chip	360	67	3	64	12
Cinnamon Crunch	510	95	3	92	12
Dutch Apple/Raisin	350	73	3	70	10
Everything	300	60	3	57	12
Morning Glory	380	71	3	68	11
Plain	290	59	2	57	11
Salad: Per Container					
Asian Chicken	410	43	4	39	26
Caesar Salad	380	22	3	19	13
Classic Café	400	12	4	8	5
Grilled Chicken/Caesar	480	23	3	20	33
Fandango	400	23	7	16	13
Greek	480	15	5	10	9

	Calories	Total Carb	Fiber	Usable Carb	Protein
Sandwiches					
Asiago Roast Beef	960	78	2	76	44
Bacon/Turkey	860	83	5	78	56
Chicken Salad on Nine Grain	600	57	5	52	35
Italian Combo on Ciabatta	1005	80	5	75	61
Peanut Butter and Jelly	440	64	3	61	16
Sierra Turkey	760	68	4	64	43
Smoked Ham & Swiss Cheese	640	49	6	43	43
Smoked Turkey on Sourdough	460	46	4	42	35
Tuna Salad on Honey Wheat	760	52	5	47	29
Tuscan Chicken	936	83	5	78	34
Garden Veggie	585	74	4	70	18
Soup: Per Container					
Baked Potato	240	20	1	19	6
Broccoli Cheddar	220	13	1	12	8
Chicken Noodle	110	15	1	14	7
Cream of Chicken w/ Wild Rice	210	18	1	17	7
Fire Roasted Veggie Bisque	180	16	2	14	4
Forest Mushroom	140	14	2	12	4
French Onion	200	21	2	19	9
Mesa Vegetable And Bean	100	18	3	15	4
Potato Cream Cheese	190	21	1	20	5
Savory Vegetable Bean	120	21	4	17	5
Vegetable & Sirloin	100	16	2	14	5
PAPA JOHN'S					
Original Large Pizza (14")					
Per Slice (⅛th Whole)					
All the Meats	390	37	2	35	18
Cheese	290	37	2	35	13
Garden Special	305	38	2	36	16
Pepperoni	310	37	2	35	13
Sausage	330	37	2	35	14
Six Cheese	435	38	2	36	23
Spinach Alfredo	335	35	1	34	17
The Works	350	38	2	36	16
Thin Crust Pizza					
All The Meats	400	22	1	21	19
Cheese	250	22	1	21	11

	Calories	Total Carb	Fiber	Usable Carb	Protein
Pepperoni	275	22	1	21	11
Sausage	290	22	1	21	12
Six Cheese	390	23	1	22	21
Spinach Alfredo	295	20	1	19	15
Extras					
Bread Sticks (1)	140	26	1	25	4
Cheese Sticks (1)	185	20	1	19	8
Cheese Sauce	*60*	*0*	*0*	*0*	*4*
Cinnapie, 1 slice	115	14	0	14	1
Garlic Sauce 1.2 oz	*235*	*0*	*0*	*0*	*0*
Pizza Sauce 1.2 oz	*30*	*3*	*2*	*1*	*0*
PIZZA HUT					
Pan Pizza: Per Slice					
(⅛ Medium Pizza)					
Beef Topping	334	29	3	26	14
Cheese	286	28	2	26	12
Chicken Supreme	276	29	2	27	13
Ham	264	28	2	26	11
Italian Sausage	343	29	2	27	13
Meat Lover's	361	29	3	26	14
Pepperoni	282	28	2	26	11
Pepperoni Lover's	334	29	2	17	14
Pork Topping	329	29	3	26	15
Super Supreme	338	30	3	27	14
Supreme	321	29	3	26	13
Veggie Lover's	268	30	3	27	10
Personal Pan Pizza: Per Pizza					
Beef	723	71	6	65	31
Cheese	648	71	6	65	28
Ham	595	70	5	65	27
Italian Sausage	759	71	6	65	31
Pepperoni	636	70	5	65	26
Pork Topping	714	71	6	65	31
Stuffed Crust: Per Slice					
(½ Large Pizza)					
Beef Topping	398	40	3	47	19
Cheese	372	39	3	36	18
Chicken Supreme	365	41	3	38	21
Ham	345	39	3	36	18
Italian Sausage	416	40	3	37	19

	Calories	Total Carb	Fiber	Usable Carb	Protein
Meat Lover's	473	40	3	37	22
Pepperoni	368	39	3	36	17
Pepperoni Lover's	433	40	3	37	21
Pork Topping	398	40	3	37	19
Super Supreme	446	41	3	38	21
Supreme	424	41	3	38	20
Veggie Lover's	358	42	3	39	16
Stuffed Crust Gold: Per Slice (½ Large Pizza)					
Beef Topping	488	44	3	41	24
Cheese	440	44	2	42	21
Chicken Supreme	438	45	3	42	24
Diced Chicken	442	44	2	42	26
Ham	409	43	2	41	21
Italian Sausage	515	44	2	42	24
Meat Lover's	545	44	3	41	27
Pepperoni	432	43	2	41	20
Pepperoni Lover's	497	44	2	42	24
Pork Topping	497	44	4	40	24
Sausage Lover's	515	44	3	41	24
Supreme	492	45	3	42	24
Veggie Lover's	422	46	3	43	19
Thin N Crispy: Per Slice (⅛ Medium Piza)					
Beef Topping	275	22	2	20	13
Cheese	209	22	2	20	10
Chicken Supreme	203	23	2	21	12
Ham	183	21	2	19	9
Italian Supreme	289	22	2	20	12
Meat Lover's	315	22	2	20	14
Pepperoni	201	21	2	19	9
Pepperoni Lover's	253	22	2	20	12
Pork Topping	266	22	2	20	13
Super Supreme	279	23	2	21	13
Supreme	257	23	2	21	12
Veggie Lover's	191	24	2	22	8
Hand Tossed: Per Slice (⅛ Medium Pizza)					
Beef Topping	330	29	3	26	16
Cheese	250	28	2	26	12
Chicken Supreme	231	29	2	27	13

	Calories	Total Carb	Fiber	Usable Carb	Protein
Ham	258	28	2	26	14
Italian Sausage	338	28	2	26	16
Meat Lover's	321	28	2	26	14
Pepperoni	281	28	2	26	13
Pepperoni Lover's	251	27	2	25	11
Pork Topping	324	29	3	26	16
Super Supreme	294	29	2	27	13
Supreme	276	29	3	26	13
Veggie Lover's	224	29	2	27	9
The Big New Yorker:					
Per Slice (⅛ Pizza)					
Beef Topping	522	47	9	38	25
Cheese	425	46	8	38	20
Ham	386	46	8	38	19
Pepperoni	409	46	8	38	18
Italian Sausage	545	47	8	39	24
Supreme	491	48	9	39	23
Veggie Lover's	500	57	10	47	19
The Chicago:					
Per Slice					
Meat Lover's	467	35	3	32	21
Pepperoni	388	34	3	31	18
Pepperoni, Italian Sausage,					
And Mushroom	414	35	3	32	19
Supreme	431	36	3	33	20
Veggie Lover's	374	36	3	33	17
The Insider: Per Slice					
(⅛ Medium Pizza)					
Cheese	365	35	2	33	18
Pepperoni	361	35	2	33	17
Supreme	413	36	3	33	20
Twisted Crust: Per Slice					
Large Pizza					
Cheese	456	58	3	55	20
Supreme	478	59	3	56	20
Ultimate Lovers Pan:					
Per Slice					
Cheese	470	47	8	39	21
Meat	581	47	9	38	24
Pepperoni	481	47	8	39	21.5
Veggie	400	50	9	41	14

	Calories	Total Carb	Fiber	Usable Carb	Protein
Ultimate Lover's Personal Pan:					
Per slice					
Cheese	331	29	2	27	15.5
Meat	370	29	2	27	14
Pepperoni	300	29	2	27	10
Veggie	270	30	3	27	10.5
Ultimate Lover's Stuffed Crust:					
Per Slice					
Cheese	400	41	3	38	16.5
Meat	472	41	3	38	18.5
Pepperoni	430	40	3	37	18
Veggie	351	42	3	39	12
Ultimate Lovers Thin n' Crispy:					
Per Slice					
Cheese	250	22	2	20	13.5
Meat	331	28	2	26	16.5
Pepperoni	251	22	2	20	11.5
Veggie	200	24	2	22	8
Ultimate Lover's Hand Tossed:					
Per Slice					
Cheese	281	28	2	26	13
Meat	331	28	2	26	16.5
Pepperoni	290	28	2	26	13
Veggie	230	30	2	28	9.5
Ultimate Big New Yorker:					
Per Slice					
Cheese	470	47	8	39	21
Meat	581	47	9	38	24
Pepperoni	481	47	8	39	21.5
Veggie	400	50	9	41	14
Sandwiches:					
Ham & Cheese	549	57	4	53	33
Supreme Sandwich	636	62	4	58	34
Dessert Pizza:					
Apple, 1 Slice	245	48	2	46	3
Cherry, 1 Slice	241	47	3	44	3
Pasta: 12.5 oz servings					
Cavatini Pasta	474	66	9	57	21
Spaghetti w/ Marinara					
Sauce, 16.6 oz	490	91	8	83	18
Spaghetti w/ Meat Sauce	601	98	9	89	23

	Calories	Total Carb	Fiber	Usable Carb	Protein
Spaghetti w/ Meatballs					
19 oz serving	844	120	10	110	37
Sides:					
Breadsticks, 1	128	20	1	19	3
Breadstick Dipping					
Sauce, 1 oz	23	4.2	0	4.2	0.4
Garlic Bread, 1	148	16	1	15	3
Hot Buffalo Wings, 4 pieces	212	4	0	4	22
Mild Wings (4)	*160*	*4*	*0*	*4*	*18.4*
POPEYE'S					
Chicken:					
Mild/Spicy 6.8 oz	530	18	1	17	46
Leg, Mild/Spicy, 2.5 oz	200	7	0	7	17
Thigh, Mild/Spicy, 4.3 oz	390	12	0	12	25
Wing, Mild/Spicy, 2.2 oz	220	10	0	10	14
Sides:					
Biscuits, 2 oz	225	25	1	24	3
Cajun Rice	180	23	2	21	8
Cinnamon Apple Pie, 1 piece	90	37	2	35	3
Coleslaw	235	20	9	11	1
Corn on the Cob	255	48	7	41	7
French Fries, 4.5 oz	380	50	4	46	5
Mashed Potatoes w/ Gravy	120	18	2	16	3
Onion Rings, 1 ser.	380	43	2	41	7
Red Beans and Rice	340	33	16	17	7
QUIZNO'S SUBS					
Sandwiches:					
Per Small Sandwich					
Honey Bourbon Chicken	360	45	3	42	24
Sierra Smoked Turkey w/					
Raspberry Chipotle	350	53	3	50	23
Turkey Lite	335	52	3	49	17
Tuscan Chick Salad	325	45	4	41	21
Veggie Lite	300	40	5	35	20
RANCH 1					
Salads					
Chicken on Gourmet Greens	350	31	5	26	32
Gourmet Greens	220	31	5	26	10
Zesty Caesar	180	31	4	27	8
Zesty Chicken Caesar	290	31	4	27	26

	Calories	Total Carb	Fiber	Usable Carb	Protein
Sandwiches					
American Ranch	390	51	3	48	25
Club American	470	53	3	50	29
Grilled Chick Philly	450	53	3	50	28
Ranch Classic	370	53	3	50	26
Spicy Grilled Chick	420	58	3	55	23
Side Kicks					
Fruit Cup	90	18	2	16	3
Ranch Fries	427	62.2	6.1	56.1	6.1
Specialties					
Baked Potato w/ Broccoli	510	117	12	105	12
w/ Cheese	790	118	11	107	23
w/ Chicken	610	114	11	103	30
Chicken Tenders	370	7	0	7	52
Grilled Chicken and Vegetables	790	129	16	113	54
Grilled Chicken Fajita	330	25	4	21	22
Grilled Chicken w/ Pasta	590	86	6	80	37

ROCKY MOUNTAIN CHOCOLATE FACTORY

Box: Per Piece					
English Toffee	350	34	2	32	3
Lucy Assorted	73	9.7	.3	9.4	.7
Square, Happy Birthday	150	13.5	0.8	12.7	1
Truffle, Regular	170	19	1	18	1
Burgundy English Toffee	90	8.7	0.7	8	0.7

ROUND TABLE PIZZA

Large Pizza: Per Slice (½ whole)					
Cheese: Thin	210	23	1	22	9
Pan	290	37	2	35	12
Chicken & Garlic Gourmet:					
Thin	230	24	1	23	11
Pan	320	38	2	36	14
Hawaiian: Thin	210	25	1	24	10
Pan	290	38	2	36	13
Gourmet Veggie: Thin	220	25	2	23	9
Pan	310	39	2	37	12
Guinevere's Garden: Thin	210	25	2	23	9
Pan	290	38	9	29	11
Hearty Bacon Supreme:					
Thin	270	22	1	21	12
Pan	360	36	1	35	15

	Calories	Total Carb	Fiber	Usable Carb	Protein
Italian Garlic Supreme: Thin	270	23	1	22	11
Pan	360	37	2	35	14
King Arthur's Supreme: Thin	270	24	2	22	11
Pan	340	38	2	36	13
Maui Zaui (Polynesian Sauce):					
Thin	240	27	1	26	11
Pan	330	41	2	39	14
Maui Zaui (Red Sauce):					
Thin	240	25	1	24	11
Pan	320	39	2	37	14
Montague's All Meat Marvel:					
Thin	290	24	1	23	12
Pan	350	37	2	35	14
Pepperoni: Thin	240	23	1	22	10
Pan	310	37	2	35	12
Pepperoni Rostadoro: Thin	270	26	1	25	12
Pan	350	40	2	38	15
Roastin Toastin Chicken Club:					
Thin	260	25	1	24	12
Pan	350	39	2	37	15
Western BBQ Chicken: Thin	240	23	1	22	11
Pan	320	37	2	35	17
16" Pizzas: Per Slice (⅛ whole)					
Aloha Vinnie	430	55	2	53	19
Big Vinnie Pepperoni	460	49	1	48	20
Maui Mama					
(Polynesian Sauce)	570	63	1	62	26
Maui Mama (Red Sauce)	560	61	1	60	27
Mama Zella	550	59	3	56	23
Personal Pizzas: Per Pizza					
Cheese: Thin	580	60	3	57	26
Pan	810	99	4	95	33
Chicken Rostadoro: Thin	680	66	4	62	35
Pan	910	112	5	107	41
Hawaiian: Thin	560	66	3	63	26
Pan	780	109	5	104	33
Gourmet Veggie: Thin	590	67	5	62	25
Pan	820	114	7	107	32
Guinevere's Garden Delight:					
Thin	550	66	5	61	23
Pan	760	110	6	104	29

	Calories	Total Carb	Fiber	Usable Carb	Protein
Hearty Bacon Supreme:					
Thin	700	59	3	56	32
Pan	940	105	4	101	38
Italian Garlic Supreme: Thin	760	63	3	60	30
Pan	990	109	5	104	37
King Arthur's Supreme:					
Thin	750	64	4	60	33
Pan	900	109	5	104	36
Maui Zaui (Polynesian Sauce):					
Thin	620	71	3	68	28
Pan	850	117	5	112	34
Maui Zaui (Red Sauce): Thin	590	66	4	62	29
Pan	820	111	5	106	35
Montague's All Meat Marvel:					
Thin	780	61	3	58	33
Pan	1010	107	4	103	39
Pepperoni: Thin	640	60	3	57	27
Pan	840	106	4	102	32
Pepperoni Rostadoro: Thin	740	70	4	66	33
Pan	970	116	5	111	39
Roastin Toastin Chicken Club:					
Thin	710	66	3	63	33
Pan	940	112	4	108	40
Western BBQ Chicken: Thin	610	61	3	58	28
Pan	840	107	5	102	34
Sides/Sandwiches					
Garlic Bread:	470	59	2	57	11
w/ Cheese	630	59	2	57	21
Garlic Parmesan Twist, 3 pcs	510	76	3	73	17
Buffalo Wings, Spicy or Honey BBQ, 3 pieces	***210***	***1***	***0***	***1***	***19***
Sandwiches:					
Chicken Club	820	75	3	72	38
Ham Club	810	76	3	73	36
RT Pizza	690	64	4	61	30
RT Veggie	680	79	5	74	23
Turkey Club	800	75	3	72	39
RUBIO'S FRESH MEXICAN GRILL					
HealthMex					
Burrito w/ Chicken	510	74	10	64	31
Burrito w/ Grilled Fish	540	74	10	64	38

	Calories	Total Carb	Fiber	Usable Carb	Protein
Taco w/ Chicken	170	23	2	21	12
Taco w/ Grilled Fish	180	24	2	22	15
Tacos: Carne Asada	250	24	2	22	14
Fish	300	28	2	26	11
Fish Taco Especial	370	30	3	27	14
Grilled Fish	310	24	2	22	18
Grilled Chicken	290	24	2	22	15
Shrimp	260	24	2	22	13
Quesadillas: Cheese	700	53	4	49	29
Grilled Chicken	810	54	4	50	49
Carne Asada	860	55	4	51	46
Lobster	770	55	4	51	41
Shrimp	760	54	4	50	39
Burritos: Baja Carne Asada	700	58	5	53	36
Baja Chicken	650	56	5	51	38
Bean & Cheese	580	74	11	63	19
Bean & Rice	600	111	13	98	15
Especial: Carne Asada	830	81	8	73	34
Chicken	780	80	8	72	37
Fish	690	70	8	62	20
Lobster	771	81	9	72	24
Shrimp	660	77	6	71	26
Los Otros: Chips	520	68	8	60	6
Nachos Grande	1270	117	22	95	33
w/ Carne Asada	1430	119	22	97	50
w/ Chicken	1380	118	22	96	53
Combo Chips & Beans	480	68	14	54	7
Chips	520	68	8	60	6
Beans	220	44	16	28	4
Rice	260	48	3	45	9
Chicken Taquitos	410	38	7	30	21
Guacamole: Small	*190*	*8*	*5*	*3*	*4*
Guacamole: Large	370	16	11	5	6
Pesky Meals: w/ Beans	130	22	8	14	3
w/ Chips	210	28	3	25	3
w/ Mini Churro	85	12	1	11	1
w/ Rice	110	21	1	20	4
Bean & Cheese Burrito	570	72	11	61	19
Cheese Quesadilla	560	48	2	46	23
Fish Taco	300	27	2	25	11
Taquitos	320	23	3	20	18

	Calories	Total Carb	Fiber	Usable Carb	Protein
Desserts: Choco Taco	300	38	1	37	4
Churro	170	23	2	21	2

Note: Rubio's uses only skinless chicken breast and lean trimmed steak. Canola oil is used—no lard or MSG.

RYAN'S FAMILY STEAKHOUSE

Menu Items: Per Serving

	Calories	Total Carb	Fiber	Usable Carb	Protein
Chicken Pot Pie	150	21	4	17	6
Clam Chowder	160	18	1	17	8
Macaroni & Cheese	340	38	1	37	16
Mashed Potatoes	100	14	1	13	3
Yeast Roll	340	68	3	65	12
Butter Pecan Frozen Yogurt					
Sugar Free/Non Fat	90	21	0	21	4

7-ELEVEN

Hot Dogs

	Calories	Total Carb	Fiber	Usable Carb	Protein
Big Bite w/ Bun	550	24	0	24	16
Hot Dog Bun Only	120	22	1	21	4
⅓ lb Big Bite					
Sausage Only	*480*	*3*	*0*	*3*	*16*
⅓ lb Big Bite Cheeseburger					
Sausage Only	*410*	*3*	*0*	*3*	*28*

Burritos

	Calories	Total Carb	Fiber	Usable Carb	Protein
The Bomb (14 oz)	940	116	12	104	32
w/ Green Chilies	940	114	12	104	30
Reynolds Jumbo Burritos (10 oz)					
Beef & Bean	680	93	10	83	27
Beef & Potato	590	82	5	77	22
Red Hot Burrito	640	88	0	88	26
Green Burrito	710	93	7	86	26

Sandwiches (7-Eleven)

Big Eats Deli Sandwiches:

	Calories	Total Carb	Fiber	Usable Carb	Protein
Chicken Salad	630	47	5	42	28
Chicken Caesar	540	47	5	42	30
Hearty Ham	570	48	3	45	26
Roast Beef/Bacon	650	47	3	44	29
Smoked Turkey	640	85	5	80	35
Stacked Turkey/Ham	630	46	3	43	24
Tuna Salad	550	56	3	53	31

	Calories	Total Carb	Fiber	Usable Carb	Protein
Stuffed Baguettes:					
Philly Steak	540	56	4	52	24
Ham/Cheese	500	58	4	54	24
Hot Pockets					
Ham/Cheese	480	55	4	51	23
Meatballs/Mozzarella	490	59	6	53	23
Giggles To Go					
Grilled Cheese	270	27	0	27	8
The Deli Market (7-Eleven)					
Breakfast Sandwiches:					
Beef, Cheese/Bacon Bite w/ Bun	390	23	0.5	22.5	22
Croissant w/ Ham, Egg, Cheese	390	34	2	32	18
English Muffin w/ Egg, Cheese & Canadian Bacon	65	29	2	27	15
Sausage, Egg, Cheese Biscuit	500	34	1	33	20
Snack Stix Treats:					
Per Stick (3.5 oz)					
BBQ Chicken	230	34	2	32	10
Cheese & Steak	290	31	1	30	14
Egg/Ham/Cheddar	280	35	2	33	11
Grilled Chicken/Cheese	270	30	2	28	12
Ham & Cheese	280	32	2	30	12
Pepperoni/Cheese	340	30	2	28	13
Supreme	280	32	2	30	11
Sausage/Cheese	300	32	2	30	12
Taquitos (Battered Tortilla)					
Beef Taco/Cheese	250	30	3	27	7
Chicken Fiesta	220	22	1	21	6
Monterey Jack Chicken	280	30	3	27	7
Fountain Drinks, Assume ¼ Ice					
Slurpees: Average All Flavors					
16 oz size	200	50	0	50	0
Fruit Coolers: 12 oz					
Orange/Cream	280	68	1	67	1
Strawberry/Cream	270	65	2	63	1
Café Coolers:					
French Vanilla	380	58	0	58	1
Mocha	350	63	0	63	1

	Calories	Total Carb	Fiber	Usable Carb	Protein
SBARRO'S					
Meals: Per Serving					
Baked Ziti, 13.6 oz	930	90	4	86	44
Chicken Parmigiana	183	6.5	0	6.5	15.5
Meat Lasagne	825	88	34	54	41
Spaghetti w/ Sauce	910	144	7	137	26
Pizza: Per Slice					
Cheeze	485	55	2	53	23
Pepperoni	590	55	2	53	29
Sausage	640	56	2	54	33
Supreme	600	59	3	56	30
Stuffed Pizza: Per slice					
Sausage Pepperoni	965	83	3	80	45
Spinach/Broccoli	825	85	6	79	33
SCHLOTZSKY'S					
Bread/Buns					
Dark Rye, Regular	327	68	3	65	10
Sourdough Regular	333	68	2	66	11
Wheat, Regular	336	66	4	62	12
Jalapeno Cheese	353	66	2	64	12
Pizza Crust	332	68	2	66	11
Original Sandwiches:					
Per Sandwich					
The Original	738	79	4	75	34
Large Original	1390	152	7	145	65
Deluxe Original	930	84	4	80	53
Ham & Cheese	749	82	4	78	44
Turkey Original	822	81	4	77	51
Sandwiches:					
Per Regular Sandwich					
Albacore Tuna	496	77	5	72	30
Albacore Tuna Melt	740	83	6	77	44
Alburquerque Turkey	919	85	5	80	53
All American Angus	898	82	5	77	57
BLT	578	70	3	67	21
Chicken Breast	499	80	4	76	36
Chicken Club	686	75	4	71	44
Corned Beef	593	78	4	74	43
Corned Beef Reuben	838	82	4	78	54
Dijon Chicken	496	74	6	68	38
Fiesta Chicken	839	79	4	75	50

	Calories	Total Carb	Fiber	Usable Carb	Protein
Pastrami & Swiss	882	81	4	77	60
Pastrami Reuben	944	83	4	79	59
Pesto Chicken	512	37	4	33	73
Roast Beef	623	78	3	75	43
Roast Beef/Cheese	586	56	3	53	39
Santa Fe Chicken	605	81	5	76	42
Smoked Turkey	498	75	3	72	34
Texas Schlotzsky	776	76	3	73	43
The Philly	840	86	4	82	57
The Vegetarian	482	79	6	73	18
Turkey/Bacon Club	834	79	5	74	52
Turkey Guacamole	643	84	3	81	36
Turkey Reuben	823	80	4	76	50
Vegetarian Club	541	76	5	71	19
Western Vegetarian	611	76	4	72	18
Soups: Per Cup (8 oz)					
Boston Clam Chowder	233	24	1	23	5
Broccoli/Cheese	252	23	1	22	7
Chicken Gumbo	110	13	2	11	4
Chicken Tortilla	167	24	3	21	10
Chicken/wild Rice	378	24	1	23	10
Minestrone	89	17	3	14	3
Old Fashion Chick Noodle	122	18	1	17	8
Pilgrim Corn Chowder	284	38	1	37	2
Potato w/ Bacon	226	31	2	29	2
Ravioli	111	21	1	20	6
Sante Fe Vegetable	120	20	5	15	5
Red Beans/Rice	167	32	4	28	8
Schlotzsky's Veggie	220	44	6	38	10
Steak/Black Bean	150	25	7	18	10
Timberline Chili	210	24	7	17	14
Veg/Beef/Barley	100	12	2	10	6
Vegetarian Vegetable	138	20	6	14	3
Wisconsin Cheese	319	26	1	25	4
Deli Salads: Per 5 oz Container					
Potato	288	35	4	31	4
Mustard Potato	250	31	4	27	4
Homestyle Cole Slaw	188	24	3	21	1
Elbow Macaroni	275	23	2	21	4
California Pasta	58	10	1	9	0
Albacore Tuna 4.4 oz	*133*	*2*	*0*	*2*	*20*

	Calories	Total Carb	Fiber	Usable Carb	Protein
Leaf Salads: w/o Dressing/ Croutons/Noodles					
Caesar	152	11	4	7	11
Chicken Caesar	254	13	4	9	28
Chinese Chicken	150	11	3	8	20
Garden	61	8	3	5	3
Greek	180	13	4	9	10
Ham/Turkey Chef	248	15	3	12	23
Smoked Turkey Chef	243	15	3	12	24
8" Sourdough Crust Pizzas					
Bacon,Tomato & Mushroom	611	78	4	74	27
Barbeque Chicken	683	93	2	91	37
Chicken & Pesto	649	78	4	74	40
Double Cheese	580	76	4	72	26
Double Cheese and Pepperoni	721	77	4	73	33
Fresh Tomato/Pesto	539	76	4	72	23
Mediterranean	524	72	3	69	21
Smoked Turkey & Jalapeno	624	80	4	76	39
Southwestern	611	76	4	72	38
Thai Chicken	663	89	5	84	40
Original Combo	625	79	5	74	26
Vegetarian Special	551	76	4	72	24
Salad Extras					
Chow Mein Noodles	74	9	1	8	2
Garlic Cheese Croutons	46	5	0	5	1
Greek Balsamic Vinaigrette	***170***	***2***	***0***	***2***	***0***
Light Italian Dressing	***90***	***3***	***0***	***3***	***0***
Old World Caesar	***260***	***1***	***0***	***1***	***2***
Ranch Dressing:					
Traditional	***270***	***1***	***0***	***1***	***0***
Spicy	***230***	***2***	***0***	***2***	***1***
Light Spicy	140	9	0	9	1
Spicy Ginger Vinaigrette	170	8	0	8	1
Thousand Island	220	6	0	6	0
Schlotzky's Deli Chips:					
1.5 oz Bag	210	26	2	24	3
Kids Deals:					
Cheese Pizza	460	72	3	69	18
Cheese Sandwich	431	50	2	48	21
Ham/Cheese	431	50	2	48	21

	Calories	Total Carb	Fiber	Usable Carb	Protein
PBJ Sandwich	470	71	4	67	15
Pepperoni Pizza	507	72	3	69	20
Cookies					
Oatmeal Raisin	150	24	1	23	1
w/ real M & M's	140	20	0	20	2
Cheesecake					
Cookies/Cream	330	36	1	35	6
NY Style	310	31	0	31	7
Strawberry	300	30	0	30	6
Fudge Brownie	410	46	0	46	5

SHONEY'S

	Calories	Total Carb	Fiber	Usable Carb	Protein
Breakfast					
All Star Breakfast	*190*	*1*	*0*	*1*	*13*
Deluxe Pancake Platter	1609	299	0	299	28.9
Half Stack Pancake Platter	930	187	0	187	15
Big Eater Steak	*629*	*1.4*	*0*	*1.4*	*59.9*
Country Fried					
Steak Breakfast	994	49	0.5	49	50
Sunrise Breakfast	973	88	2	86	22
Sausage Biscuit	539	42	1	41	16
Burgers					
All-American	688	44	2	42	54
Bacon/Cheeseburger	891	44	3	41	66
Mushroom Swiss	970	49	4	45	64
Famous Patty Melt	946	40	5	35	59
Half O-Pound	1351	129.6	1	128.6	88.9
Sandwiches					
Blackened Chicken	885	122.1	0.4	121.7	54.4
Charbroiled Chick	894	121.9	1	120.9	54.5
Chicken Parmesan	751	79.7	3.6	76.1	42.1
Corned Beef Reuben	793	37	5	32	40
Fish Sandwich	827	127	0.5	126.5	44
Fried Chicken	561	77	4	73	32
Original Slim Jim	1004	122.7	0.2	122.5	54
French Dip	498	53	2	51	41
Turkey Club	952	47	3	44	71
Ultimate Grilled Cheese	896	77	4	73	42
Steaks					
BBQ Ribs	1520	124	5	119	80
Choice Sirloin, 6 oz	1224	128	5	123	63

	Calories	Total Carb	Fiber	Usable Carb	Protein
Half-O-Pound					
w/ Grilled Onions	1337	133	7	126	84
w/ Mushrooms	1317	127	6	121	84
Southwest	1304	83	3	80	85
Ribeye, 8 oz	1481	128	5	123	73
T-Bone, 12 oz	1809	28	5	23	96
Surf & Turf:					
Ribeye & 5 Fried Shrimp	1639	138.5	5.1	133.4	84.8
Ribeye & 6 Grilled Shrimp	1589	128.2	4.9	123.3	85.4
Sirloin & 5 Fried Shrimp	1385	139	5.1	133.9	76
Sirloin & 6 Grilled Shrimp	1330	128	4.9	123.1	76
T-Bone & 5 Fried Shrimp	1967	138.5	5.1	133.4	108.6
T-Bone & 6 Grilled Shrimp	1918	128.2	4.9	123.3	109.2
Rib Combos, w/ Fries:					
¼ Rack/ BBQ Chicken	1228	104	4	100	80
¼ Rack /Tenderloins	1372	120.5	4.4	116.1	64.9
¼ Rack/Fried Shrimp	1144	113.4	4	109.4	58.4
¼ Rack/Grilled Shrimp	1125	103.2	3.8	99.4	59
Blue Plate Specials					
Cajun Whitefish	480	56.2	0.2	56	39.7
Baked Whitefish	507	58	0.5	57.5	48
Grandma's Meatloaf					
w/ Glaze	1092	93	0.5	92.5	72
w/ Gravy	1089	87.4	0.8	86.6	72.3
Original Country Fried Steak	1151	103.1	0.6	102.5	47.2
Grilled Liver/Onions	711	79	2	77	49
Ham Steak Dinner	667	60	0.5	59.5	48
Roast Beef Platter	880	96	5	91	59
Pasta					
Chicken Alfredo	1705	170.5	5.5	165	85
Italian Feast	1435	203.9	7.7	196.2	64
Pasta Ya-Ya	1847	175.5	6.8	168.7	110.4
Shrimp Alfredo	1781	171.6	5.5	166.1	87.1
Seafood					
Fish n' Shrimp	1098	129.3	5.8	123.5	53
Fried Fish Platter	1049	123	6	117	49
Grilled Salmon	749	95	0.5	94.5	50
Grilled Salmon Lite	*181*	*0*	*0*	*0*	*37.1*
Grilled Cod Lite	*201*	*0.5*	*0*	*0.5*	*38.9*
Grilled Shrimp	720	96	0.5	95.5	39
Grilled Shrimp Lite	218	29.6	0.5	29.1	28.3

	Calories	Total Carb	Fiber	Usable Carb	Protein
Shrimpers Feast	1032	127.7	5.7	122	39.1
Shrimp Stir Fry	873	131	5	126	41
Sides					
Baked Potato, Plain	344	67	5	62	6
French Fries, 4 oz	213	25	3	22	3
Onion Rings, (7)	500	83	4	79	12
Chicken					
Chicken Stir Fry	1200	172.1	4.7	167.4	48.4
Charbroiled: Blackened	831	99.8	1	98.8	47.4
Chicken Breast	797	99	0.5	98.5	47
Fried Tenderloins	1157	121.2	5.9	115.3	30.3
Monterey Chicken	909	84	3	81	53
Smothered Chicken	890	90	2	88	56
Junior Meals:					
Fish 'n Chips	308	29	3	26	20
All American Junior Burger	235	20	0	20	14
Junior Chicken	189	12	0.5	11.5	13
Spaghetti	250	32	0	32	13
Desserts, Ice Cream, Sundaes					
Apple Pie á la Mode	1203	173.7	8.7	165	12.4
w/ Nutrasweet	454	64.3	2.6	61.7	4.2
Cheesecake	364	23.1	0.4	22.7	5
Hot Fudge Sundae	599	74.9	0.2	74.7	9.5
Original Strawberry	332	44.5	2.3	42.2	2.1
Ultimate Hot Fudge Cake	875	126.3	3.4	122.9	13.7
Peach Pie w/ Nutrasweet	479	68.2	3.9	64.3	4.2
Caramel Sundae	621	83.2	0.2	83	9.6
Chocolate Milk Shake	1082	141.3	3.8	137.5	25.1
Strawberry Sundae	609	85.3	0.6	84.7	9.2
Walnut Brownie á la mode	584	60.6	0	60.6	9.6

SKYLINE CHILI

	Calories	Total Carb	Fiber	Usable Carb	Protein
Menu Items: Per Serving					
Chili (Regular)					
½ Pint	250	4	2	2	24
w/ beans, ½ pint	260	17	5	12	23
Chili Spaghetti	400	44	4	42	25
w/ beans	480	57	9	48	30
w/ onions	410	47	5	42	25
w/ beans and onions	490	60	9	51	30

	Calories	Total Carb	Fiber	Usable Carb	Protein
Burritos: Regular	570	42	6	36	28
Deluxe	640	47	7	40	29
Skyliner Cheese Coneys	350	23	1	22	20
Chili Sandwich	190	25	1	24	14
w/ Cheese	300	18	1	17	21
Black Beans/Rice	330	44	8	36	11
3-Way (Spagh, Chili, Cheese)	710	39	4	35	45
4-Way (3-Way + Onions)	720	41	4	37	45
4-Way (3-Way + Beans)	780	52	8	44	50
5-Way (3-Way + Onions + Beans)	790	54	9	45	50
Salads: Garden Salad	*80*	*4*	*1*	*3*	*5*
Greek Salad	370	9	3	6	6
Nacho Salad	450	40	8	32	17

SMOOTHIE KING

	Calories	Total Carb	Fiber	Usable Carb	Protein
Weight Gain Smoothies:					
Per 20 oz					
Hulk Chocolate	846	128.6	5.6	123	23
Strawberry	953	156	5.7	150.3	24
Malts	887	118.5	0.1	118.4	2.5
Peanut Power	502	71.5	3.5	68	14.5
Peanut Power Plus:					
Grape	703	119	3.5	115.5	16
Strawberry	632	105	5	100	15.5
Shakes	875	117	0	117	16.5
Lowfat Smoothies: Per 20 oz					
Angel Food	330	79	3.5	75.1	5.6
Blackberry Dream	343	86	3	83	2.4
Blueberry Heaven	260	58	2	56	7
Celestial Cherry High	285	69	3.6	65.4	0.8
Cherry Picker	360	98	2.1	95.9	6
Cranberry Cooler	538	132	2.6	129.4	0.6
Grape Expectations	399	96	2.4	93.6	3
Hearty Apple	380	81	2.0	79	12
Immune Builder	333	80	3.5	76.5	5
Instant Vigor	359	87.5	2	85.5	2
Lemon Twist Banana	339	82	2.4	79.6	2.6
Strawberry	399	97	2.3	94.7	2.7
Light & Fluffy	389	98	3.5	94.5	2.5
Muscle Punch	339	80	3.5	76.5	5.8
Orange Ka-Bam	320	104	3	101	2

	Calories	Total Carb	Fiber	Usable Carb	Protein
Peach Slice	341	80	3	77	4.6
Peach Slice Plus	471	113	4.7	108.3	5.5
Pep Upper	334	80	4.5	75.5	3.5
Pineapple Pleasure	313	76	4	72	1.6
Pineapple Surf	440	104	4	100	8
Raspberry Sunrise	335	84.5	4.3	80.2	3
Slim/Trim:					
Chocolate	270	55	3	52	12
Strawberry	357	78.5	3.3	75.2	6.7
Vanilla	227	51.5	2.2	49.3	6
Strawberry Kiwi	300	70	2	68	4
Strawberry X-treme	370	91	4	87	3
Youth Fountain	267	65	4.6	60.4	3.3
Specialty Smoothies: Per 20 oz					
Banana Boat	520	93	5	88	11
Coconut Surprise	457	99	4.5	94.5	8.3
Mo'cuccino	420	71	1	70	9
Pina Colada Island	550	102	6	96	16
Workout Smoothies: Per 20 oz					
Activator:					
Banana/Chocolate/Vanilla	429	90	3.6	86.4	19.4
Strawberry	559	123	5.4	117.6	20.3
Power Punch	430	102	3.5	98.5	6
Power Punch Plus	499	113	3.5	109.5	10
Super Punch	425	95	5.5	89.5	1.6
Super Punch Plus	516	118	5.5	112.5	1.6
High Protein Smoothies: Per 20 oz					
Almond Mocha	402	45	4.3	40.7	31
Chocolate	401	45	4.2	40.8	31
Banana	412	44	5.5	38.5	34
Lemon/Pineapple	390	41	3.3	37.7	29

SNAPPY TOMATO

Large Pizza: Per Slice (½ Pizza)					
Cheese Pizza	160	21	1	20	7
Sausage	190	22	1	21	8
Pepperoni	200	21	1	20	9

SOUPER SALAD

Cornbread, 1 piece	266	49	2	47	4
Blueberry Bread	257	49	1	48	4
Focaccia Bread	387	69	3	66	12

	Calories	Total Carb	Fiber	Usable Carb	Protein
Gingerbread	295	46	0.5	45.5	3
Salad Dressings: Per 2 Tbsp					
Fat Free Ranch	32	9	0.5	8.5	0
Fat Free Cranberry Vinaigrette	48	12	0	12	0

SOUPLANTATION

	Calories	Total Carb	Fiber	Usable Carb	Protein
Soups: Per 1 cup					
Chicken Tortilla	*100*	*5*	*1*	*4*	*12*
Chesapeake Corn Chowder	280	30	2	28	7
Cream /Mushroom	290	15	2	13	10
Irish Potato Leek	250	23	1	24	5
Minestrone w/ Italian					
Sausage	210	14	5	9	13
Navy Bean w/ Ham	340	30	6	24	35
Vegetarian Harvest	190	23	4	19	5
Chili: Per cup					
Arizona Chili	220	25	7	18	14
Cheatin Heart Chili	300	23	6.	17	18
Deep Kettle House	230	26	7	19	15
Breads: per piece					
Buttermilk Corn	140	27	2	25	3
Sourdough	150	27	0	27	9
Focaccia:					
Garlic Parmesan	100	15	1	14	2
Pepperoni	160	19	1	18	5
Fresh Tossed Salads, Per 1 cup					
Antipasto	*140*	*6*	*2*	*4*	*5*
BBQ Julienne	190	20	3	17	5
Caesar	190	10	1	9	5
Won Ton Chicken	150	12	2	10	6
Prepared Salads: Per ½ cup					
Artichoke Rice	160	21	2	19	3
Aunt Doris' Red Pepper Slaw	70	18	3	15	1
Baja Bean & Cilantro	180	29	5	25	9
BBQ Potato Salad	160	20	2	18	2
Carrot Raisin	90	17	2	15	1
Chinese Krab	160	19	3	16	5
Dijon Potato w/ garlic					
Dill Vinegar	150	9	3	6	1
Greek Couscous w/					
Feta Cheese	170	19	3	16	6

	Calories	Total Carb	Fiber	Usable Carb	Protein
Oriental Ginger Slaw	*70*	*8*	*4*	*4*	*2*
Southern Dill Potato	120	20	2	18	4
Thai Noodle w/					
Peanut Sauce	170	17	3	14	5
Hot Tossed Pastas: Per cup					
Bruschetta	260	41	3	38	10
Creamy	360	43	3	40	12
Garden Vegetable					
w/ Meatballs	270	42	3	39	11
w/ Italian Sausage	300	42	3	39	12
Vegetarian Marinara					
w/ Basil	260	44	3	41	10
Muffins: Per Muffin					
Regular					
Apple Raisin	150	22	1	21	2
Banana/Cherry/Nut	150	22	1	21	2

SOUTHERN TSUNAMI

	Calories	Total Carb	Fiber	Usable Carb	Protein
Sushi: Per Serving					
California Roll, 9 pieces	289	54	3	51	7
Califorina Roll &					
Inari, 7 pieces	324	58.5	2.1	56.4	9.1
California Salad					
Roll, 6 pieces	570	82.9	4.5	78.4	15.1
Combos:					
Seaside, 12 pieces	303	48.8	1.6	47.2	19
Shoreline, 10 pieces	473	84	2.4	81.6	21.5
Stardust, 11 pieces	307	57.8	2.2	55.6	12.2
Vegetable, 9 pieces	232	45	1	44	4
Cream Cheese Roll:					
(Per 9 Pieces unless indicated)					
w/ imitation Crab	529	59.3	2.4	56.9	15.7
w/ Salmon	569	53.1	2.4	50.7	23.1
w/ Tuna	548	53.1	2.4	50.7	25.3
Crunchy Shrimp	650	83	4	79	36.8
Dragon Roll	643	62.9	7.3	55.6	21.9
Eel Roll	467	55.5	2.2	53.3	20.4
Full Moon, 6 Pieces	307	50.1	2.2	47.9	11.2
Futomaki, 6 pieces	314	68	3	65	7
Green River	491	55.5	4.5	51	21.8
Grilled Salmon Roll	349	54.4	3.3	51.1	18.4
Inari, 4 pieces	261	46	1	45	8

	Calories	Total Carb	Fiber	Usable Carb	Protein
Mix & Match (M & M Rolls)					
Per 12 Pieces Unless Indicated:					
Eel & Carrot	314	51.6	2.1	49.5	11.2
Imitation Crab and Carrot	245	53.1	2.1	51	6.7
Tuna & Cucumber	247	49.4	1.7	47.7	10.6
Shrimp & Avocado	281	50.4	2.5	47.9	10.4
Marina Plate, 6 pieces	272	48	2	46	11
Meteor Special, 11 pieces	371	66.7	2.1	64.6	18.9
Nigiri: Per Piece					
Eel	85	13.4	0.1	13.3	3
Octopus	66	12.4	0.1	12.3	3.4
Salmon	64	12	0.1	11.9	2.6
Yellowtail	64	12	0.1	11.9	2.9
Shrimp	88	12	0.1	11.9	8.2
Snapper	60	12	0.1	11.9	2.6
Squid	60	12.3	0.1	12.2	2.2
Tuna	62	12	0.1	11.9	3.1
Nigiri: Per 9 Pieces					
Ocean Crab Roll	345	53.6	3.9	49.7	14.2
Orange Roll	395	65	3.9	61.1	16.2
Small Roll: Per 12 Pieces					
Avocado	292	51.9	3.6	48	5.4
Carrot	238	53.1	2.8	50.3	5
Cucumber	224	49.9	1.8	48.1	4.8
Eel	392	50.3	1.5	48.8	17.5
Imitation Crab	251	53.2	1.5	51.7	8.4
Salmon	327	47	1.5	45.5	21.4
Shrimp	266	48.8	1.5	47.3	15.3
Tuna	258	47	2	45	14
Yellowtail	290	48.8	1.5	47.3	16.4
Snack Pack: Per 12 Pieces					
Avocado	293	52	3.6	48.4	5.4
Carrot-Cucumber	231	51.5	2.3	49.2	4.9
Carrot	238	53.1	2.8	50.3	5
Cucumber	225	50	1.8	48.2	4.8
Imitation Crab & Cucumber	238	51.6	1.6	50	6.6
Spicy Rolls: Per 9 Pieces					
Shrimp	335	52.4	2.4	50	18.9
Yellowtail	364	52.4	2.4	50	20.4
Salmon	362	52.4	2.4	50	18.3
Tuna	290	45	3	42	14

	Calories	Total Carb	Fiber	Usable Carb	Protein
Sunshine Platter, 15 pieces	815	154.1	7.9	146.2	19.4
Tofu Roll, 9 pcs	251	48	3	45	8
Tsunami Roll, 9 pcs	480	63.2	2.7	60.5	22
Salads					
Calamari Salad, 4 oz	182	20.2	0	20.2	20.2
Edamame, 4 oz	*60*	*4.5*	*0.6*	*3.9*	*3.4*
(Soybeans), 4 oz	172	12.5	4.8	7.7	14
Harusame, 2 oz	59	13.2	0	13.2	0.7
Seabreeze, 2 oz	57	11.3	0	11.3	0
Sauce: AFC Spicy, 2 oz	*49*	*2.6*	*0*	*2.6*	*0.1*
STARBUCK'S					
Hot Beverages: Grande (16 fl. oz.)					
Caffe Americano	*15*	*3*	*0*	*3*	*1*
Caffe Latte: w/ whole milk	260	21	0	21	14
w/ nonfat milk	160	24	0	24	16
Caffe Misto/Au Lait:					
w/ whole milk	140	11	0	11	8
w/ nonfat milk	90	13	0	13	9
Cappuccino: w/ whole milk	150	13	0	13	8
w/ nonfat milk	100	14	0	14	9
Carmel Apple Cider	300	72	0	72	0
w/ whipped cream	410	76	0	76	0
Carmel Mocha:					
w/ whole milk	470	63	2	61	13
w/ nonfat milk	410	65	2	63	14
Carmel Macchiato:					
w/ whole milk	320	37	0	37	12
w/ nonfat milk	230	40	0	40	14
Cinnamon Spice Mocha :					
w/ whole milk	330	45	1	44	13
Drip Coffee	*10*	*2*	*0*	*2*	*0*
Espresso, solo	*5*	*1*	*0*	*1*	*0*
Espresso, Doppio	*10*	*2*	*0*	*2*	*1*
Espresso Macchiato: Solo	*10*	*1*	*0*	*1*	*1*
Hot Chocolate w/ whole milk	440	44	2	42	15
Steamed Milk: Whole	270	21	0	21	15
Nonfat	160	23	0	23	16
Steamed Cider	230	57	0	57	0
Tazo Chai	290	50	0	50	8
White Hot Chocolate					
w/ whole milk	580	65	0	65	17

	Calories	Total Carb	Fiber	Usable Carb	Protein
White Chocolate Mocha:					
w/ whole milk	510	58	0	58	14
w/ nonfat milk	440	60	0	60	16
Starbucks on Ice:					
Grande (16 fl. oz.)					
Iced Caffe Americano	*20*	*3*	*0*	*3*	*1*
Iced Caffe Latte:					
w/ whole milk	160	13	0	13	8
w/ nonfat milk	100	14	0	14	9
Iced Mocha: w/ whole milk	350	37	2	35	9
w/ nonfat milk	310	38	2	36	9
White Chocolate Mocha					
w/ whole milk	490	58	0	58	11
w/ nonfat milk	450	59	0	59	11
Iced Tazo Chai					
w/ whole milk	270	48	0	48	7
Ice Blended Drinks:					
Grande (16 fl. oz.)					
Frappucino:					
Caramel	430	61	0	61	6
Caramel Brownie	510	72	2	70	7
Coffee	260	52	0	52	5
Espresso	230	46	0	46	5
Mocha	420	61	0	61	6
Mocha Coconut	550	80	2	78	7
Crème Frappuccino					
Chocolate	530	75	1	74	18
Malt	610	90	2	88	15
Vanilla	480	66	0	66	15
Tazo Tea Frappuccino:					
Tazoberry	190	49	1	48	1
Tazoberry Cream	460	76	1	75	6
Tazo Chai Cream	500	72	0	72	15
Beverage Additions: Per Serving					
Mocha Syrup	25	6	0	6	1
Whipped Cream	*130*	*2*	*0*	*2*	*0*

SUBWAY

7 Under 6" Sandwiches
Figures based on Italian bread
and: Lettuce, tomato, onion,
green peppers, olives and pickles.

	Calories	Total Carb	Fiber	Usable Carb	Protein
Ham	290	46	4	42	18
Roast Beef	293	45	4	41	19
Roast Chick Breast	318	47	58	42	23
Subway Club	323	46	4	42	24
Turkey Breast	281	46	4	42	18
Turkey Breast/Ham	293	46	4	42	20
Veggie Delite	226	44	4	40	9
Breakfast Sandwiches (6")					
Based on Italian bread					
Bacon & Egg	451	42	3	39	28
Cheese & Egg	447	42	3	39	27
Ham & Egg	437	42	3	39	29
Steak & Egg	466	43	4	39	33
Vegetable & Egg	420	44	4	40	25
Western Egg	437	44	4	40	27
Classic Sandwiches (6")					
Figures based on Italian bread					
and following toppings: Lettuce,					
tomato, onion, green peppers,					
olives, pickles, cheese, oil,					
vinegar, salt and pepper.					
Cold Cut Trio	441	47	4	43	21
Italian BMT	480	47	4	43	23
Meatball	527	53	5	48	23
Seafood & Crab	405	52	5	47	16
Steak & Cheese	389	48	5	43	24
Subway Melt	408	46.8	4.0	42.8	24.9
Tuna	445	36	3	33	13
Deli Sandwiches (6")					
Ham	210	35	3	32	11
Roast Beef	223	35	3	32	13
Tuna	325	36	3	33	13
Turkey Breast	215	36	3	33	13
Select Sandwiches (6")					
Figures based on Italian bread					
and: Lettuce, tomato, onion,					
green peppers, and select sauce.					
Dijon Horseradish Melt	470	48	5	43	26
Honey Mustard Ham	311	52	4	48	18
Red Wine Vinaigrette Club	350	53	4	49	24

	Calories	Total Carb	Fiber	Usable Carb	Protein
Chipotle Southwest					
Turkey Bacon	407	48	4	44	22
Sweet Onion					
Chicken Teriyaki	374	59	4	55	26
Select Sauces:					
Per 1.5 Tablespoon on 6" Sub					
Fat Free: Honey Mustard	30	7	0	7	0
Red Wine	30	6	0	6	0
Sweet Onion	40	9	0	9	0
Chipotle Southwest	*90*	*2*	*0*	*2*	*0*
Dijon Horseradish	*90*	*1*	*0*	*1*	*0*
7 Under 6" Salads: Figures					
include lettuce, tomato,					
onion, green peppers, olives					
and pickles.					
Ham	112	11	3	8	11
Roast Beef	117	10	3	7	12
Roasted Chicken Breast	140	12	3	9	16
Subway Club	146	12	3	9	17
Turkey Breast	105	11	3	8	11
Turkey Breast/Ham	117	11	3	8	13
Veggie Delite	50	9	3	6	13
Classic Salads: Figures include					
lettuce, tomato, onion, green					
peppers, olives, pickles and					
cheese.					
Cold Cut Trio	230	12	3	9	14
Italian BMT	275	12	3	9	16
Meatball	320	18	3	15	16
Seafood & Crab	200	17	4	13	9
Steak & Cheese	181	13	4	9	17
Subway Melt	200	12	3	9	18
Tuna	240	11	3	8	13
Salad Dressings: Per 2 oz					
Fat Free French	70	17	0	17	0
Fat Free Italian	*20*	*4*	*0*	*4*	*0*
Fat Free Ranch	60	14	0	14	0
Soup: Per cup					
Black Bean	180	27	15	12	9
Brown & Wild Rice					
w/ Chicken	190	17	2	15	6

	Calories	Total Carb	Fiber	Usable Carb	Protein
Cheese w/ Ham & Bacon	230	13	2	11	8
Chicken Dumplings	130	16	1	15	7
Chili Con Carne	240	28	9	19	17
Cream of Broccoli	130	15	2	13	5
Cream of Potato w/ Bacon	210	20	4	16	5
Golden Broccoli Cheese	*180*	*12*	*9*	*3*	*6*
Minestrone	70	11	2	9	3
New England Style Clam Chowder	140	19	7	12	5
Potato Cheese Chowder	210	22	2	20	7
Roasted Chicken Noodle	90	7	1	6	7
Tomato Bisque	90	15	3	12	1
Vegetable Beef	90	14	2	12	5
Breads:					
6" Hearty Italian	210	41	3	38	8
6" Honey Oat	250	48	4	44	10
6" Italian Herb/Cheese	254	40	3	37	10
6" Italian (White)	200	38	3	35	7
6" Monterey Cheddar	240	39	3	36	10
6" Parmesan Oregano	210	40	3	37	8
6" Roasted Garlic	230	45	4	41	8
6" Sourdough	210	41	3	38	8
6" Wheat Bread	200	40	3	37	8
Deli Style Roll	170	32	3	29	6
Condiments & Extras:					
Bacon, 2 strips	*45*	*0*	*0*	*0*	*3*
Cheese (Per 2)	*40*	*0*	*0*	*0*	*2*
Pepperjack	*40*	*0*	*0*	*0*	*2*
Cheddar	*60*	*0*	*0*	*0*	*4*
Provolone	*25*	*0*	*0*	*0*	*2*
Swiss	*50*	*0*	*0*	*0*	*4*
Mayonnaise:					
Regular, 1 Tbsp	*110*	*0*	*0*	*0*	*0*
Light, 1 Tbsp	*45*	*1*	*0*	*1*	*0*
Mustard, all types	*5*	*1*	*0*	*1*	*0*
Olive Oil Blend per tsp	*45*	*0*	*0*	*0*	*0*
Vinegar, 1 tsp	*0*	*0*	*0*	*0*	*0*
Cookies; Per Cookie					
Chocolate Chip	210	30	1	29	2
Chocolate Chunk	220	30	1	29	2
Double Chocolate	210	30	1	29	2

	Calories	Total Carb	Fiber	Usable Carb	Protein
Peanut Butter	220	26	1	25	4
Oatmeal Raisin	200	30	2	28	3
Sugar	230	28	0	28	2
White Macadamia	220	28	1	27	2
Fruizle Express (Small)					
Berry Lishus	110	28	1	27	1
Berry Lishus With Banana	140	35	2	33	1
Peach Pizazz	100	26	0	26	0
Pineapple Delite	130	33	1	32	1
Pineapple Delite w/ Banana	160	40	2	38	1
Sunrise Refresher	120	29	1	28	1
TACO BELL					
Burritos					
7-Layer Burrito	530	67	10	57	18
Bean Burrito	370	55	8	47	14
Burrito Supreme Beef	440	51	7	44	18
Chicken	410	50	5	45	21
Steak	420	50	6	44	19
Chili Cheese	390	41	4	37	16
Fiesta Beef	390	50	5	45	14
Fiesta Chicken	370	48	3	45	18
Fiesta Steak	370	48	4	44	16
Grilled Stuft Beef	730	79	10	69	28
Grilled Stuft Chicken	680	76	7	69	35
Steak	680	76	8	68	31
Tacos					
Regular	170	13	3	10	8
Supreme	220	14	3	11	9
Soft Beef	210	21	2	19	10
Soft Chicken	190	19	0.5	18.5	14
Soft Beef Supreme	260	22	3	19	11
Soft Chick Supreme	230	21	1	20	15
Soft Grilled Steak	280	21	1	20	12
Double Decker	340	39	6	33	15
Double Decker Supreme	380	40	6	34	15
Gorditas					
Baja Beef	360	31	4	27	14
Baja Chicken	340	29	2	27	17
Baja Steak	340	29	2	27	15
Supreme Beef	320	30	3	27	14
Supreme Chicken	300	28	2	26	17

	Calories	Total Carb	Fiber	Usable Carb	Protein
Supreme Steak	300	28	2	26	16
Nacho Cheese/Beef	310	32	3	29	13
Nacho Cheese/Chicken	290	30	2	28	16
Nacho Cheese/Steak	290	30	2	28	14
Chalupas					
Baja Chicken	390	30	2	28	17
Baja Steak	390	30	2	28	15
Supreme Beef	370	31	3	28	14
Supreme Chicken	350	30	1	29	17
Supreme Steak	350	29	2	27	15
Nacho Cheese/Beef	360	33	3	30	12
Nacho Cheese/Chicken	340	31	1	30	16
Nacho Cheese/Steak	340	31	2	29	14
Breakfast					
Gordita	400	28	2	26	14
Burrito	530	48	6	42	22
Burrito, Steak	530	40	3	37	26
Quesadilla	420	38	3	35	17
Steak Quesadilla w/ green sauce	470	39	3	36	24
Nachos and Sides					
Nachos, 3.5 oz	350	33	2	31	5
Nachos Supreme	470	42	7	35	13
Nachos Bell Grande	760	80	12	68	20
Pintos/Cheese, 4.5 oz	180	20	7	13	9
Mexican Rice, 4.6 oz	190	21	0.5	20.5	5
Cinnamon Twists, (1)	150	27	0.5	26.5	1
Specialties					
Tostada	250	29	7	22	11
Cheese Quesadilla	490	39	3	36	19
Chicken Quesadilla	550	40	3	37	28
Enchirito, Chicken	350	33	5	28	23
Enchirito, Beef	370	35	6	29	19
Enchirito, Steak	350	33	5	28	21
Meximelt	290	23	3	20	15
Mexican Pizza	550	46	7	39	21
Taco Salad w/ Salsa & Shell	830	73	13	60	31
Taco Salad w/ Salsa no shell	410	33	11	22	24
Southwest Steak Bowl	660	73	13	60	30
Zesty Chicken Border Bowl	720	65	12	53	23
without dressing	460	60	12	48	22

	Calories	Total Carb	Fiber	Usable Carb	Protein
TACO JOHN'S					
Tacos					
Bravo	360	40	6	34	15
Burger	280	29	1	28	14
Crispy	190	13	0	13	9
El Grande	481	30	1	29	24
El Grande, Chicken	327	24	1	23	17
Sierra Taco Beef	500	39	2	37	18
Sierra Taco Chicken	430	37	3	34	18
Softshell	230	23	3	20	11
Softshell Chicken	170	21	4	17	11
Burritos					
Bean Burrito	380	53	12	41	12
Beefy Burrito	440	44	6	38	22
Chicken Fajita	320	41	7	34	18
Chicken and Potato	455	56	1	55	15
Combination	410	49	9	40	18
El Grande	730	69	8	61	33
El Grande Chicken	630	66	8	58	33
Meat and Potato	500	58	8	50	15
Ranch Burrito Beef	440	43	7	36	16
Chicken	380	41	7	34	16
Smothered	540	57	11	46	25
Super Burrito	450	51	10	41	19
Favorites					
Bean Tostada	160	17	3	14	6
Cheese Crisp 2 oz	220	9	0	9	10
Chilito, 6.1 oz	440	41	7	34	21
Double Enchilada	780	58	8	50	38
Mexi Rolls, 9.6 oz	670	53	2	51	28
Mexican Pizza	560	47	4	43	23
Quesadilla, Regular	460	41	7	34	18
Chicken	430	42	7	35	20
Tostada	200	13	0	13	9
Specialties					
Chicken Festiva Salad	690	39	5	34	22
w/o dressing	370	27	5	22	21
Chicken Nachos	810	57	7	50	26
Potato Oles Bravo	570	55	6	49	9
without Nacho Cheese	530	50	4	46	7
Sierra Chicken Sandwich	480	37	2	35	25

	Calories	Total Carb	Fiber	Usable Carb	Protein
Super Nachos	900	68	10	58	23
Taco Salad	770	55	3	52	24
w/o dressing	600	50	3	47	24
Platters					
Beef/Bean Chimi	740	82	10	72	26
Beef Enchilada	830	79	11	68	34
Chicken Enchilada	690	71	10	61	27
Smothered Burrito	880	101	17	84	35
Sides					
Green Chili	223	20	2	18	10
Mexican Rice	250	44	0	44	6
Nachos	440	35	4	31	7
Refried Beans	360	45	15	30	18
Side Salad	290	15	2	13	3
Texas Style Chili	380	23	4	19	21
Desserts					
Apple Grande	258	40	1	39	5
Choco Taco	311	37	1	36	3
Churros	158	13	1	12	2
Cookies, 1 Bag	70	6	0	6	2
Taco John's Cinnamon					
Mint Swirl	60	14	0	14	1
TACO TIME					
Burritos					
Casita Burrito, Beef	647	54	16	38	40
Crisp Burrito: Bean	427	53	9	44	15
Meat	552	39	7	32	34
Chicken	422	32	2	30	17
Double Soft Bean	506	77	19	58	23
Double Soft Combo	615	66	18	48	39
Double Soft Meat	725	55	17	38	57
Value Soft Bean Single	380	58	13	45	16
Value Soft Beef Single	490	48	12	36	31
Veggie	490	70	10	60	21
Tacos					
Crisp Taco	295	16	5	11	22
Natural Super Meat	625	60	14	46	41
Rolled Soft Flour	510	46	12	34	33
Soft Chicken	387	41	7	34	21
Soft Super Shredded Beef	370	38	7	31	12
Taco Cheeseburger	635	48	7	41	31

	Calories	Total Carb	Fiber	Usable Carb	Protein
Value Soft Taco	315	23	5	18	24
Specialties					
Crustos, 3.5 oz	375	47	0	47	9
Empanada, Cherry	250	37	0	37	5
Mexi Fries, Regular	265	26.9	0	26.9	3.0
Mexican Rice	160	30	1	29	3
Nachos	680	61	11	50	26
Quesadilla, Cheese	205	17	1	16	11
Refritos, 7 oz	325	44	13	31	18
Salads: Per Serving					
Chicken Taco No Dressing	370	27	3	24	19
Taco Salad No Dressing	480	30	7	23	30
Tostada Delight Salad Meat	630	48	13	35	36
Fillings & Extras:					
Chips, 2 oz	265	35	3	32	4
6" Taco Shell	110	14	2	12	2
Cheddar Cheese ¾ oz	*85*	*0*	*0*	*0*	*5*
Chicken 2.5 oz	*110*	*2*	*0*	*2*	*11*
Enchilada Sauce, 1 oz	*10*	*3*	*1*	*2*	*0*
Lettuce, ½ oz	*2*	*0*	*0*	*0*	*0*
Shredded Beef, 2.5 oz	*70*	*1*	*0*	*1*	*1*
Taco Meat, 2.5 oz	*210*	*7*	*5*	*2*	*22*
TOGO'S					
Salads: Per Serving					
Chicken Caesar, 9 oz	315	13	3	10	37
Oriental Salad, 21.3 oz	390	53	12	41	29
Farmer's Market, 9 oz	120	18	5	13	5
Taco Salad, 24.5 oz	1050	79	14	65	35
Dressings:					
Per 2.75 oz or Packet					
Ranch	*100*	*3*	*0*	*3*	*1*
Oriental Sesame	70	7.5	0	7.5	0
Caesar	125	9	0	9	2
Sandwiches: Per 6" Sandwich					
on White Roll					
Albacore Tuna	455	69	5	64	22
Avocado & Turkey	690	78	11	67	34
BBQ Beef	525	64	4	60	38
California Chicken	620	68	4	64	54
Chunky Chicken Salad	1087	92.8	5.8	87	39.1
Egg Salad	610	69	5	64	20

	Calories	Total Carb	Fiber	Usable Carb	Protein
Hot Pastrami	810	72	6	66	36
Hummus	807	104	5	99	28
Salami/Cheese	760	70	5	65	37
The Italian	745	68	5	63	35
Meatball	690	80	7	73	41
Reuben	660	69	5	64	40
Roast Beef	670	68	5	63	50
Turkey/Cheese	600	71	5	66	38
Turkey/Ham/Cheese	600	70	5	65	37
UNA MAS					
Burritos:					
Bean & Cheese	649	80	17	63	32
El Cheapo	553	98	15	83	22
Fajita:					
Chicken	715	89	11	78	41
Steak	737	89	11	78	36
Fish Cabo Style	488	53	3	50	36
Gallito	591	62	2	60	47
Thai Chicken	498	62	2	60	28
Vegetariano	539	69	6	63	22
Una Mas Chicken	584	76	8	68	36
Una Mas Steak	606	76	8	68	31
Tacos:					
Crispy Chicken	239	12	2	10	9
Fish Cabo Style	267	36	3	33	18
Una Mas Chicken	339	48	5	43	18
Una Mas Steak	346	48	5	43	16
Una Mas Veggie	273	45	4	41	11
Favoritos:					
5-Layer Dip	343	25	8	17	15
Chicken Enchiladas	480	37	2	35	39
Nachos	1219	91	13	78	36
Quesadilla Grande	634	49	5	44	36
Quesadilla Chica	353	28	1	27	19
TJ Caesar Salad	356	29	1	28	7
w/ Chicken	522	30	1	29	28
Tortilla Soup: cup	*201*	*4*	*2*	*2*	*16*
Tostada Salad	473	50	6	44	19
w/ Chicken	640	53	4	49	38
Verde Salad	211	19	1	18	7

	Calories	Total Carb	Fiber	Usable Carb	Protein
Side Orders:					
Beef, 3 oz	*188*	*1*	*0*	*1*	*16*
Black Beans, 5 oz	149	23	4	19	8
Chicken, 3 oz	*166*	*1*	*0*	*1*	*21*
Corn Tortilla	8	17	1	16	2
Fish, 4 oz	*195*	*0*	*0*	*0*	*28*
Flour Tortilla (12")	150	25	1	24	5
Fresh Guacamole, 2 oz	*78*	*4*	*2*	*2*	*1*
Monterey Jack Cheese	*100*	*1*	*0*	*1*	*7*
Pinto Beans, 5 oz	168	29	8	21	9
Refried Beans, ½ C	100	18	6	12	6
Rice, 5 oz	160	31	1	30	3
Sour Cream, 1 oz	*62*	*1*	*0*	*1*	*1*
The Works	*159*	*5*	*2*	*3*	*5*
Tortilla Chips 1 oz	142	18	2	16	2
Salsa & Dressing:					
Chipotle Sauce	*3*	*1*	*0*	*1*	*0*
Salsa Fresca, 1 oz	*3*	*1*	*0*	*1*	*0*
Mild Sauce, 1 oz	*7*	*2*	*0*	*2*	*0*
Ceasar Dressing, 2 oz	*140*	*2*	*0*	*2*	*0*
Jalapeno Vinaigrette, 2 oz	140	16	0	16	3
WENDY'S					
Sandwiches					
Big Bacon Classic	580	46	3	43	34
Chicken Breast	435	46	2	44	27
Chicken Club	480	47	2	45	30
Classic Single with					
Everything	415	37	2	35	24
Grilled Chicken	305	36	2	34	24
Kids' Meal:					
Jr. Hamburger	270	33	2	31	14
Jr. Cheeseburger	310	34	2	32	17
Deluxe	360	37	2	35	17
Jr. Bacon Cheeseburger	380	34	2	32	20
Spicy Chicken	430	47	3	44	27
French Fries:					
Medium	395	56	6	50	4
Chicken Nuggets:					
5 Piece	220	13	0	13	11
4 Piece (Kids)	175	10	0	10	9
Salads:					

	Calories	Total Carb	Fiber	Usable Carb	Protein
Caesar Side	285	12	1	11	9
w/o Croutons and Dressing	*70*	*2*	*1*	*1*	*7*
Side Salad w/o Dressing	*35*	*7*	*3*	*4*	*2*
Garden Sensations Salads:					
Chicken BLT	660	30	4	26	35
w/o Croutons/Dressing	315	10	4	6	33
Mandarin Chicken					
w/ Almonds/Noodles	590	50	5	45	26
w/o Dressing	340	31	5	26	25
Spring Mix w/ Pecans	530	25	7	18	13
w/o Dressing	335	17	7	10	13
Taco Supremo	670	61	10	51	32
w/o Sour Cream, Salsa,					
and Chips	375	29	8	21	27
Dressings & Sauce:					
Per packet					
Barbecue Sauce	45	10	0	10	1
Blue Cheese	*260*	*2*	*0*	*2*	*2*
Caeser	*150*	*1*	*0*	*1*	*1*
Creamy Ranch	230	5	0	5	1
Reduced Fat	100	6	1	5	1
French, Fat Free	85	21	0	21	0
Honey Mustard	280	11	0	11	1
Low Fat	110	21	0	21	0
House Vinaigrette	195	8	0	8	0
Oriental Sesame	250	19	0	19	1
Hot Stuff Baked Potato					
Plain	315	72	7	65	7
Bacon & Cheese	585	79	7	72	18
Broccoli & Cheese	485	81	9	72	9
Sour Cream/Chives	375	73	7	66	7
Country Crock Spread	*60*	*0*	*0*	*0*	*0*
Chili: Per Serving					
Small	205	21	5	16	17
Hot Chili Seasoning	*10*	*2*	*0*	*2*	*0*
Cheddar Cheese					
Shredded, 2 Tbsp	*75*	*1*	*0*	*1*	*4*
Saltine Cracker	*13*	*2*	*0*	*2*	*0.5*
Frosty Dairy Dessert: Per cup					
Junior, 6 oz	165	28	0	28	4
Small, 12 oz	330	56	0	56	8

	Calories	Total Carb	Fiber	Usable Carb	Protein
Medium, 16 oz	435	73	0	73	11
WHATABURGER					
Burgers/Sandwiches					
Whataburger	607	53.3	3.3	50	30.8
small bun/no oil	427.2	31.1	2.3	28.8	26.8
w/ bacon/cheese	809.5	53.5	3.3	50.2	42.1
Whatachick, 2 pc	813.6	37.7	2	35.7	28
Whataburger Jr.	314	29.2	1.7	27.4	16.4
Grilled Chicken	473	49.2	3.9	45.3	30.4
small bun, no oil	334.4	37.3	2.3	35.0	28.4
Chicken Strips, 2 pieces	382.3	22	4	18	18.7
3 pieces	573	33	6	27	28.1
4 pieces	765	44	8	36	37.4
Sides					
French Fries: small	257	33	2.6	30.4	4.3
Onion Rings: medium	201	23.3	1	22.3	3.2
Chicken & Salads					
Garden Salad	48.8	10.3	4.1	6.3	2.8
w/ cheddar cheese	217.8	10.3	4.1	6.3	12.7
w/ cheddar/bacon	292.8	10.5	4.1	6.5	17.6
Grilled Chicken Salad	228.8	18.7	4.6	14.0	24.6
w/ cheddar cheese	397.8	18.7	3.8	14.9	34.5
Dressings: per 2 oz					
Ranch	**310**	**3**	**0**	**3**	**1**
Low Fat	66.2	9.5	2	7.5	1.9
Thousand Island	150	11	0	11	0
Low Fat Vinaigrette	35	6	0	6	0
Shakes, small, 20 oz.					
Chocolate	616.2	100.2	0	100.2	13.1
Vanilla	559	81.7	0	81.7	12.9
Desserts					
Hot Apple Pie	240	31	1.2	29.8	2
Chocolate Chunk Cookie	210	33	2	31	3
White Chocolate Macadamia Nut	230	30	1	29	3
Breakfast					
Bacon	**75**	**.2**	**0**	**.2**	**4.9**
Biscuit: Plain	300	34	0	34	5
w/ bacon	375.2	34.2	0	34.2	9.9
w/ bacon/egg/cheese	520.6	35.2	0	35.2	19.4
w/ egg/cheese	445.6	35	0	35	14.5

	Calories	Total Carb	Fiber	Usable Carb	Protein
w/ sausage	517.2	34	1.1	32.9	16
w/ sausage gravy	490.7	46.9	0.2	46.8	8.3
w/ sausage/egg/cheese	662.6	35	1.1	33.9	25.5
Breakfast-On-A-Bun					
w/ bacon	397.5	28.2	2.0	26.2	20.4
w/ sausage	539.5	28	2.1	25.9	26.5
Breakfast Platters					
(Biscuit/Eggs/Hash Browns):					
w/ bacon	698	51.8	2.8	49	23.3
w/ sausage	840	51.6	3.9	47.7	29.4
Cinnamon Roll	860	126	4	122	12
Egg Sandwich	322.5	28	1	27	15.5
Hash Browns	140	16	2.8	13.2	0
Pancakes: Plain	614	117.6	3.4	114.2	18.8
w/ bacon	689	117.8	3.4	114.4	23.7
w/ sausage	831	117.6	4.5	113.1	29.8
Taquitos:					
Bacon & Egg	387.2	25.4	1.0	24.4	19
Bacon/Egg/Cheese	432.2	25.4	1.0	24.4	21.5
Potato/Egg	382.2	33.2	3.8	29.4	14.1
Sausage/Egg	389.5	25.5	1.9	24.3	16.6
WHITE CASTLE					
Hamburgers					
Hamburger	140	11	2	9	6
Cheeseburger	160	11	2	9	7
Bacon Cheeseburger	200	12	3	9	10
Double Hamburger	240	16	4	12	11
Double Cheeseburger	290	16	5	11	14
Sandwiches					
Chicken	299	15	1	14	5
Fish	180	27	1	26	5
Breakfast Sandwich	340	17	0	17	14
French Fries, small	115	15	2	13	0

ABOUT THE AUTHOR

Dana Carpender is the author of the national best-seller *500 Low-Carb Recipes*, *15-Minute Low-Carb Recipes*, and *How I Gave Up My Low-Fat Diet and Lost Forty Pounds*. She appears frequently on television and radio, and is the author of *Lowcarbezine!*, the popular internet newsletter. Dana lives in Bloomington, Indiana and has been eating a low-carb diet for the last eight years, with nothing but great health to show for it.

ALSO BY DANA CARPENDER

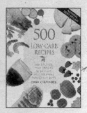

500 Low-Carb Recipes
ISBN 1-931412-06-5
$19.95; Paperback, 500 pages
Fair Winds Press, 2002

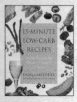

15-Minute Low-Carb Recipes
ISBN 1-59233-041-X
$17.95; Paperback, 260 pages
Fair Winds Press, 2003

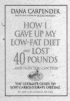

How I Gave Up My Low-Fat Diet and Lost Forty Pounds
ISBN: 1-59233-040-1
$14.95; Paperback, 312 pages
Fair Winds Press, 2003